Register Now ~~~~~~ ~~~~~~~~ to Yo~~

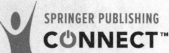

SPRINGER PUBLISHING
C⏻NNECT™

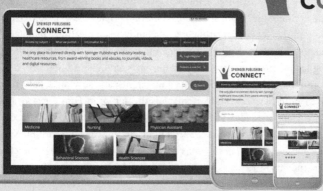

Your print purchase of *School Nursing* **includes online access to the contents of your book**—increasing accessibility, portability, and searchability!

Access today at:
http://connect.springerpub.com/content/book/978-0-8261-3537-7
or scan the QR code at the right with your smartphone
and enter the access code below.

PYJGVCWV

Scan here for quick access.

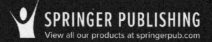

SPRINGER PUBLISHING
View all our products at springerpub.com

Janice Loschiavo, MA, RN, NJ-CSN, is an adjunct instructor at William Paterson University Graduate Nursing Division and serves as a field supervisor for New Jersey City University. She had 26 years of experience as a school nurse before retiring from those positions in 2007. Ms. Loschiavo has received recognition for excellence both in teaching and as a school nurse, including the New Jersey Distinguished Alumni Award (2014), the Governor's Teacher Recognition Award in 2006–2007, the nominee for Disney Teacher of the Year (2002), the New Jersey State School Nurse of the Year (1994–1995), the Bergen County School Nurse of the Year (1994–1995), and the state nominee for National School Nurse of the Year (1994–1995). While a school nurse, she was responsible for participating in Child Study Team meetings, maintaining health records, conducting health screenings, and providing first aid to students; teaching health classes; conducting faculty in-service training (anaphylaxis, child abuse, and first aid); organizing health fairs; running workshops for teachers and parents; and serving as liaison to the Division of Youth and Family Services. Ms. Loschiavo is the author of *Fasts Facts for the School Nurse*, now in its third edition, and contributed to *Health Counseling: A Microskills Approach for Counselors, Educators, and School Nurses*, Second Edition, edited by Richard Blonna. Mrs. Loschiavo also wrote and published *Life's Lessons for Children*, which provides character education lesson plans for students K-12.

SCHOOL NURSING

The Essential Reference

Janice Loschiavo, MA, RN, NJ-CSN

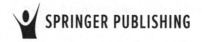 SPRINGER PUBLISHING

Springer Publishing Company, LLC
11 West 42nd Street, New York, NY 10036
www.springerpub.com
connect.springerpub.com/

Acquisitions Editor: Adrianne Brigido
Compositor: S4Carlisle Publishing Services

ISBN: 978-0-8261-3536-0
ebook ISBN: 978-0-8261-3537-7

A Multiple-Choice Review Question supplement is available at http://connect.springerpub.com/content/book/978-0-8261-3537-7

Multiple-Choice Review Questions ISBN: 978-0-8261-8282-1
DOI: 10.1891/9780826135377

20 21 22 23 24 / 5 4 3 2 1

The author and the publisher of this Work have made every effort to use sources believed to be reliable to provide information that is accurate and compatible with the standards generally accepted at the time of publication. Because medical science is continually advancing, our knowledge base continues to expand. Therefore, as new information becomes available, changes in procedures become necessary. We recommend that the reader always consult current research and specific institutional policies before performing any clinical procedure or delivering any medication. The author and publisher shall not be liable for any special, consequential, or exemplary damages resulting, in whole or in part, from the readers' use of, or reliance on, the information contained in this book. The publisher has no responsibility for the persistence or accuracy of URLs for external or third-party Internet websites referred to in this publication and does not guarantee that any content on such websites is, or will remain, accurate or appropriate.

Library of Congress Cataloging-in-Publication Data

Names: Loschiavo, Janice, author.
Title: School nursing : the essential reference / Janice Loschiavo.
Description: New York, NY : Springer Publishing Company, [2021] | Includes
    bibliographical references and index.
Identifiers: LCCN 2020035283 (print) | LCCN 2020035284 (ebook) | ISBN
    9780826135360 (cloth) | ISBN 9780826135377 (ebook)
Subjects: MESH: School Nursing | Nurse's Role | Nurse-Patient Relations |
    School Health Services
Classification: LCC RT41 (print) | LCC RT41 (ebook) | NLM WY 113 | DDC 610.73–dc23
LC record available at https://lccn.loc.gov/2020035283
LC ebook record available at https://lccn.loc.gov/2020035284

Contact sales@springerpub.com to receive discount rates on bulk purchases.

Publisher's Note: **New and used products purchased from third-party sellers are not guaranteed for quality, authenticity, or access to any included digital components.**

Printed in the United States of America.

This book is dedicated to all school nurses—past, present, and future. May we always remember: Children do not interrupt our work; they are our work.

*And to **Jeanne J. Kiefner**, RN, MEd, FNASN, and **Judith A. Woop**, MEd, RN, NJ-CSN, whose wisdom and commitment to school nursing serve as a beacon for those who follow and share the vision that children must always be our first priority.*

CONTENTS

CONTRIBUTORS

HUGH BASES, MD Clinical Associate Professor of Pediatrics, Program Director, Fellowship in Developmental-Behavioral Pediatrics, New York University School of Medicine, Bellevue Hospital Center, Department of Pediatrics, New York, New York

MARY ELLEN ULLMER BOLTON, MA, RN, NJ-CSN, SAC, CPM Adjunct Faculty, Department of Graduate Nursing, William Paterson University, Wayne, New Jersey

MATTHEW BOLTON, EdD, MS, BS Principal, Edison Intermediate School, Westfield, New Jersey

JOHN M. DEWITT, MA Director of Student Services, Glen Ridge Board of Education, Glen Ridge, New Jersey

ANNEMARIE J. DELLE DONNE, MS, BSN, RN, NCSN Colts Neck School Nurse, Colts Neck, New Jersey; DNP Student, Marjorie K. Unterberg School of Nursing & Health Studies, Monmouth University, West Long Branch, New Jersey

CARLEA D. M. DRIES, PsyD, ABSNP School Psychologist, Allendale Public Schools, Allendale, New Jersey; Adjunct Professor, School of Psychology and Counseling, Fairleigh Dickinson University, Metropolitan Campus, Teaneck, New Jersey

LAURA A. GUERRA, EdD, MS, MS, MBA, CHES Research Associate, Laurie M. Tisch Center for Food, Education, and Policy, Program in Nutrition, Department of Health and Behavior Studies, Teachers College, Columbia University, New York, New York

JANET HALDER, MS, BS, BSN, RN, NJ-CSN, Clinical Supervisor, Department of Graduate Nursing, William Paterson University, Wayne, New Jersey

LAURA T. JANNONE, EdD, MSN, MS, BSN, RN, CSN-NJ, FNASN Associate Professor and Coordinator, School Nurse Program, Marjorie K. Unterberg School of Nursing and Health Studies, Monmouth University, West Long Branch, New Jersey

LUCILLE A. JOEL, APN, EdD, FAAN   Distinguished Professor, School of Nursing, Rutgers, The State University of New Jersey, Newark/New Brunswick, New Jersey

DAPHNE JOSLIN, PhD, MPH   Faculty, Marymount Manhattan College at Bedford Hills Correctional Facility, Faculty, Hudson Link for Higher Education in Prison, Professor Emerita, Department of Public Health, William Paterson University, Wayne, New Jersey

WILLIAM DAVID KERNAN, EdD, MPA, MCHES   Professor Department of Public Health, William Paterson University, Wayne, New Jersey

SEAN LARE, MSW, LCSW-C   Social Worker and Consultant in Private Practice, Sean Lare Counseling and Consulting, Columbia, Maryland

MARIA TORCHIA LOGRIPPO, PhD, RN, MSN, NE-BC   Practice Associate Professor, Department of Family and Community Health and Associated Faculty, Assistant Dean of Curricular Affairs and Innovation, University of Pennsylvania School of Nursing, Philadelphia, Pennsylvania

JANICE LOSCHIAVO, MA, RN, NJ-CSN   Adjunct Faculty, Graduate Department of Nursing, William Paterson University, Wayne, New Jersey

BRENDA MARSHALL, EdD, APRN, PMHNP-BC, ANEF, FAANP   Professor, Department of Nursing, William Paterson University, Wayne, New Jersey

LEWIS W. MARSHALL Jr., MS, MD, JD, FACP, FACHE   Fulbright Scholar Specialist, Disaster Medicine Specialist, Clinical Assistant, Professor of Medicine, New York University School of Medicine, New York, New York

DAVID NASH, Esq.   Legal One Director, Foundation for Educational Administration, Monroe Township, New Jersey

KATHERINE J. ROBERTS, EdD, MPH, MCHES, CPH   Adjunct Professor Department of Health and Behavior Studies, Teachers College, Columbia University, New York, New York

WAYNE A. YANKUS, MD, FAAP   School Physician for Ridgewood and Leonia Boards of Education, American Academy of Pediatrics, Children's Aid and Family Services of New Jersey, Bergen County, New Jersey

PREFACE

This textbook was developed out of need. As a practicing school nurse for more than 25 years and adjunct instructor at the university level for the past 20 years, I have witnessed firsthand the changes in today's school-age child. These many changes drove me to edit a comprehensive reference, which had to include basic information needed by every school nurse, as well as provide insight into emerging issues in childhood, society, and education to help prepare future school nurses for the challenges ahead and ensure their continuing professional growth.

Due to the complexity of the role of the school nurse, I was certain that alone I could not do every area justice. I sought and was able to assemble the most knowledgeable experts to speak where I felt I could not. I am honored by every author's willingness to give their valuable time to help children through the hands of the school nurse.

Each chapter includes comprehensive, updated information on the author's area of expertise. Objectives are clearly noted and relevant questions posed to aid in the student's evaluation. Most of the authors I know personally and have worked alongside as a nurse or instructor. All have taught and inspired me. I now offer their wisdom and wise counsel to you so each current and prospective school nurse can benefit as I have from their knowledge.

School Nursing: The Essential Reference contains the following information, in summary:

Part I shares the exciting history of school nursing. You will meet nursing heroes, learn how school nursing is defined today, and recognize how it has evolved while still remaining grounded in public health principles. The overriding goal of helping children achieve their highest level of wellness so they can learn and thrive remains constant—exactly as it was more than 100 years ago when school nursing began. The distinction between prevention and intervention, various levels, scope of prevention practice, and specific measures the school nurse can employ to implement them are identified. Part I also introduces basic health education principles, theories, and practices that can advance the well-being, academic success, and lifelong health behaviors of students. By utilizing prevention concepts and these health principles, each school nurse can help raise the wellness level of every child, each school community, and, ultimately, our nation.

Part II acquaints the reader with the role of the school nurse in building healthy communities. The *Framework for the 21st Century School Nursing Practice,* as put forth by the National Association of School Nurses, is explored and clarified. The varied role is explained. The Health Office is discussed, including how it can be a refuge and resource for many students. This is where therapeutic interventions are applied in the school day. With this information, we then look closely at those children who most frequently visit the school nurse. Serving special needs children, brain functions, and specific helpful strategies are discussed. Acute and chronic conditions commonly seen in the school-aged child are reviewed, including recommendations for preventing illnesses/injuries and when to summon help. New terminology and available resources pertaining to the role of the school nurse are reviewed.

Part III deals exclusively with issues that tend to marginalize today's student. This section explores mental health disorders, cultural diversity, substance abuse, gender identity, eating disorders, and bullying. All areas are discussed by the experts who not only have the academic expertise, but also identify, work with, and counsel these children.

Part IV leads us into the future of school health practice. Topics include legal aspects, school-based clinics, special education, school violence, crisis management, ethical issues/legal guidance, technology, and the ever-shifting paradigm for school health.

In light of the global pandemic that has inflicted extensive pain and suffering, an additional chapter was added. Chapter 26, Pandemics and Plagues, gives the reader an historical perspective of the scope of pandemics as well as specific information on coronavirus. It puts the current crisis in perspective and provides realistic strategies to deal with the reopening of schools. This is an essential read for all school personnel.

This unique reference takes the reader on a journey from the humble beginnings of the school nurse profession through today's expanded role. It culminates with an exciting look at the potential that lies before us. Join me and my noble colleagues as we reflect on our past, learn, grow and explore the future. This is how we can improve our school nurse practice for the children we serve today and the school nurses who will follow in our footsteps.

Janice Loschiavo,
MA, RN, NJ-CSN

ACKNOWLEDGMENTS

I would like to thank Adrianne Brigido, Executive Director, Springer Publishing Company, for helping me put together this new book. She clearly has an understanding of the profession of nursing and skillfully held my hand through the writing process. Adrianne helped to make this book the valuable resource we so needed.

I remain ever grateful to my friend Lucille Joel for her faith in me and encouragement to reach further to do more and better throughout my career. She continues to serve as my role model, not only as a nurse, but also as a wife, mother, and grandmother.

This book would not have been possible without the support of the many authors who graciously gave their valuable time to contribute to this book. I am especially grateful to Dr. Wayne Yankus, not only for his contribution, but also for his ongoing support and appreciation for the role of the school nurse. Dr. Yankus radiates professionalism and sincere love for children.

I thank my many school nurse colleagues and especially my students who continue to impress me with their knowledge and perseverance; in doing so, they have kept me humble.

I thank the members of my writing group, Paula Mate, Jane Paterson, and Tina Segali, for their enthusiastic encouragement and provocative ideas.

I thank my children, Lori, Jill, and Rick, for their understanding when they so often had to share their mother. I also thank them for the gift of grandchildren: Ryan, Ashley, Richard, Luke, Preston, and Austin. These bright, beautiful babies keep me focused on what truly matters in life.

Most of all, I thank my husband, Rich. Rich has learned to tolerate piles of papers and often a most distracted, preoccupied wife. After 53 years of marriage, he continues to hold my hand and heart as well.

1

20TH CENTURY SCHOOL HEALTH PRACTICE

SCHOOL NURSING: EARLY BEGINNINGS AND THE UNFOLDING OF A NEW NURSING SPECIALTY

JANICE LOSCHIAVO

LEARNING OBJECTIVES

- Recognize the historical role of women as caregivers.
- Define school nursing.
- Describe how school nursing evolved from public health roots.
- State three ways in which school nursing differs from other nursing subspecialties.
- Compare today's level of school health services with that of the past.

▧ Introduction

The profession of school nursing has an exciting history. Commencing at the turn of the 20th century in an effort to support the requirement for mandatory school attendance, a group of astute women linked the horrific results of illness and poverty to school absenteeism and the profession of school nursing was born.

These women immediately recognized that help was needed to improve living conditions of poor, malnourished, immigrant families, so that children could attend school and become healthy, educated, American citizens.

Their story is that of:

- ■ A new country which quickly recognized the need for children to be educated
- ■ Brave, insightful women who made many sacrifices to help impoverished immigrants find a safe, healthy home in America
- ■ Legendary nurses who courageously revealed inhumane living conditions and the pervasive impact of poverty

- ■ Seldom-acknowledged heroes like Lillian Wald who fought politicians and advocated tirelessly for maltreated children

- ■ Insightful pioneers such as Lina Rogers, our first school nurse who, through education, created an atmosphere of acceptance and wellness so children could learn and thrive

- ■ The emergence of a new nursing specialty, grounded in public health principles

- ■ The school nurse of today who upholds our founders original goal to help each child attain the highest level of wellness

In this chapter, you will learn how nursing grew out of women's position as caregiver in the home and evolved into a larger role within the community. Once women were recognized outside of the home as competent caregivers, they quickly were also accepted as pioneers in the healthcare delivery system. Armed with an historical insight, today's school nurse can once again take up the challenge to create greater opportunities and a better world for our children.

Now, meet the heroes of our profession whose work will inspire you. Join those who came before us by adding your contribution as the story of school nursing continues to unfold. It is hoped that you will be motivated by their accomplishments. Although books may not be written about you, each and every one of you will be called upon to do work that is extraordinary.

■ Our History: Women as Nurturers and Caregivers

Early Beginnings

If one looks back on the history of caring for the ill, it is apparent that women have always assumed the responsibility for healing. With no formal education available and spurred on solely by intuition and observations, women delivered babies, cared for sick children, and tended to the elderly and those in need within the home setting. Nursing was considered a natural extension of motherhood (Joel, 2018, pp. 3–7).

First reports of nursing go back to the Romans in 300 AD, who attempted to have a hospital in every town under the rule of the Empire. Nurses were known to work alongside doctors. As Rome came under the Byzantine Empire, hospitals were created in Constantinople. These early hospitals were known to have both male and female nurses (Nursing School Hub, n.d.)

The Middle Ages

The development of the nursing profession has been heavily influenced by religion and wars (Wold, 1981, pp. 4–18). Starting around 500 AD, hospitals existed in Merida, Spain, that were run by Catholic priests. These early institutions cared for all people, regardless of nationality or religion. From the 10th to 11th century, nursing expanded and monasteries began to house hospitals on their premises.

During the years from 1500 to 1850, nurses were often viewed as *wayward* women. Some who were poor or homeless were offered positions as nurses in lieu of going to jail. Those without immediate family or caring relatives became nurses. Lacking a family or home of their own, this left them with little choice. Nursing was seen as dirty work and the lowest of positions in the social hierarchy.

During the Middle Ages, early Christians viewed nursing care as an act of mercy and expression of faith. Women of religious and secular orders tended to the sick in institutional settings. Churches built adjacent hospitals, and nuns cared for the sick and dying.

The Age of Modern Nursing

Florence Nightingale, *the lady with the lamp*, earned her title from nightly checks on soldiers injured in the Crimean War of 1854. A well-educated daughter of wealthy British parents, Nightingale chose to become a nurse despite the strong social convention that asserted this was not a respectable career for well-bred ladies (D'Antonio, n.d.) She later went on to open a school to train women to care for men in battle.

Born in 1820, Florence Nightingale became an English social reformer and the founder of modern nursing. Authoring over 150 books, she is credited with making hospitals cleaner and safer. Nightingale is also acknowledged as the creator of the first PIE Chart for nursing: *Problem, Intervention, and Evaluation* (Alexander, 2018).

Today we have modified PIE and use the Nursing Process: Assessment, Diagnosis, Planning, Implementation, and Evaluation.

It is believed that modern nursing in the United States commenced in 1873, when the first three training schools for nurses opened in an attempt by women reformers to formalize training and pass on their knowledge. These women were looking for meaningful work, which led to a new healthcare professional—the trained nurse.

The Age of Nurse's Training

As the United States' population grew in numbers, so likewise did their health needs. Many hospitals were still affiliated with religious groups and established their own schools in order to staff an ever growing number of patients. Schools developed under the control of hospitals where nurses learned by a hands-on approach to caring. In exchange for lectures and clinical instructions, students provided hospitals with skilled, free nursing care while they *trained,* usually for several years. Prospective nurses were housed in a residence located on the hospital grounds, and daily hospital duties were part of their nursing preparation.

Upon completion of a prescribed program, the student nurse was permitted to take a state examination, passage of which certified the candidate as a registered nurse

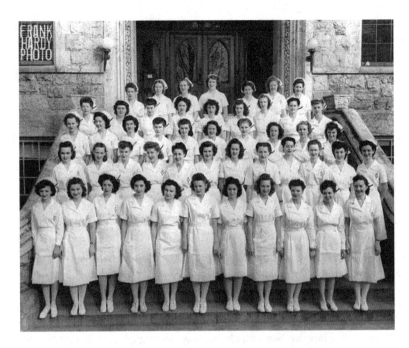

FIGURE 1.1 Sacred Heart School of Nursing Graduates, Pensacola, Florida (1947).

SOURCE: Courtesy of Frank Hardy Photography.

in that state. After being properly trained and passing the exam, the student usually remained at the hospital that prepared her and served as a staff nurse (Figure 1.1).

Once training was completed, nurses proudly donned their caps, white uniforms, shoes and stockings set about to care for those in need and begin their career as a professional nurse.

The Age of Educational Preparation

Today, nurses attend a college or university to obtain an associate's or bachelor's degree in nursing. Hospital experience is not as extensive in the preparation. Much of the bedside care is rendered by health assistants with the nurse supervising or preparing to work in specialty areas of the hospital.

The 20th century paved the way for a more expanded role and introduced distinct areas of specialization for nurses. Entering as a nurse with general preparation means further educational preparation is needed if one wishes to go on to specialize in one field of nursing. This usually occurs at the bachelor's or master's level.

As with most professions, specialization is the current way. The nurse who chooses to work exclusively in one area must seek additional educational preparation before doing so. Such is the specialty of school nursing.

Today's Nursing Profession

From these humble beginnings, the profession of nursing has grown in staggering leaps. Nursing is now the largest and most diverse of all healthcare professions. With true demographic representation remaining an elusive goal, nursing does have a higher proportional representation of racial and ethnic minorities than other healthcare professions (D'Antonio, n.d.).

In 2019, for the 18th consecutive year, nurses were voted as the most trusted professionals (Daily Nurse, 2020). Mother Teresa, our most famous nurse of modern times, eloquently stated, "the world's problems have risen because we all recognize a family that is too small." As nurses, we include many more in our families. We make our circle much larger as we care for strangers with the same devotion our predecessors gave solely to family members.

Today nurses no longer wear white caps and uniforms. These have been replaced with lab coats, slacks, and pins. Moreover, more men are becoming registered nurses and, fortunately, all ethnic groups are growing in representation. Instead of a capping ceremony, graduation program consists of a *pinning* signifying completion of the course of study.

The nurse of today is a registered professional nurse who most likely holds a bachelor's degree. Today's nurse is better educated than ever and is seen as a leader in a hospital or any chosen health field. In most instances, the nurse will select an area of specialty to focus on such as school nursing.

Definition of School Nursing

The Board of Directors of the National Association of School Nurses gives us the following definition:

> School nursing, a specialized practice of nursing, protects and promotes student health, facilitates optimal development, and advances academic success. School nurses, grounded in ethical and evidence-based practice, are the leaders who bridge healthcare and education, provide care coordination, advocate for quality student-centered care, and collaborate to design systems that allow individuals and communities to develop their full potential. (Adopted by the NASN Board of Directors, February 2017)

A History of School Nursing: The Path to and from Henry Street

School nursing began to appear in Europe as early as 1892. As educational opportunities were made available to all, schools and student enrollment grew. Once children gathered, it did not take long to recognize that malnourishment and/or illness and the ability to learn were linked. In order for children to learn, they had to be in school and well. Absenteeism could not be corrected without looking at the underlying causes.

Amy Hughes, the first European school nurse was hired in London in 1892. Her job was to investigate the nutritional status of school children (Table 1.1). Once the

TABLE 1.1 SCHOOL NURSING HISTORICAL TIMELINE

1892	London Amy Hughes is hired to investigate the nutritional status of schoolchildren in the school setting. This is the first recorded employment of a school nurse.
1893	Belgium Brussels is the first city to employ a school physician and establish organized, citywide inspection of schools.
1894	Boston School health services are initiated to identify and exclude students with serious communicable diseases, such as pertussis, measles, mumps, scarlet fever, and parasitic diseases, including lice, ringworm, and scabies.
1902	New York The Henry Street Settlement is organized, modeled after an English program. Lillian Wald, head nurse, appoints Lina Rogers as the nation's first school nurse. The goal is to decrease absenteeism following implementation of mandatory school attendance. Between 1902 and 1903 the number of absentees decreases from 10,567 to 1,101. Twenty-five more nurses are then hired and paid by the New York City Board of Education.
1920s	This decade sees the expansion of the school nurse's role. Health education is added and medical examinations begin in schools to identify physical defects.
1930s	Individual states begin to require specific education for school nurse practice.
1940s	With war present in much of the world, leaders in the United States realize the importance of the maximum degree of health for all to serve in the armed forces and support the country at home. Health as a school subject begins to include an emphasis on physical fitness. Educators recognize the correlation between health teaching and practice.
1950s	The role of the school nurse is expanded to focus on prevention. Screenings in dental health, vision, and hearing are followed up and fewer students are left with chronic diseases. Health counseling is introduced.
1960	Some states require nurses to have teaching degrees.
1965	Federal laws begin to take shape, ensuring that all children, whether handicapped or not, are to be appropriately educated. These laws further strengthen the position of the school nurse, whose presence now is required to perform treatments and give medications in the school setting. These laws continue to be revised, renamed, and enhanced to further benefit all children with special needs.
1968	The NEA establishes the DSN. A nationwide survey is conducted to establish school nurse credentials for each state. The DSN begins to form committees, develop policies, and elect officers.
1979	The DSN separates from NEA to form the NASN, which now serves as the hub for all the state organizations.

(continued)

TABLE 1.1 SCHOOL NURSING HISTORICAL TIMELINE (*CONTINUED*)

Today	School nursing continues to flourish as a separate discipline. Through NASN, school nurses partner with national health organizations, publish a journal and reference books, formulate position statements, and hold nationwide conventions to disseminate information and foster communication. NASN also employs a Washington, DC–based representative to lobby for school nursing issues and interact with Congress on the organization's behalf.

NASN, National Association of School Nurses; NEA, National Education Association; DSN, Department of School Nurses.

SOURCE: Reproduced from Loschiavo, J. (2019). *Fast facts for the school nurse* (3rd ed., pp. 8–9). New York, NY: Springer Publishing Company.

awareness was raised in Europe, those who were receptive, were ready to take action in the United States.

In 1894, the city of Boston began to recognize the seriousness of communicable disease in children and made efforts to exclude students with symptoms of illness. Shortly after that, New York City also sought to address the problem of school illness and the resulting absenteeism.

■ The Henry Street Settlement

Between the years 1880 and 1920, approximately 19 million immigrants arrived in New York City. Most settled on the east side, and were poor, malnourished, lived in squalid, deplorable conditions. Illness was rampant and people suffered and died due to poor living accommodations.

The Henry Street Settlement was the idea of Lillian Wald (1867–1940), one of the most influential and respected humanitarians and social reformers of the 20th century (Henry Street Settlement, n.d.). Born into a wealthy family of Jewish professionals, Wald was a trained nurse and a visionary.

Lillian Wald developed a community-based nursing practice on the Lower East Side of New York City where the need was greatest. She hand-picked a small group of nurses capable of working independently. Lina Rogers was one of them. Lillian Wald and Lina Rogers, both prominent women, are credited with bringing nurses into schools in the United States.

Not only was Wald a dedicated nurse, but she also proved be a savvy politician. Wald recognized the needs of people and knew how and where to go to make things happen. Her awareness came about by accident.

In March of 1893, Lillian Wald was just 25 years old and a student enrolled in the Women's Medical College. Wald was in the middle of teaching a class to immigrant mothers at the Louis Technical School on the Lower East Side of New York City when a little girl interrupted crying, begging for help for her mother. Wald followed the girl to her home on Ludlow Street. Entering the tenement, Wald noted courtyard out-houses, with missing doors and overflowing with feces. She located the apartment the family lived in and was appalled to learn that it was also inhabited by other families who shared rooms at different times of the day.

Wald saw that the young mother had hemorrhaged while in labor and been abandoned by her doctor, due to her inability to pay his fee.

Wald called the experience her "Baptism of Fire." She was ashamed to live "in a society that permitted such conditions to exist" (Levine, 2018).

At that time, there was no such thing as shelters. The homeless went to police stations. There were no child labor laws or playgrounds and little access to clean milk or pure water. One out of 10 infants died. School was not mandatory and many small children were kept at home to care for infants so both parents could work. Poverty caused the inhumane living conditions and the living conditions caused disease. Wald recognized that she was not only dealing with the illness but the conditions which caused it.

Wald knew then what most people were totally unaware of, that she not only had to help the sick patient but must also first address poverty and the social issues that caused the diseases and illness.

Wald wrote: Tuberculosis was "pre-eminently a disease of poverty, and can never be successfully combatted without dealing with its underlying economic causes: bad housing, bad workshops, undernourishment and so on" (Wald, Henry Street Settlement).

Little government support was offered and many maintained the illusion that poor were poor because of their own moral failures. The attitude of officials was one of indifference and arrogant condemnation.

As a political activist, Wald firmly believed that a democratic government must first help to alleviate poverty. She saw and understood that social justice work was democracy in action and maintained that working as a nurse on the Lower East Side was a way for her to "assert by deed [her] faith in democracy."

Lillian Wald moved into the Lower East Side neighborhood and lived and worked among the impoverished. The nurses charged patients on a sliding scale according to what they could pay. The nurses' residence became known as the Henry Street Settlement. Besides providing nursing services, Wald's nurses gave English language lessons, served meals, provided music enrichment classes, and made a safe playground in the yard for children. Wald pioneered what we know now as public health nursing, strived for housing reform, supported the movement for the advancement of colored people, fought for world peace and women's rights, and emerged as a political leader (Figure 1.2).

"Our basic idea was that the nurse's peculiar introduction to the patient and her organic relationship with the neighborhood should constitute the starting point for a universal service to the region… We planned to utilize, as well as to be implemented by all agencies and groups of whatever creed which were working for social betterment, private as well as municipal. Our scheme was to be motivated by a vital sense of the interrelation of all these forces. We consider ourselves best described by the term public health nurses." (Wald, Henry Street Settlement)

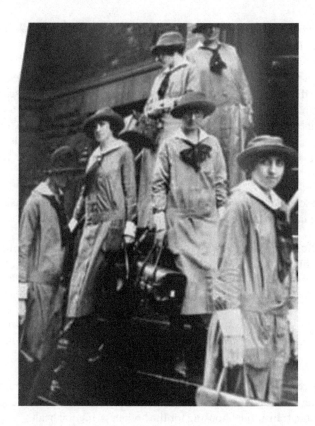

FIGURE 1.2 The Henry Street Settlement, First Public Health Nurses, Circa 1902.

SOURCE: Getty Images/Bettmann.

The Challenge

In 1897, the city of New York hired 150 physicians to help control the large number of school absentees. They examined and excluded children with cases of lice, impetigo, and tuberculosis. By excluding quickly, it was hoped that the child would recover, not further spread disease, and be able to return to a healthier school environment sooner (Working Nurse, 2019). This attempt proved to be totally ineffective. Once home, children never returned to school. Diseases continued to spread since many families could not afford medical care, were severely malnourished, and remained living in crowded conditions.

In 1902, an article appeared in the *American Journal of Nursing* identifying the major problem to the New York City Board of Health and Board of Education. An experiment was to be conducted to address the large number of children absent from school. School attendance had become mandatory yet many children did not attend school. Wald offered the services of one of her nurses, Lina Rogers, to address the absentee problem.

Thus, on October 1, 1902, after the failure of the physicians to decrease absentee rate, Lina Rogers was placed in the school setting. Rogers was assigned to the four schools with the highest level of absenteeism, a total of over 10,000 children. An agreement was struck with the city officials that if Rogers succeeded in reducing absenteeism, the city would henceforth pay for nurses to be placed in schools.

In 1 month, the absentee rate was significantly decreased. Within 6 months, absenteeism fell by 90% and 27 more nurses were assigned to New York City schools.

Lina Rogers succeeded because she developed formal protocols for various health issues and carefully documented nursing interventions. She wrote in her journal:

> A sensible school nurse, with good judgment, discretion and enthusiasm, may be a powerful factor in the general improvement of a community. (Hanink, 2019)

In 1914, Rogers married one of the school physicians, William Struthers, and in 1917, she authored the first school nurse textbook, *The School Nurse: A Survey of the Duties and Responsibilities of the Nurse in Maintenance of Health and Physical Perfection and the Prevention of Disease Among School Children*. Her introduction states:

> School nursing is still in its infancy, and many changes in methods are to be expected, but the underlying essentials – child love and preservation of child health – will exist as long as child life.

Now declared a National Historic Landmark, the Henry Street Settlement is recognized as laying the foundation for child labor laws, playground construction, battered women's shelter, transitional housing for the homeless, mental health services, senior citizen lunch programs, and many other services the poor benefit from today.

School Nursing Today

As you ponder the accomplishments of those who came before us, do not do so in terms of our world as it exists today. One must bear in mind that the 19th Amendment of the Constitution which granted women the right to vote, was not passed until 1920. Our female predecessors not only were founding mothers but political activists who made their voices heard decades before women had any status.

Today, many states can boast a school nurse in almost every school. All teach one-on-one with students and serve as the health expert in their respective schools. Many school nurses are also certified teachers of health and have formal, teaching schedules.

There is a State School Nurses Association in each of the 50 states and, in 1979, the National Association of School Nurses (NASN) was organized. NASN serves as the hub for all state organizations as well as providing numerous educational programs, formulates position papers, offers professional journals, and sets the standards for all school nurses through the Framework for 21st Century School Nurse Practice.

Today's school nurse recognizes that we should not only care for people when they are ill but that the real power lies in our ability to change unhealthy lifestyle choices through education. Pain, disease, and illness, in many instances, can be lessened or totally prevented.

■ Legislation Impacting Schools

The role of the school nurse was significantly impacted by legislation supporting those children with special needs. No longer ignored, these children now have rights. The school nurse is involved with seeing that the laws are implemented.

The Individual with Disabilities Education Act is a federal law that protects students with disabilities. Adopted in 1975 and amended in 2004, the law clearly states that every child is entitled to a Free Appropriate Public Education (FAPE). Provisions include:

- ■ Emphasis must be placed on those children with disabilities and providing them with related services.
- ■ Children must receive appropriate evaluations by a team of knowledgeable and trained evaluators.
- ■ Each child must have an Individualized Education Plan to ensure access to a FAPE.
- ■ Children must be placed in the *least restrictive environment*.
- ■ All efforts must be made to keep the child in a general education setting.
- ■ Classroom modifications, teaching aids, and alternate methods must be explored.
- ■ If classroom presence proves inappropriate, with parental participation, other placements can be explored (Saleh, n.d.).

No longer isolated in special schools, more children now receive medications and treatments in the mainstream school setting. This can only be accomplished by the school nurse. The school nurse plans their care so all, regardless of need, have a place in the school community.

Current Issues Facing School Nurses

Recognizing that the specialty of school nursing continues to evolve, there are a number of issues that confront the school nurse of today. These include:

Lack of Uniform, State, Educational Requirements

Since passage of the 10th Amendment to the Bill of Rights in 1791, all aspects of education are left to the individual states to determine. Some states require school nurses to have a bachelor's degree in nursing and certification. Other states may only require a few courses in child development to qualify as a school nurse. There is no continuity in requirements. This creates confusion as nurses frequently move from one state to another. The better educated the nurse is the better prepared to teach and render care.

Poor Pay

In many instances, the school nurse will be paid on a teacher's salary guide. Usually, this is far less than hospital wages. After completing a program of study to become a school nurse, the nurse will be faced with greater responsibility for far lower pay.

Growing Number of Medically Fragile Students

Since passage of the Individuals with Disabilities Act (1973), children with chronic conditions needing medications and/or treatments are part of the mainstream. Children with diabetes, severe allergies, seizure disorders, etc., require intense planning and care in order to allow them to blend into the mainstream and learn in the least restrictive environment. Only the school nurse can make this happen. These plans necessitate a working knowledge of the health issue and require many hours of intense preparation.

Resistance of Parents to Immunize Children

The school nurse is the gatekeeper for immunization requirements. Until the child registers for school, parents can choose not to immunize. Since there are a growing number of children unprotected against highly communicable diseases, the school nurse must be alert to protect all students. Religious, medical, and/or philosophical exemptions are granted in most states.

Acceptance of the Needs of the Marginalized Child

Today, nurses have a greater awareness of the student who is marginalized because of the challenges they face. These include students who are mentally ill, transgender, culturally different, dependent on illegal substances transient, morbidly obese, etc. Moreover, teachers are not always prepared to deal with issues as they develop in the classroom. The school nurse must be cognizant of these special needs children and work to help them find their place in the school community.

High Risk Area

For the most part, the school nurse works independently. In almost all other nursing settings, nurses work as part of a team so if a difficult decision must be made, the team or someone in charge will make the decision. Also, when a shift is completed, another nurse comes in to pick-up where the prior nurse left off. Additionally, in school nursing, you make decisions with little or no diagnostic tools.

The school position involves many varied tasks including nursing, teaching, record- keeping, medications, treatments, and health counseling, all high risk areas. Even the smallest error can be libelous if misconstrued.

No Substitutes

School nurses will report that this is their number one concern. Qualified substitutes are almost nonexistent. If one does manage to recruit a substitute, most likely that person will quickly be offered a full-time position.

Substitute pay is comparable to what teachers get which is far less than the nurse can make per diem in a hospital setting or through an agency.

▨ Summary

To know the history of the nursing profession is to know the foundation on which school nursing was built. To know the foundation is to know how necessary it is to continue to affirm and grow our profession.

Recognized as the most trusted profession, nursing carries tremendous responsibilities and challenges as well. School nursing will provide unique opportunities through education to make significant changes in lifestyle which will continue to have a lifetime impact on children.

This is an exciting time for school nursing. Our role is broader and encompasses much more than ever (NASN Framework, 2018).

The school nurse of today possesses innate qualities which identify and separate us from other nursing specialties. Walking proudly with one foot in nursing and the other in education, we recognize the importance of teaching and community involvement. This common thread, when accepted and affirmed, will allow all of us and our school nursing profession to grow and flourish for many years to come.

▨ References

Alexander, K. (2018). *Florence Nightingale. Woman's history museum*. Retrieved from www.womanshistory.org

D'Antonio, B. (n.d.). *Nursing medical profession*. Retrieved from https://www.britannica.com/science/nursing

Daily Nurse. (2020) Gallup's 2019 most trusted professions. Retrieved from dailynurse.com/gallups-2019-most-trusted (2020)

Hanink, E. (2019). Lina Rogers, the first school nurse. Providing healthcare to keep kids in school. *Working Nurse*. Retrieved from https://www.workingnurse.com/articles/lina-rogers-the-first-school-nurse

Henry Street Settlement. (n.d.). *Lillian Wald*. Retrieved from https://www.henrystreet.org

Joel, L. (2018). *Advanced practice nursing* (pp. 3–7). Philadelphia, PA: F.A. Davis Company.

Levine, L. (2018, November). *Lillian Wald's lower east side: From visiting nurse service to the Henry Street Settlement*. Retrieved from https://www.6sqft.com/lillian-walds-lower-east-side

Loschiavo, J. (2019). *Fast facts for the school nurse* (3rd ed., pp. 8–9). New York, NY: Springer Publishing Company.

National Association of School Nurses. (2016). *Definition of school nursing*. Retrieved from https://www.nasn.org/advocacy/aboutnasn

National Association of School Nurses. (2018). *Framework for 21st century school nursing practice*. Retrieved from https://www.nasn.org/nasn/nasn-resources/professional-topics/framework

Nursing School Hub. (n.d.). *The history of nursing*. Retrieved from www.nursingschoolhub.com

Rogers, L. (1917). *The school nurse: A survey of the duties and responsibilities of the nurse in maintenance of health and physical perfection and the prevention of disease among school children*. New York, NY: G.P. Putnam's Sons.

Saleh, M. (n.d.). *Smart kids, your child's right: 6 principles of IDEA*. Retrieved from www.smartkidswithld.org

Wold, S. (1981). *School nursing: A framework for practice* (pp. 4–18). Minnesota, MN: Sunrise River Press.

Further Readings

Ehrenreich, B. (1973). *Witches, midwives, and nurses; A history of women healers*. Old Westbury, NY: The Feminist Press.

Hallet, C. (2010). *Celebrating nurse: A visual history*. London, England: Barrons.

2

PREVENTION CONCEPTS IN SCHOOL NURSING

JANICE LOSCHIAVO

LEARNING OBJECTIVES

- Compare the prevention approach to health care with that of intervention.
- Recognize the important role the school nurse has in primary prevention through education.
- Identify one specific example of primary, secondary, and tertiary prevention
- Assess the level of wellness today as compared with a century ago.

▣ Introduction

Most Americans would readily agree that the past few decades have brought enormous advancements in healthcare. This is due, in part, to the fact that we have been educated to recognize the many risk factors that cause cancer and heart disease, the two leading causes of death. Americans now live longer, much more productive lives (Nicolos, 2019). When we consider the dual role of the school nurse as both nurse and teacher, it is obvious that we play, and must continue to play, a vital role in the on-going advancement of healthcare. Through a systematic educational process, our goal is to improve or maintain the health status of children so they can get the greatest benefit from the school experience and make wise decisions as adults.

If the school nurse does their job well there will be far fewer accidents, illnesses, and long-range health problems. This is why the school nurse's work is so challenging. This is also why their work can be most rewarding.

In this chapter you will learn the distinction between prevention and intervention, various levels of prevention, scope of prevention practice and specific measures the school nurse can use to implement them.

By utilizing prevention concepts, you will help raise the wellness level of each child, your school community and our nation.

Prevention Versus Intervention

School nursing differs from all other subspecialties of nursing because our major thrust is *PREVENTION* as opposed to *INTERVENTION.*

To *prevent* means to stop something from happening. The implication is that the "something" to be avoided could prove harmful in the present or the future. *Primary prevention* is done through education. Since all children are required to attend school, we are given the opportunity to impact students' decisions at an early age.

Intervention is the act of interfering with the outcome or course of a condition. In a hospital setting, the child has already experienced an accident or illness and now requires intervention.

This may in the form of a specific treatment or medication. Along with a team of other health professionals, the nurse plans the strategies to *intervene* and restore wellness.

A portion of the school nurse's job is to intervene as accidents occur; however, the main thrust is education. Through a comprehensive school health education program, the school nurse strives to *prevent* the illness or accident from occurring.

Categories of Health Prevention

Primary Prevention

In primary prevention the effects of disease or illness are halted before symptoms manifest. This is done through education on issues such as vaccinations and risky behaviors like smoking, poor diet, lack of exercise and the abuse of substances known to be associated with life-threatening conditions.

Secondary Prevention

Secondary Prevention involves screening to identify diseases at the earliest possible state, before the onset of symptoms. School screenings such as blood pressure, height, weight, BMI, audiometrics, vision, oral, scoliosis, and so forth are now common and serve to warn the individual of possible long-range problems.

Tertiary Prevention

Once the disease has manifested itself, the goal is to slow, control, or stop the progression. In the school setting, the objective is to allow the child to blend and participate in the same educational experience as their peers to the best of their ability (Centers for Disease Control and Prevention [CDC] Prevention, n.d.). Today's educators recognize that children learn from each other and a nurturing, mainstreamed classroom environment is best for the student and cost-effective for the school district.

Children with chronic illnesses must have an Individualized Healthcare Plan with strategies in place to deal with symptoms as they present during the school day. The student can be treated for respiratory illnesses, monitored for diabetes and cared for during a seizure by the competent school nurse. Once the problem is addressed, in most instances, the child can return to the classroom and join their peers to complete the school day.

Primary Prevention and Education

The most effective and least costly way to prevent illness and maintain wellness is through education. As with other disciplines, most states have specific standards for health education.

We also have national standards which were developed by The Joint Committee. These National Health Education Standards serve to establish, promote, and support health-enhancing behaviors for students from pre-kindergarten through grade 12.

The National Health Education Standards are written expectations for what students should know and be able to do by grades 2, 5, 8, and 12 to promote personal, family, and community health (Box 2.1). These standards provide a foundation on which to build a comprehensive health curriculum and assess student learning. From these broad areas, specific lessons on risk factors, dietary habits, exercise, substance abuse, mental health, infection control, and so forth can be developed and implemented.

BOX 2.1

NATIONAL HEALTH EDUCATION STANDARDS

STANDARD 1

Students will comprehend concepts related to health promotion and disease prevention to enhance health.

STANDARD 2

Students will analyze the influence of family, peers, culture, media, technology and other factors on health behaviors.

STANDARD 3

Students will demonstrate the ability to access valid information, products and services to enhance health.

STANDARD 4

Students will demonstrate the ability to use interpersonal communication skills to enhance health and avoid or reduce health risks.

STANDARD 5

Students will demonstrate the ability to use decision-making skills to enhance health.

(continued)

STANDARD 6

Students will demonstrate the ability to use goal-setting skills to enhance health.

STANDARD 7

Students will demonstrate the ability to practice health-enhancing behaviors and avoid or reduce health risks.

STANDARD 8

Students will demonstrate the ability to advocate for personal, family, and community health (CDC, 2019a).

Primary Prevention and Immunizations

Until the child is required to attend school, parents may refuse all immunizations. However, education is required for all students in the United States and few parents elect to home school their children. In most schools, the nurse is given the task of monitoring compliance for immunizations. This means that the school nurse, when registering the child, will be the first person to confront a resistant parent. Do not get into an argument with the parent who refuses to immunize their child. Explain the options and legal recourse. Remind them that you are a mere agent of the Board of Education and must uphold the state requirements. Note your conversation in writing and forward the information to the building principal for school attorney review.

Immunization Exemptions

There are three types of exemptions: medical, religious, and philosophical. States will vary as to terms and conditions for each.

Medical

A medical exemption can be given when the immunization is medically contraindicated. The private physician or advanced practice nurse must put in writing the reason and time period the child is to be exempt. When the child's health condition permits, the exemption is terminated.

Religious

A parent/guardian must submit to the school a written statement requesting an exemption on the grounds that the immunization interferes with the pupil's religious rights.

Philosophical

A parent may request a philosophical exemption based on personal, moral or other beliefs.

All 50 states require specific vaccines for students. Currently, all states permit medical exemptions. Washington, DC, and 45 states permit religious exemptions and 15 states allow philosophical exemptions (National Conference of State Legislatures, 2019).

Provisional Admission

In some states, provisional admission may be granted for up to 30 days for the student transferring from out of state or country. If the documents are not produced after 1 month, then one dose of each age-appropriate vaccine must be given and the entire immunization series must be repeated.

Documents Acceptable as Proof of Immunizations

Most states agree that the following documents may be acceptable as proof of immunization provided that the type of immunization and date of administration is in compliance with immunization requirements:

- *An official school record:* If the student is transferring from another school, you may accept the immunizations records from that school. The information should be presented on a school/district letterhead with appropriate signatures.

- *A record from a public health department:* Immunizations are frequently given at a town-sponsored clinic. The location, type of immunization, vaccine number, dates, and signature of who administered the vaccine should be included.

- *A physician-signed certificate:* The physician must be licensed to practice medicine or osteopathy and the certificate must be presented on an official office letterhead.

- *A certificate signed by an advanced practice nurse:* This must be presented on an official letterhead.

- *An official state or national record:* If transferring from out-of-state or country, the immunization dates will be listed on a document which clearly indicates that it is a national or state approved document.

Immunization Provisions

School immunization records are to be considered educational documents and are covered under the provisions of the Family Educational Rights and Privacy Act (FERPA). This Act states that all educational institutions (elementary, high school, and college) that receive any funds for programs administered by the United States Department of Education are covered by FERPA.

FERPA also allows for the sharing of information with parents and students over 18 years of age and prevents the disclosure of personally identifiable information without the consent of a parent (Association of State and Territorial Health Officials, 2019).

These health records are to be retained by the district for a specified period of time, usually 100 years.

All dates must be recorded to include the month, date, and year. Be cognizant of the fact that foreign countries may list the date differently—day, month, and year.

Immunizations are to be recorded on a permanent record and made available to local or state officials for the purpose of auditing. These health records are to be retained by the district for a specified period of time, usually 100 years. Many states will also require each school to submit an Annual Immunization Report. This document is used to assess the immunization compliance level.

Immunization Requirements

Requirements may vary from state to state and year to year. For an accurate, updated list of age-appropriate vaccines, check your individual state requirements; for CDC recommendations, accesswww.cdc.gov/vaccines/schedules/hcp/imz/child-adolescent.html.

Secondary Prevention and Screenings

There is no question that there is a strong link between a child's mental and physical well-being and their ability to learn. Ideally, students should all have access to preventive medical care. However, even when it is available, many do not see a physician on a regular basis. Since all children must attend school, the school is the right place for a healthy start. Today we recognize seven *Health Barriers to Learning*:

- Uncorrected vision problems
- Unaddressed hearing loss
- Uncontrolled asthma
- Dental pain
- Persistent hunger
- Untreated mental and behavioral health problems
- Lead exposure (Children's Health Fund, 2017)

As discussed previously, health screenings are an example of secondary prevention. Through systematic screenings, the school nurse will be able to detect early stages of health defects, address them appropriately, and thereby avoid serious, future problems which might impact learning.

What screenings are required and when is determined by your local/state policy though most school nurses will agree that those entered in this chapter are necessary for all children. They include: Height/Weight, Vision, Audiometrics, Blood Pressure, Oral Screening, and Scoliosis.

■ Suggestions for Screening Implementation

Have all equipment calibrated yearly or as recommended by the manufacturer. Budget equipment replacements 1 year in advance.

■ Request that you *not* be disturbed during screening times except for an emergency.

Define what an emergency is. The student deserves your full attention and you deserve to not be interrupted. You may choose to do all vision at once, then all audio, and so forth. This will allow you to see all children several times a year. Or you may schedule each student for a 10- to 15-minute time slot and do all screenings at once.

Perform screenings using the procedure that works best for you and provides the least interruption to teachers and students.

Consider arranging screenings to coincide with seasons. In the fall, do audio screenings before cold season. Do blood pressure screenings in warm weather when students are likely to be sleeveless.

Follow-up on all referrals according to district policy. Carefully document all notices and keep administration informed of parents not following-up with referrals. *There is no point in screening if there is no follow-up.*

Stress that screenings are just that—*screenings*—and should never be considered the same as a thorough, professional examination by a physician. The diagnosis must be made by the physician.

If the child does not pass the initial screening, retest in 1 to 2 weeks. If the same problem is noted, refer.

■ Once a possible problem has been detected, a referral must be made for physician follow-up.

■ Height/Weight Screening

Every child should have their growth and development checked annually to be certain that they are thriving. Both low weight and excessive weight gain can indicate medical or emotional problems.

Procedure for Height and Weight Screenings

■ Shoes and heavy sweaters or jackets should be removed

■ Students must stand on the scale with their back toward the ruler

■ Measure height from the highest point on the back of the head with the chin forward.

■ Calculate weight while the student is motionless

■ Screen for height and weight approximately the same time every year.

■ Record findings on the student's permanent health record.

Body Mass Index

An objective measurement of body fat is the Body Mass Index (BMI). This is a weight-to-height ratio, computed by dividing the weight by the square of height. The comparative percentile figure you get is an indicator of obesity or underweight (Table 2.1). A quick reference can be found using the CDC's BMI Calculator Charts for Boys or Girls (www.cdc.gov/healthyweight/bmi/calculator.html). Students found to be below the 5th percentile (underweight) or above the 95th percentile (overweight) are at risk for immediate and long-term impacts on their physical, social, and emotional health.

When to Refer

All students who are less than 5% and over than 85% for weight or BMI should be referred.

When checking a child's height and weight, discretion is urged. Do not announce the child's height and weight so another student can hear. It is best not to tell any child this information while measuring. Ask them to see you after school if they wish to know their height and weight.

Advise any assistant(s) to likewise be discreet.

Consider calling the parent before sending a mailed, written notice for BMI referral. Parents are easily offended if they think you are criticizing their child. Be aware that morbid obesity or extreme underweight may have nothing to do with food. Frequently, there is an underlying problem that must be identified before the child can be helped.

TABLE 2.1 PERCENTILE RANGES FOR WEIGHT STATUS CATEGORIES

WEIGHT STATUS CATEGORY	PERCENTILE CATEGORY
Underweight	Less than the 5th percentile
Normal or healthy weight	5th percentile to less than the 85th percentile
Overweight	85th to less than the 95th percentile
Obese	Equal to or greater than the 95th percentile

SOURCE: Centers for Disease Control and Prevention. (2010). *Defining childhood obesity.* Retrieved from https://www.cdc.gov/obesity/childhood/defining.html

▓ Vision Screening

Good vision is essential to a child's academic success and overall well-being. Unless a child can see clearly, they will not be able to read books, laptops, or materials posted. Learning will dramatically be compromised since much of what is learned is accomplished through visual processing.

The school nurse must be cognizant of the fact that often the changes are subtle and go unnoticed until academic problems emerge. The school nurse is responsible for promoting secondary prevention by screening children for visual deficits and identifying those who need some type of correction.

By age 8 years, vision maturity is complete. Therefore, it is essential to screen and implement corrective measures as early as possible.

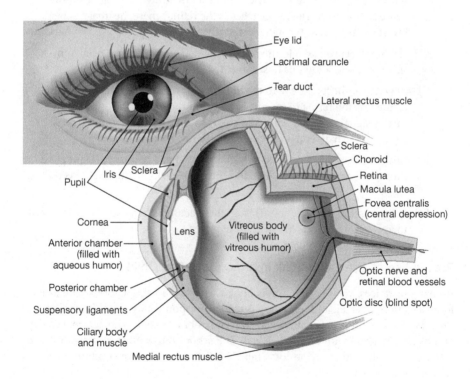

FIGURE 2.1 Anatomy of the eye.

SOURCE: Reproduced from Gawlik, K. S., Melnyk, B. M., & Teall, A. M. (2020). *Evidence-based physical examination: Best practices for health and well-being assessment.* New York, NY: Springer Publishing Company.

The Parts of the Eye and How We See (Figure 2.1)

Cornea: Clear front window of the eye that transmits and focuses light into the eye. Light must first enter the eye through the cornea. The cornea's refractive power bends the light rays. The cornea also keeps foreign bodies from harming the delicate eye.

Iris: Colored part of the eye that helps regulate the amount of light that enters. The iris works like a shutter in a camera. It can enlarge or shrink the image depending on how much light is entering the eye.

Pupil: Dark aperture in the iris. From the cornea, the light passes through the pupil. The amount of light passing through is regulated by the iris.

Lens: Transparent structure inside the eye. The light then hits the lens, which focuses light rays onto the retina.

Retina: Thin layer of nervous tissue that lines the back of the eye. The retina senses light, and creates electrical impulses that travel through the optic nerve to the brain. The image reaches the retina where the image appears inverted. As soon as the light reaches the retina, the process of vision begins.

Macula: Small central area in the retina. The macula contains special light-sensitive cells and allows us to see fine details clearly.

Optic nerve: Connects the eye to the brain and carries the electrical impulses formed by the retina to the visual cortex of the brain. The optic nerve carries signals of light, dark, and colors to the area of the brain (the visual cortex), which assembles the signals into images (vision).

Vitreous gel: Clear substance that helps keep the shape of the eye. Light passes through the vitreous gel which fills the globe, helping the eye to keep its shape

Fovea: Depression in the retina. This is where acuity is highest (Canadian Keratoconus Foundation, 2015).

Prevalence of Eye Conditions in the School-Age Child

In many instances, vision screening is done exclusively in the school setting; therefore, detection, referral, and follow-up is a major responsibility. Once identified, it is the school nurse, in collaboration with the classroom teacher, who can make adaptations for the child with a vision deficit. The school nurse must be a strong advocate for the child with a vision loss. Table 2.2 lists common eye conditions seen in school-age children.

Symptoms of Visual Deficits

Be alert for a number of symptoms with which the child might present. A teacher might report that the student frequently rubs their eyes, has chronic tearing, squints, or covers one eye to read. The child might also struggle with reading and have a poor

TABLE 2.2 COMMON EYE CONDITIONS SEEN IN THE SCHOOL-AGE CHILD

Vision loss	3%	Even with corrective lenses, some children under 18 years old remains completely blind or significantly visually impaired.
Amblyopia (lazy eye)	2%	6 months to 6 years—Vision is compromised due to poor neural connections. Eye function is otherwise normal. Most often only one eye is involved. One of the most common cause of vision loss in children
Strabismus (crossed-eyes)	2%–4%	Under 6 years Condition occurs when eyes are not aligned properly and point in different directions due to muscle dysfunction. Early patching is recommended to force the affected eye muscle to properly align.
Refractive errors	4%	Myopia 6–72 months (nearsightedness) The eye structure is too long and light cannot focus correctly.
	9%	Myopia 5–17 years Visual images come in focus in front of the retina resulting in defective distant images; close vision is sharp and clear; can become worse with age.
	21%	Hyperopia 6–72 months (farsightedness)
	13%	5–17 years Visual images come in focus beyond the retina. Distant objects are seen clearly, close ones do not come into proper focus.
Astigmatism	15%–28%	5–17 years A condition where the eye is not completely round causing vision to be blurred.
Color blindness	8% Males	Cannot see colors in a normal way—genetic predisposition.
	1% Females	

SOURCE: Data from Prevent Blindness. (2019). *Prevalence and impact of vision disorders in U.S. children*. Retrieved from https://www.preventblindness.org/.../prevalence-and-impact-vision-disorder

attention span. On external examination, one eye might turn in a different direction. Sometimes, abnormal eye movements can be noted or the child will turn their head, favoring one position.

The school nurse might also find that the child frequently complains of headaches following close visual activities like reading.

Any report of the symptoms in Table 2.1 should begin with a screening and immediate referral if deficiency exists (Salvin, 2014).

Types of Vision Screenings

It is important to remember that the school nurse is *not* a physician and does *not* have the necessary skills or equipment for a thorough eye examination. Parents who request such should be referred to appropriate medical personnel or facility. All injuries, foreign bodies, abrasions need to be referred out. Do not attempt any invasive eye procedure.

Screenings can consist of:

- *Visual acuity*: Done with a wall chart placed 20 feet away or appropriate slides in a machine such as a Titmus.
- *Color blindness test*: Accomplished with a book or appropriate machine slides where the color blind cannot see numbers or shapes within dot patterns.
- *Eye alignment:* Done to evaluate the movement of your eye muscles. Have the student follow a colorful object such as a pencil eraser, from the nose circling each ear.

Procedure for Vision Screenings

Vision screening is best done as soon as possible once the child enters school. Unless noted on the school entrance examination, do not assume that the child has been evaluated for vision defects. Age-appropriate screening tools are available for children as young as 3 years of age. They include:

- E chart: Have student cover one eye at a time, stand 20 feet away, and indicate if the E is up, down, right, or left.
- Preschool charts: Student must say if E is pointing to boy, girl, toy, or dog.
- Titmus: Have student read appropriate slides for different tests.

When to Refer

Refer if acuity is less than 20/40, or there is any problem with color perception, alignment, or motility, or in compliance with district or state guidelines.

■ Audiometric Screening

Hearing loss is the most common developmental disorder seen at birth. Since hearing is almost fully developed at birth, most states now mandate newborn tests for early detection of hearing loss. Often the number of children identified with hearing defects will increase during the school years.

This gives the school nurse an important role for early detection, referral, and implementation of strategies to assist the child. The goal is to identify and remedy the problem before academic, social, language, or emotional issues arise.

Parts of the Ear and How We Hear (Figure 2.2)

Sound is caused by vibrations that travel through the air. These vibrations are gathered up by the outer ear. Early hearing aid devices were designed to enlarge the pinna

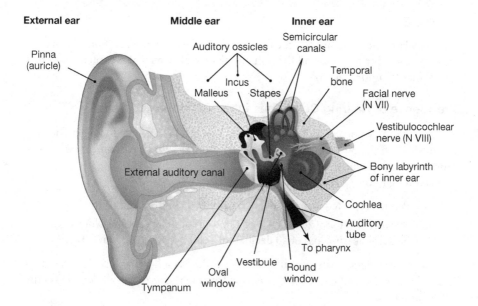

FIGURE 2.2 Anatomy of the ear.

SOURCE: Reproduced from Gawlik, K. S., Melnyk, B. M., & Teall, A. M. (2020). *Evidence-based physical examination: Best practices for health and well-being assessment.* New York, NY: Springer Publishing Company.

or auricle to allow for greater accumulation of sounds from the air. The vibrations stimulate the nerve endings of the cochlea and communicate directly to the brain for interpretation.

Outer Ear

Pinna or auricle: When sound is made, the auricle gathers the sound and sends vibrations through the ear canal which strike the eardrum or tympanic membrane.

Middle Ear

Tympanic membrane or eardrum: The tympanic membrane separates the outer from the middle ear. It helps to equalize the pressure in the middle ear which is needed for the proper transfer of sound waves. When the eardrum vibrates it passes the vibration to the ossicles.

> *Ossicles:* The ossicles are three small bones—malleus, incus and stapes—that transmit the sound waves to the inner ear. Sound is converted to electrical impulses which the auditory nerve sends to the brain. The ossicles amplify the sound and send sound waves to the cochlea in the inner ear.

> *Brain:* The brain translates these impulses as sound.

Inner Ear

The bony labyrinth contains the cochlea, nerves for hearing, the vestibule which contains receptors for balance, and the semicircular canals which also contain receptors for balance (Stanford, 2015).

Prevalence of Hearing Conditions in the School-Aged Child

Most cases of newborn or childhood hearing loss can be attributed to a genetic predisposition. Of the 50% to 60% of diagnosed children, 20% have some type of syndrome such as Down.

According to the CDC:

■ Parents reported hearing loss in 5 per 1,000 children, ages 3 to 17
■ Between 1991 and 2010, 1.4% of 1,000 children 8 years and older have a bilateral hearing loss of 40 decibels or more (CDC Data, May 2017).

It is not sufficient to just identify that the child has a hearing loss. It is essential that the type or cause be identified since the treatment approach will depend on the nature of the loss.

Types of Hearing Loss

■ Conductive Hearing Loss

This is hearing loss caused by something that stops sounds from getting through the outer or middle ear.

■ Sensorineural Hearing Loss

Sensorineural loss occurs when there is a problem in the way the inner ear or auditory nerve functions.

■ Mixed Hearing Loss

This is hearing loss that includes both a conductive and a sensorineural hearing loss.

■ Auditory Neuropathy Spectrum Disorder

This is hearing loss that occurs when sound enters the ear normally, but because of damage to the inner ear or the hearing nerve, sound isn't organized in a way that the brain can understand (CDC Data, 2017).

Symptoms of Hearing Loss

Hearing loss can develop at any age for a variety of reasons. Sensorineural damage can be progressive in the inner ear or can have a conductive cause due to repeated otitis or excessive cerumen buildup.

Frequently, a parent will be the first to notice that the child is not hearing adequately. The parent will mention that the volume on the television is too high, or the child might withdraw from conversations or avoid social settings. In school, the teacher might note that the child's speech is not clear, understanding words is difficult, or the child tries to read lips.

Types of Screenings

Pure tone: Sounds are initiated by the school nurse and travel through the outer and middle ear, inner ear and to the brain. The student indicates when they hear the sound. Sound is measured in decibels (loudness) and Hertz (pitch). Normal speech is 50 to 70 dB. A 3,000-Hertz tone of 0 dB is the softest level a person can hear.

Conduction: This type of testing is used when something, such as wax or fluid, is blocking the outer or middle ear so the sound does not reach the inner ear or hearing nerves. The brain is unable to recognize the sound in a way that can be understood (CDC Data, 2017).

Procedure for Auditory Screening

- Audiometric testing is done with the use of an audiometer and head set.
- Place the clean head set over the child's ears. Make sure it fits properly.
- Seat the child at least 6 feet away with their back to you and the audiometer.
- Instruct the child to raise their hand when they hear the sound.
- If child has difficulty with first sounds, readjust the headset and try again.
- Begin with 1,000 Hertz at 40 decibels and gradually reduce to 20 or 25 and screen from 1,000 to 4,000.

When to Refer for Auditory Defects

If a child fails one or more frequencies within the speaking range, 1,000 to 4,000 decibels, retest in 1 to 2 weeks. If the student fails at the same level when re-screened, refer.

If school policy permits, you may use an otoscope to check the ear canal for excessive wax buildup. Do not remove the wax. Notify the parent for physician's recommendation for removal.

Blood Pressure Screening

Hypertension in children appears to be on the increase, especially as it relates to obesity. All children should be checked annually in hopes of avoiding long-term complications.

Blood pressure is considered elevated when it is the same or higher than 95% of children who are the same sex, age, and height as the child. In young children hypertension is related to other health conditions or hormonal disorders. Older children who are overweight will most likely to be hypertensive.

How High Blood Pressure Occurs

Blood pressure is the force of blood as it flows through the body's vessels. The heart is the pump; its vessels widen and contract to keep the blood flowing as it should. If the heart has to work too hard, the pressure builds up in the vessels causing high blood pressure.

Prevalence of Hypertension

The latest CDC report which included over 12,000 participants indicated that more than 1 in 7 U.S. youths, 12 to 19 years old, had hypertension or elevated blood pressure (U.S. Department of Health and Human Services [DHHS], 2007). Symptoms of hypertension include fast or pounding heat beat, seizures, chest pains, shortness of breath, headaches, and vomiting.

Procedure for Blood Pressure Screening

- Blood pressure screening can begin as early as 3 years of age.
- Use the proper cuff size. Use proper size cuff. Place on upper arm allowing room for the stethoscope head.
- Right arm should be used.
- Allow the child to be seated, rested and relaxed.
- Blood pressure by auscultation is the gold standard (DHHS, 2007)

Refer

Recheck after 15 minutes if elevated. Refer all elevations to private MD.

Ranges can be found in *A Pocket Guide to Blood Pressure Measurement in Children* (DHHS, 2007; www.nhlbi.nih.gov/health-topics/all-publications-and-resources/pocket-guide-blood-pressure-measurement-children)

▓ Oral Screening

Tooth decay is believed to be the most prevalent chronic condition among children in the United States. Cavities are one of the most common diseases of childhood.

Untreated cavities cause pain and infections that may lead to problems with eating, speaking, playing, and learning. Children who have poor oral health often miss more school and receive lower grades than children who do not (CDC Oral Health, May 2019). Dental screening laws exist in 14 states and Washington, DC (Children's Dental Health Project, 2019).

Prevalence of Oral Disease

Oral disease is seen in children of all ages. Often it is tied into poor diet and lack of generally good health habits including brushing, fluoride treatments, and appropriate professional care. The short- and long-term effects of neglect are staggering:

- 1 of 5 (20%) of children aged 5 to 11 years have at least one untreated, decayed tooth.
- 1 of 7 (13%) of adolescents aged 12 to 19 years have at least one untreated, decayed tooth.
- Children aged 5 to 19 years from low-income families are twice as likely (25%) to have cavities, compared with children from higher-income households (11%) (CDC Oral Health, May 2019).

Symptoms of Oral Disease

Dental disease is easily noted in children. Teeth will appear cracked or broken with visible decay. The school nurse or teacher might also see the student in obvious pain when chewing.

Sometimes decay is so advanced that there will be red, irritated gums, a swollen jaw, or excessive bleeding. When these symptoms present, an immediate referral is warranted.

Procedure for Oral Screening

Here again, a screening will not replace a qualified, dental expert's evaluation. It would be best to work with school administrators to add this requirement prior to school starting.

- Check to see if your district requires a dental exam by a qualified dental expert prior to school entrance and periodically throughout the school experience.
- With administrative approval, arrange for a local dentist or students from a school of dentistry to come to screen all students.
- If necessary, with administrative and parental consent, you may do a superficial screening.

When to Refer for Oral Disease

Send a referral home to all who say they have never seen a dentist or show evidence of possible dental disease. Arrange clinic services if necessary.

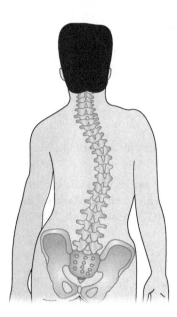

FIGURE 2.3 Spine curvature of scoliosis.

SOURCE: Reproduced from Gawlik, K. S., Melnyk, B. M., & Teall, A. M. (2020). *Evidence-based physical examination: Best practices for health and well-being assessment.* New York, NY: Springer Publishing Company.

Scoliosis Screening

The goal of a scoliosis screening is to detect a curvature of the spine at the earliest possible stage so there is an opportunity for a less invasive method of treatment and surgery can be avoided (Figure 2.3).

About half of U.S. states have mandatory scoliosis screening in schools. Screenings are done on children 10 to 18 years.

Some children mature faster than others. There is no harm in checking children at 9 years of age.

Prevalence of Scoliosis

- Affects 2% to 3% of the population
- Can develop in infancy or early childhood
- Primary age of onset is 10 to 15 years, occurring in both genders
- Idiopathic scoliosis occurs 10 times more often in girls than boys over 10 years old
- Girls more likely to develop severe curves (American Association of Neurological Surgeons, n.d.)

Procedure for Scoliosis Screening

Be cognizant of the fact that many boys have some breast development and are very self-conscious about their bodies. Privacy is needed for girls, as well.

This screening is especially challenging for school nurses. We fear making an unnecessary referral. Rest assured, after looking at dozens or even hundreds of children's backs, you will become very accomplished at identifying even minor curvatures.

Notify parents in advance of your plans to screen and allow them to exclude their child.

- Demonstrate how you will check their back.
  - Have the child stand straight, arms at sides, back to you. Then have them bend forward as if diving in a pool, clap hands, and bend forward to 45 degree angle. (The clap is an auditory reminder to bend appropriately.) Look at the back from rear and front. Have the child stand straight again and look at arm distance from hip and scapula symmetry.
- Provide as much privacy for *both* boys and girls.
- Allow girls to wear halter tops or body suits.
- Have student remove shirt and shoes.
- Place chalk marks on floor where you want them to place their feet.
- Have them stare at a designated point on the wall.
- Look at child's back, have them bend, look from the front, have them stand, and check back again.

When to Refer

If in doubt, recheck the child at the earliest convenience. Refer any questionable observations.

■ Medications and Tertiary Prevention

Children who have a diagnosed chronic condition are now part of the mainstream. For these children the school nurse provides tertiary prevention in hopes that their symptoms will be slowed, controlled or stopped completely.

It is estimated that about 25% of children in the United States aged 2 to 8 years have a chronic health condition. The healthcare needs of these children are complex and continuous. They must be managed on a daily basis as well as cared for during an emergency (CDC, 2018).

Medication administration is a major part of the school nurse's responsibilities and considered an area of high risk. Many children would not be able to attend school without being medicated.

Administering medication in the school setting is a challenging task for any nurse.

The registered, professional school nurse is responsible for medication administration in the school setting and for leading the development of written medication administration policies and procedures that focus on safe and efficient medication administration at school. Well-written policies and procedures will enable schools to fulfill their obligations to provide health-related services to all children, especially those with healthcare needs included under the Individuals with Disabilities Education Improvement Act (2004) and Section 504 of the Rehabilitation Act (1973) as amended through the Americans with Disabilities Amendment Act in 2008.

The school nurse is the professional with the clinical knowledge and understanding of the complex issues surrounding the safe administration of medication and the responsibility to protect the health and safety of students (American Academy of Pediatrics, 2016). As the health leader in the school setting, the school nurse promotes current evidence-based practices so students requiring medication during the school day can safely have their needs met and remain in school ready to learn (Maughan, 2016).

Policies and procedures for medication administration must be clearly written and adhered to.

This is a high risk area in that errors can occur and the nurse and district will be liable.

School nurses have the responsibility to develop, promote, and implement clearly written policies and procedures for medication administration, storage, and documentation. Each district must have:

- Physician orders indicating the child's name, medication, when to be given and possible side effects
- Appropriate storage for all medications: refrigeration, double lock for controlled substances
- Charting procedure
- Medication labeled in the original container
- Policy for medications given on field trips
- Proper disposal procedures of unused medication
- Orders for over-the-counter medications
- Student confidentiality plans
- Procedure for reporting errors
- Policy for herbal remedies
- Delegation procedures (when permitted by state law). The training, supervision and evaluation must be done by the school nurse. Emergency medications such as epinephrine, albuterol, diastat, and glucagon may be delegated to non-nursing personnel.

- Staff medications policies
- Communication protocols for parents and classroom teachers.

Treatments and Tertiary Prevention

In order for them to remain in school, some children may require a specific treatment on a regular or acute need basis. Some of these treatments include:

- Nebulizer inhalation
- Tube feedings
- Catheterizations

Again, it is the school nurse's responsibility to meet with parents and students to develop an Individualized Healthcare Plan centered around the private physician's orders.

The Prevention Framework (CDC Prevention, n.d.)

In order to achieve the best possible outcomes, prevention strategies must take place at different levels.

Individual Prevention—These strategies include:

- Educating teachers and staff
- Implementing a health education program reflective of the National Health Education Standards
- Strengthening individual knowledge and reducing the risk factors through proper diet and exercise

Local Prevention—These strategies include:

- Awareness of and action on local, environmental health issues
- Attempts to decrease the number of liquor stores in an area
- Recognition of community-based organizations to sponsor health education programs
- Inspections of food establishments, day care facilities
- Promote community education
- Offer school breakfast and lunch programs

State Prevention—These include:

- Careful monitoring of waste disposal sites
- Supporting state sponsored efforts to offer health screenings
- Initiating anti-smoking campaigns
- Influencing policy making

National Prevention—These include:

- Regulatory programs and policies to reduce the presence of and exposure to harmful agents in the environment (Clean Water Act, National Tobacco Control Program)
- National Asthma Control
- The Environmental Protection Agency Dept. of Agriculture (CDC Prevention, n.d.)

References

American Academy of Pediatrics. (2016, June). Role of the school nurse in providing school health services (Policy Statement). *Pediatrics, 137*(6), 1–6. doi: 10.1542/peds.2016-0852

American Association of Neurological Surgeons. (n.d.). *Scoliosis*. Retrieved from https://www.aans.org/Patients/Neurosurgical-Conditions-and-Treatments/Scoliosis

Association of State and Territorial Health Officials. (2019). *Comparison of FERPA and HIPAA Privacy Rule for accessing student health data: Fact sheet*. Retrieved from https://www.astho.org/programs/preparedness/public-health-emergency-law/public-health-and-schools-toolkit/comparison-of-ferpa-and-hipaa-privacy-rule/

Canadian Keratoconus Foundation. (2015). *Anatomy of the eye*. Retrieved from http://keratoconuscanada.org/about-keratoconus/about-the-eye

Centers for Disease Control and Prevention. (2010). *Defining childhood obesity*. Retrieved from https://www.cdc.gov/obesity/childhood/defining.html

Centers for Disease Control and Prevention. (2017, May). *Data and statistics about hearing loss in children*. Retrieved from https://www.cdc.gov/ncbddd/hearingloss/data.html

Centers for Disease Control and Prevention. (2018). *Managing chronic health conditions in schools*. Retrieved from https://www.cdc.gov/healthyschools/chronicconditions.htm

Centers for Disease Control and Prevention. (2019a). *CDC Healthy Schools: National Health Education Standards*. Retrieved from https://www.cdc.gov/healthyschools/sher/standards/index.htm

Centers for Disease Control and Prevention. (2019b, May). *Children's oral health*. Retrieved from https://www.cdc.gov/oralhealth/basics/childrens-oral-health/index.html

Centers for Disease Control and Prevention. (n.d.). *BMI percentile calculator for children and teen*. Retrieved from https://www.cdc.gov/healthyweight/bmi/calculator.html

Centers for Disease Control and Prevention. (n.d.). *Oral health*. Retrieved from https://www.cdc.gov/healthyschools/npao/oralhealth.htm

Centers for Disease Control and Prevention. (n.d.). *Prevention*. Retrieved from https://www.cdc.gov/pictureofamerica/pdfs/picture_of_america_prevention.pdf

Centers for Disease Control and Prevention. (n.d.). *Table 1. Recommended child and adolescent immunization schedule for ages 18 years or younger, United States, 2020.* Retrieved from https://www.cdc.gov/vaccines/schedules/hcp/imz/child-adolescent.html

Centers for Disease Control and Prevention. (n.d.). *2 to 20 years: Boys. Body mass index-for-age percentiles.* Retrieved from https://www.cdc.gov/growthcharts/data/set1clinical/cj41l023.pdf

Centers for Disease Control and Prevention. (n.d.). *2 to 20 years: Girls. Body mass index-for-age percentiles.* Retrieved from https://www.cdc.gov/growthcharts/data/set1clinical/cj41l024.pdf

Children's Dental Health Project. (2019, Jan 30). *State dental screening laws for children: Examining the trend and impact.* Retrieved from https://www.cdhp.org/resources/341-state-dental-screening-laws-for-children-examining-the-trend-and-impact

Children's Health Fund. (2017, January). *The prevalence and educational consequences in disadvantaged children.* Retrieved from https://www.childrenshealthfund.org/wp-content/uploads/2017/01/Health-Barriers-to-Learning.pdf

Gawlik, K. S., Melnyk, B. M., & Teall, A. M. (2020). *Evidence-based physical examination: Best practices for health and well-being assessment.* New York, NY: Springer Publishing Company.

Maughan, E. (2016, Spring). Building strong children. Why we need nurses in schools. *American Educator.* Retrieved from https://www.aft.org/sites/default/files/ae_spring2016school-nursing.pdf

National Conference of State Legislatures. (2019, June 14). *States with religious and philosophical exemptions from school immunization requirements.* Retrieved from https://www.ncsl.org/research/health/school-immunization-exemption-state-laws.aspx

Nicolos, H. (2019). What are the leading causes of death in the US? *Medical News Today.* Retrieved from https://www.medicalnewstoday.com/articles/282929

Prevent Blindness. (2019). *Prevalence and impact of vision disorders in U.S. children.* Retrieved from https://wisconsin.preventblindness.org/prevalence-and-impact-of-vision-disorders-in-u-s-children/

Salvin, J. (2014). Your child's vision. *KidsHealth.* Retrieved from https://kidshealth.org/en/parents/vision.html

Stanford Children's Health. (2015). *Anatomy and physiology of the ear.* Retrieved from https://www.stanfordchildrens.org/en/topic/default?id=anatomy-and-physiology-of-the-ear-90-P02025

United States Department of Health and Human Services. (2007, May). *A pocket guide to blood pressure measurement in children.* Retrieved from https://www.nhlbi.nih.gov/health-topics/all-publications-and-resources/pocket-guide-blood-pressure-measurement-children

▨ Further Readings

American Academy of Pediatrics, American Public Health Association, & National Resource Center for Health and Safety in Child Care and Early Education. (2011). *Caring for our children: National health and safety performance standards; Guidelines for early care and education programs* (3rd ed.). Elk Grove Village, IL: American Academy of Pediatrics; Washington, DC: American Public Health Association.

American Academy of Pediatrics, American Public Health Association, & National Resource Center for Health and Safety in Child Care and Early Education. (2011). *Caring for our children: National health and safety performance standards; Guidelines for early care and education programs* (3rd ed.). Elk Grove Village, IL: American Academy of Pediatrics; Washington, DC: American Public Health Association.

Centers for Disease Control and Prevention. (2019, May 9). *BMI percentile calculator for children and teen.* Retrieved from https://www.cdc.gov/healthyweight/bmi/calculator .html

Centers for Disease Control and Prevention. (n.d.). *About child & teen BMI.* Retrieved from https://www.cdc.gov/healthyweight/assessing/bmi/childrens_bmi/about_childrens _bmi.html

Centers for Disease Control and Prevention. (n.d.). *Growth charts.* Retrieved from https:// www.cdc.gov/growthcharts/index.htm

Department of Defense Education Activity. (n.d.). *Health education: Standards.* Retrieved from https://www.dodea.edu/Curriculum/healthEducation/standards.cfm

National Institute on Deafness and Other Communication Disorders. (n.d.). *How do we hear?* Retrieved from https://www.nidcd.nih.gov/health/how-do-we-hear

Raising Children Network. (n.d.). *Suitable for 0–18 years: Scoliosis.* Retrieved from https:raisingchildren.net.au/guides/a-z-health-reference/scoliosis

United States Department of Health and Human Services. (n.d.). *FERPA and HIPPAA.* Retrieved from https://www.hhs.gov/hipaa/for-professionals/faq/ferpa-and-hipaa/ index.html

Webb, C. (2018, Jan 29). *Tackling health barriers to learning—Does your state mandate student health screenings?* Retrieved from https://ccf.georgetown.edu/2018/01/29/ tackling-health-barriers-to-learning-does-your-state-mandate-student-health -screenings/

3

THE INTERSECTION OF HEALTH EDUCATION AND SCHOOL NURSING

KATHERINE J. ROBERTS

LEARNING OBJECTIVES

- Describe different behavior change theories used in health education.
- Identify characteristics of effective health education curricula.
- Utilize the National Health Education Standards to promote health-enhancing behaviors.
- Advocate for effective school health education policies and practices.

■ Introduction

The advantages of having nurses work in schools have long been recognized. At the turn of the 20th century, it was shown that there was a reduction in school absenteeism by having a nurse provide direct care to students. Over the past one hundred years, the role of the school nurse has expanded to include providing preventive and screening services, immunization against preventable diseases, as well as general health education. Effective health education programs and practices have often been delivered in the classroom by trained non-nursing professionals, such as school health educators. However, given the scope and complexity of the health problems of today's students, it is ever more critical that school nurses also be skilled in delivering effective health education, not only on the individual level but also across multiple school settings. If well-versed in health education, a school nurse can be an informed voice in shaping school health policies and programs. This chapter introduces basic health education principles, theories, and practices that can advance the well-being, academic success, and lifelong health behaviors of students.

Role of the School Nurse in Health Education

The role of school nurse traditionally was in population health, tasked with keeping students healthy and in school. In 1902, the first school nurse was placed in New York City, which resulted in reduced school absenteeism and improved health through the decrease in treatable illnesses (Bergren, 2017). By 1913, there were 176 school nurses in the city providing routine inspection of all students to detect diseases and encouraging families to seek and follow through with treatment (Allensworth, Wyche, Lawson, & Nicholson, 1995). Due to their positive effect on school outcomes, this school nursing model was promptly replicated in communities across the country.

During the 1960s, the number of school nurses tripled due to a number of initiatives (Allensworth et al., 1995) including the Elementary and Secondary Education Act of 1965 which provided federal funds to schools with children from low-income families. A new nursing role, the school nurse practitioner, also began, which expanded the clinical functions of school nurses to include primary care services. Having a nurse provide primary care services can reduce health care disparities since children from families of low socioeconomic status often have poorer health outcomes due to difficulty accessing, understanding, and utilizing health care services (Pettit & Nienhaus, 2010). Today, school nurses continue to have an influence on student health outcomes and student absenteeism through multiple avenues, including reducing illness rates through education, early recognition of disease processes, and improving chronic disease management (Maughan, 2003).

The National Association of School Nurses (NASN, 2016) recommends that every child have access all day, every day, to a full-time school nurse. School nurses play an important role in ensuring that students are healthy, safe, and ready to learn. Healthier students are better learners; they are better able to concentrate, achieve higher test scores, and miss fewer classes (Basch, 2011). Health-risk behaviors, such as unhealthy dietary behaviors, inadequate physical activity, violence, risky sexual behaviors, and substance use, have an inverse relationship with indicators of academic achievement (Bradley & Greene, 2013). The school nurse can promote health behaviors and support student success by providing assessment, intervention, and follow-up for all children within the school setting (NASN, 2016).

History of Health Education

The definition and scope of health education have evolved over time. The early emphasis of health education was directed toward the individual, providing them with educational activities to convince them to practice optimum health behaviors (Griffiths, 1972). Later, a broader context of health education in relation to policy, systems, and environmental changes began to emerge, encompassing health promotion to increase optimal health outcomes, not just prevention of death and disease. Today, health education not only includes instructional activities to change individual behavior, but also organizational efforts, policy directives, economic supports, environmental activities, and mass media and community-level programs (Glanz, Rimer, & Viswanath, 2014).

The Joint Committee on Health Education and Promotion Terminology (2012) defines health education as "any combination of planned learning experiences using evidence-based practices and /or sound theories that provide the opportunity to acquire knowledge, attitudes, and skills needed to adopt and maintain health behaviors" (p. 12). The Nursing Interventions Classification defines health education as "developing and providing instruction and learning experiences to facilitate voluntary adaptation of behavior conducive to health in individuals, families, groups, or communities" (Butcher, Bulechek, Dochterman, & Wagner, 2018, p. 5510). Today's school nurse has much broader roles and responsibilities which are increasingly shifting toward the area of health promotion (Whitehead, 2009). Therefore, the school nurse must be skilled in delivering effective health education to multiple audiences and across multiple settings.

Behavior Change Theories

Theories are useful in understanding and explaining behavior and can guide the planning, implementation, and evaluation of health education curricula and interventions. There are a multitude of theories that address health behavior change with different theories best suited for different practices, target audiences, and environments. For example, one theory may be best used to motivate an individual to adopt a new health behavior, while another theory may be more useful in explaining how an individual maintains that behavior change over time (Nigg, 2002). Many theories have similarities and overlapping constructs; however, each theory is unique in articulating the specific factors considered to be important (Glanz et al., 2014). The three most established theories in health behavior research are the Transtheoretical Model/Stages of Change (TTM), Social Cognitive Theory (SCT), and the Health Belief Model (HBM; Painter, Borba, Hynes, Mays, & Glanz, 2008). These health behavior theories can help to explain factors that influence health-related behaviors among youth.

Transtheoretical Model/Stages of Change

The TTM suggests that health behavior change involves progress through six stages of change: precontemplation, contemplation, preparation, action, maintenance, and termination (Prochaska & Velicer, 1997). The TTM focuses on the decision-making of the individual and assumes behavior change does not occur quickly. Often behavior change is not linear, meaning people do not systematically progress from one stage to the other. For each stage of change, different intervention strategies are used to move the individual onto the next stage.

As mentioned, the TTM posits that individuals move through six stages of change:

1. **Precontemplation**—People do not intend to take action in the foreseeable future, usually measured as within the next 6 months. People at this stage may be unaware that their behavior is problematic or that there are negative consequences to their behavior. Or they may have tried to change their behavior multiple times and become demoralized.

2. **Contemplation**—People intend to start the healthy behavior in the next 6 months. They are more aware of the pros and cons of changing the behavior, with an equal emphasis placed on both. People may feel ambivalent toward changing their behavior and be stuck in this stage for long periods of time.

3. **Preparation**—People are ready to take action soon, within the next month. They have a plan of action, and they believe changing their behavior can lead to a healthier life.

4. **Action**—People have made specific, overt modifications in their lifestyles within the past 6 months. They intend to keep moving forward with that behavior change. People may exhibit this by modifying their problem behavior or acquiring new healthy behaviors.

5. **Maintenance**—People have sustained their behavior change for more than 6 months and are working to prevent relapse.

6. **Termination**—People have no desire to return to their unhealthy behaviors and are sure they will not relapse. Termination may not be a practical reality for most people as they tend to stay in the maintenance stage; therefore, this stage is often not considered in health promotion programs.

Social Cognitive Theory

SCT suggests that learning occurs in a social context with a dynamic and reciprocal interaction between people, behavior, and the environment (Bandura, 1989, 1997, 2004). SCT considers the way in which individuals acquire and maintain behavior, while also considering the social environment in which individuals perform the behavior. This theory is particularly valuable in teaching health education in that it suggests that people learn and are influenced by observing what others do, whether it is positive behavior or negative behavior. Self-efficacy is also a central component of this theory, which is important to promote in youth.

Concepts of SCT include:

- **Reciprocal determinism**—Environmental factors influence individuals and groups, but individual groups can also influence their environment and regulate their behavior.

- **Outcome expectations**—Beliefs about the likelihood and value of the consequences of behavioral choices.

- **Self-efficacy**—Defined as "the conviction that one can successfully execute the behavior required to produce the outcomes" (Bandura, 1997).

- **Collective efficacy**—Beliefs about the ability of a group to perform concerted actions that bring desired outcomes.

- **Observational learning**—Learning to perform new behaviors by exposure to interpersonal or media displays of them, particularly through "modeling" of behaviors. If people see successful demonstration of a behavior, they are more likely to complete the behavior successfully.

- ■ **Incentive motivation**—The use and misuse of rewards and punishments to modify behavior.
- ■ **Facilitation**—Providing tools, resources, or environmental changes that make new behaviors easier to perform.
- ■ **Self-regulation**—Controlling oneself through self-monitoring, goal-setting, feedback, self-reward, self-instruction, and enlistment of social support.
- ■ **Moral disengagement**—Ways of thinking about harmful behaviors and the people who are harmed that make infliction of suffering acceptable by disengaging self-regulatory moral standards.

Health Belief Model

The HBM is one of the first models that adapted behavioral sciences theory to health problems (Glanz et al., 2014). It was developed in the early 1950s in order to understand why people do not participate in programs to prevent and detect disease. The HBM suggests that a person's belief in a personal threat of an illness or disease, along with a person's belief in the effectiveness of that health behavior, predicts the likelihood the person will adopt the behavior.

There are six constructs of the HBM:

1. **Perceived susceptibility**—A person's s belief about the threat of an illness or disease. A person must believe there is a possibility they are susceptible to an illness or disease.

2. **Perceived severity**—A person's feelings on the seriousness of contracting an illness or of leaving the illness or disease untreated and possible social consequences (e.g., family life, social relationships). The combination of susceptibility and severity is labeled a threat.

3. **Perceived benefits**—A person's perception of the effectiveness of various actions available to reduce or prevent the threat of illness or disease. A person would not accept the recommended health action unless they also perceive the action to be beneficial in reducing the threat.

4. **Perceived barriers**—A person's feelings on the obstacles to performing a recommended health action. It is a type of cost–benefit comparison, where a person weighs the expected benefits with perceived barriers. Barriers can include that the health action is unpleasant, time-consuming, or inconvenient.

5. **Cue to action**—The stimulus needed to trigger the decision-making process to accept a recommended health action. These cues can be bodily events (tiredness, wheezing, etc.) or environmental events (e.g., new events, social media postings).

6. **Self-efficacy**—As defined in SCT, "The conviction that one can successfully execute the behavior required to produce the outcomes" (Bandura, 1997). Self-efficacy is a construct in many behavioral theories as it is important in initiation and maintenance of behavior change.

▓ Characteristics of Effective Health Education

Health education is considered humanistic, promoting informed and shared decision-making, not dictating and prescribing behaviors (Glanz et al., 2014). The emphasis of health education should not be increasing knowledge since we have learned that knowledge alone does not change behavior (Kelly & Barker, 2016). Similar to changes in the medical field, the traditional doctor–patient relationship of paternalism, where the doctor imparted knowledge and made decisions on behalf of their patients, is outdated. Today, it is patient-centered and person-centered care where there is engagement, collaboration, and shared decision-making (Håkansson Eklund et al., 2019). Much of the shift away from solely teaching facts in both the medical field and in health education has come from the emergence of the Internet, which provides access to an unprecedented amount of information.

The school nurse often delivers health education on a one-to-one basis, providing information and skills that students need to make quality health decisions, including self-management skills that can enable students to better manage their health conditions and to make life decisions. However, providing health education to students in the classroom provides the opportunity to see students in a more natural setting, rather than during a health crisis and allows students to become acquainted with the nurse (Denehy, 2001). The school nurse, along with certified health educators and teachers, can be an essential member of an interdisciplinary team assigned to select or develop appropriate and effective health education curricula and programs. Therefore, they need to be aware of the characteristics of effective health education curriculum (Centers for Disease Control and Prevention [CDC], 2012) which should emphasize functional health knowledge and develop essential health skills necessary to adopt, practice and maintain healthy behaviors. In addition, the curriculum should help to shape personal values that support healthy behaviors and shape group norms that value a healthy lifestyle. An effective curriculum has instructional strategies and learning experiences built on theoretical approaches that have effectively influenced health-related behaviors among youth. Knowledge and skill expectations should be subsequent and increase in complexity over time.

Functional Knowledge

Providing functional knowledge allows students to assess risk, clarify attitudes and beliefs, correct misperceptions about social norms, identify ways to avoid or minimize risky situations, examine internal and external influences, make behaviorally relevant decisions, and build personal and social competence. Functional knowledge is considered to be useful and essential information that is directly related to behavioral outcomes. There should not be an emphasis on teaching scientific facts which are not crucial and will not influence health behaviors. Below are examples of scientific knowledge compared to functional health knowledge:

> **EXAMPLE:** Learning that there are over 400 chemicals in marijuana. How is this going to change behavior? All plants are made up of hundreds of chemicals. **Better:** Examine data on the number of students who smoke mar-

ijuana, which can correct inaccurate perceptions and help students learn that the social norm is that most students do not smoke marijuana or use drugs.

EXAMPLE: Learning the signs and symptoms of various tropical diseases. How is this going to change behavior? *Better:* Learn ways of preventing getting a tropical disease or if you are sick, learn how to seek out a medical expert.

Develops Essential Health Skills

Building students' skills can help them to make informed decisions, solve problems, think critically and creatively, communicate effectively, build healthy relationships, empathize with others, and cope with and manage their lives in a healthy and productive manner (CDC, 2012). Important health skills include communication, refusal, assessing the accuracy of information, decision-making, planning and goal-setting, self-control, and self-management. When teaching a health skill, it is helpful to follow the behavioral skill training (BST) method of instruction; that is, modeling, rehearsal, and feedback (Ward-Horner & Sturmey, 2012). Detailed steps include:

- Discuss the importance of the skill, its relevance, and relationship to other learned skills and explain the steps required to perform the skill.
- Model the skill. If there are steps, demonstrate each one so that the student can follow along and gain confidence in their ability to conduct the skill.
- Practice and rehearse the skill using real-life scenarios. When students practice the skill in a safe environment and become proficient, they will be better able to use the skill when they are forced to react in a high-risk situation.
- Provide feedback and reinforcement so that students feel comfortable and confident that they can use the skill.

Building students health skills is an important aspect of health literacy, which is applicable across many aspects of life. Health literacy entails people's knowledge, motivation, and competences to access, understand, appraise, and apply health information in order to make judgments and decisions in everyday life (Sørensen et al., 2012).

Shapes Personal Values

Fostering attitudes, values, and beliefs that support positive health behaviors is an important aspect of health education. Students should be provided with instructional strategies and learning experiences that allow them to examine personal perspectives critically, consider new arguments that support health-promoting attitudes and values while generating positive perceptions about protective behaviors and negative perceptions about risk behaviors (CDC, 2012).

Shapes Norms

Helping students correct misperceptions of peer and social norms is especially important when addressing behaviors in youth. Social norms are unwritten codes and informal understandings that define what we expect of other people and what they expect of us; they are behavioral patterns, collective attitudes, and individuals' beliefs about others' behaviors and attitudes (Young, 2015). Social norm theory suggests that our behaviors are influenced by our perceptions, or misperceptions, about how our peers think and act (Tankard & Paluck, 2016). The role of perceived normative peer behaviors and attitudes have emerged as key predictors of health behaviors (Dempsey, McAlaney, & Bewick, 2018). Therefore, it is critical to promote health behaviors in a positive manner that challenge commonly held normative misperceptions of various health-related behaviors. Misconceptions have been associated with a range of behaviors, including increased substance use as well as sexual and dietary practices (Dempsey et al., 2018). Social norms initiatives that portray the actual norms and provide resources and services have been demonstrated to be effective in reducing alcohol use in youth by changing the perceived norms (Marshall, Roberts, Donnelly, & Rutledge, 2011).

Health Education Curriculum Analysis Tool

The Health Education Curriculum Analysis Tool (HECAT) can be used to help select or develop appropriate and effective health education curricula, enhance existing curricula, and improve the delivery of health education (CDC, 2012). This tool, which is found online at www.cdc.gov/healthyyouth/hecat, builds on the characteristics of effective health education curricula and the National Health Education Standards (NHES). It addresses a comprehensive array of health topics, including alcohol and other drugs, healthy eating, mental and emotional health, personal health and wellness, physical activity, safety, sexual health, tobacco, and violence prevention.

National Health Education Standards

The NHES were developed to establish, promote, and support health-enhancing behaviors in students (Joint Committee on National Health Education Standards, 2007). The standards provide expectations for what health education should entail in school. The school nurse can use these standards to guide instruction, select curriculum, and assess students in health education. All but the first standard focuses on life skills development (Box 3.1).

Whole School, Whole Community, Whole Child

The Whole School, Whole Community, and Whole Child (WSCC) model (CDC, n.d.) was established in 2014 through a collaboration between the CDC and the ASCD® (formerly known as the Association for Supervision and Curriculum Development). The WSCC combines and builds on elements of the traditional coordinated school health approach and ASCD's whole child framework. The model emphasizes a coordinated school-wide approach to learning and health, with the school being a

BOX 3.1

NATIONAL HEALTH EDUCATION STANDARDS

STANDARD 1. CORE CONCEPTS

Students will comprehend concepts related to health promotion and disease prevention to enhance health.

Rationale

The acquisition of basic health concepts and functional health knowledge provides a foundation for promoting health-enhancing behaviors among youth. This standard includes essential concepts that are based on established health behavior theories and models.

STANDARD 2. ANALYZE INFLUENCES

Students will analyze the influence of family, peers, culture, media, technology, and other factors on health behaviors.

Rationale

Health is affected by a variety of positive and negative influences within society. This standard focuses on identifying and understanding the diverse internal and external factors that influence health practices and behaviors among youth including personal values, beliefs, and perceived norms.

STANDARD 3. ACCESS INFORMATION, PRODUCTS, AND SERVICES

Students will demonstrate the ability to access valid information, products, and services to enhance health.

Rationale

Accessing valid health information and health-promoting products and services is critical in the prevention, early detection, and treatment of health problems. This standard focuses on how to identify and access valid health resources and to reject unproven sources. Application of the skills of analysis, comparison, and evaluation of health resources empowers students to achieve health literacy.

STANDARD 4. INTERPERSONAL COMMUNICATION

Students will demonstrate the ability to use interpersonal communication skills to enhance health and avoid or reduce health risks.

Rationale

Effective communication enhances personal, family, and community health. This standard focuses on how responsible individuals use verbal and nonverbal skills to develop and maintain healthy personal relationships. The ability to organize and to convey in-

(continued)

formation and feelings is the basis for strengthening interpersonal interactions and reducing or avoiding conflict.

STANDARD 5. DECISION-MAKING

Students will demonstrate the ability to use decision-making skills to enhance health.

Rationale

Decision-making skills are needed in order to identify, implement, and sustain health-enhancing behaviors. This standard includes the essential steps that are needed to make healthy decisions as prescribed in the performance indicators. When applied to health issues, the decision-making process enables individuals to collaborate with others to improve quality of life.

STANDARD 6. GOAL SETTING

Students will demonstrate the ability to use goal-setting skills to enhance health.

Rationale

Goal-setting skills are essential to help students identify, adopt, and maintain healthy behaviors. This standard includes the critical steps needed to achieve both short-term and long-term health goals. These skills make it possible for individuals to have aspirations and plans for the future.

STANDARD 7. SELF-MANAGEMENT

Students will demonstrate the ability to practice health-enhancing behaviors and avoid or reduce health risks.

Rationale

Research confirms that the practice of health-enhancing behaviors can contribute to a positive quality of life. In addition, many diseases and injuries can be prevented by reducing harmful and risk-taking behaviors. This standard promotes the acceptance of personal responsibility for health and encourages the practice of healthy behaviors.

STANDARD 8. ADVOCACY

Students will demonstrate the ability to advocate for personal, family, and community health.

Rationale

Advocacy skills help students promote healthy norms and healthy behaviors. This standard helps students develop important skills to target their health enhancing messages and to encourage others to adopt healthy behaviors.

SOURCE: The Joint Committee on National Health Education Standards. (2007). *National health education standards: Achieving excellence* (2nd ed.). Washington, DC: The American Cancer Society.

reflection of the larger community. It highlights the connection between health and academic achievement and the importance of evidence-based school health policies and practices. Six of the 10 components address the health needs of students (physical education and physical activity; nutrition environment and services; health education; health services; counseling, psychological, and social services; and employee wellness). The other four components are cross-cutting and help support student healthy behavior (social and emotional school climate, physical environment, family engagement, and community involvement).

School nurses are ideally situated to advocate for improvements in school health practices, procedures, policies, and curriculum. Indeed, advocacy is a professional expectation of school nurses (NASN, 2017). However, it may be that additional education and training is needed to improve school nurses' knowledge and confidence in advocacy skills (Gormley, 2018). However, within the context of the WSCC, the school nurse does not work alone; the school nurse works collaboratively with other stakeholders to advocate collectively for comprehensive health education that is theory-based with evidence supporting its effectiveness.

■ References

Allensworth, D., Wyche, J., Lawson, E., & Nicholson, L. (Eds.). (1995). *Defining a comprehensive school health program: An interim statement.* Washington, DC: National Academy of Sciences.

Bandura, A. (1989). Social cognitive theory. In R. Vasta (Ed.), *Annals of child development* (*Vol. 6*, pp. 1–60). Greenwich, CT: JAI Press. doi:10.1037/13273-005

Bandura, A. (1997). *Self-efficacy: The exercise of self-control.* New York, NY: W. H. Freeman and Company.

Bandura, A. (2004). Health promotion by social cognitive means. *Health Education and Behavior, 31*, 143–164. doi:10.1177/1090198104263660

Basch, C. E. (2011). Healthier students are better learners: A missing link in school reforms to close the achievement gap. *Journal of School Health, 81*, 593–598. doi:10.1111/j.1746-1561.2011.00632.x

Bergren, M. D. (2017). School nursing and population health: Past, present, and future. *Online Journal of Issues in Nursing, 22*, 3. doi:10.3912/OJIN.Vol22No03Man03

Bradley, B. J., & Greene, A. C. (2013). Do health and education agencies in the United States share responsibility for academic achievement and health? A review of 25 years of evidence about the relationship of adolescents' academic achievement and health behaviors. *Journal of Adolescent Health, 52*, 523–532. doi:10.1016/j.jadohealth.2013.01.008

Butcher, H. K., Bulechek, G. M., Dochterman, J. M., & Wagner, C. M. (Eds.). (2018). *Nursing interventions classification (NIC)* (7th ed.). St. Louis, MO: Elsevier.

Centers for Disease Control and Prevention. (2012). *Health education curriculum analysis tool, 2012.* Atlanta, GA: Author.

Centers for Disease Control and Prevention. (n.d.). *Whole school, whole community, whole child (WSCC).* Retrieved from https://www.cdc.gov/healthyschools/wscc

Dempsey, R. C., McAlaney, J., & Bewick, B. M. (2018). A critical appraisal of the social norms approach as an interventional strategy for health-related behavior and attitude change. *Frontiers in Psychology, 9*, 2180. doi:10.3389/fpsyg.2018.02180

Denehy, J. (2001). Health education: An important role for school nurses. *Journal of School Nursing, 17*(5), 233–238. doi:10.1177/10598405010170050101

Glanz, K., Rimer, B. K., & Viswanath, K. (2014). *Health behavior: Theory, research, and practice.* San Francisco, CA: Jossey-Bass.

Gormley, J. M. (2018). School nurse advocacy for student health, safety, and school attendance: Impact of an educational activity. *Journal of School Nursing, 35*(6), 401–411. doi:10.1177/1059840518814294

Griffiths, W. (1972). Health education definitions, problems, and philosphies. *Health Education Monographs, 31,* 12–14. doi:10.1177/109019817200103103

Håkansson Eklund, J., Holmström, I. K., Kumlin, T., Kaminsky, E., Skoglund, K., Höglander, J., … Summer Meranius, M. (2019). "Same same or different?" A review of reviews of person-centered and patient-centered care. *Patient Education and Counseling, 102,* 3–11. doi:10.1016/j.pec.2018.08.029

The Joint Committee on Health Education and Promotion Terminology. (2012). Report of the 2011 Joint Committee on health education and promotion terminology. *American Journal of Health Education, 43*(2), S1–S19. doi:10.1080/19325037.2012.11008225

The Joint Committee on National Health Education Standards. (2007). *National health education standards: Achieving excellence* (2nd ed.). Washington, DC: American Cancer Society.

Kelly, M. P., & Barker, M. (2016). Why is changing health-related behaviour so difficult? *Public Health, 136*(4), 109–116. doi:10.1016/j.puhe.2016.03.030

Marshall, B. L., Roberts, K. J., Donnelly, J. W., & Rutledge, I. N. (2011). College student perceptions on campus alcohol policies and consumption patterns. *Journal of Drug Education, 41*(4), 345–358. doi:10.2190/DE.41.4.a

Maughan, E. (2003). The impact of school nursing on school performance: A research synthesis. *The Journal of School Nursing, 19*(3), 163–171. doi:10.1177/1059840503019 0030701

National Association of School Nurses. (2016). *The role of the 21st century school nurse* (Position Statement). Silver Springs, MD: Author.

National Association of School Nurses. (2017). *School nursing: Scope and standards of practice* (3rd ed.). American Nurses Association.

Nigg, C. R. (2002). Theory-comparison and multiple-behavior research: Common themes advancing health behavior research. *Health Education Research, 17*(5), 670–679. doi:10.1093/her/17.5.670

Painter, J. E., Borba, C. P. C., Hynes, M., Mays, D., & Glanz, K. (2008). The use of theory in health behavior research from 2000 to 2005: A systematic review. *Annals of Behavioral Medicine, 35*(3), 358–362. doi:10.1007/s12160-008-9042-y

Pettit, M., & Nienhaus, A. (2010). The current scope of health disparities in the U.S.: A review of literature. *The Health Educator, 42*(2), 47–55. Retrieved from https://files.eric.ed.gov/fulltext/EJ942538.pdf

Prochaska, J. O., & Velicer, W. F. (1997). The transtheoretical model of health behavior change. *American Journal of Health Promotion, 12*(1), 38–48. doi:10.4278/0890-1171-12.1.38

Sørensen, K., Van Den Broucke, S., Fullam, J., Doyle, G., Pelikan, J., Slonska, Z., & Brand, H. (2012). Health literacy and public health: A systematic review and integration of definitions and models. *BMC Public Health, 12,* 80. doi:10.1186/1471-2458-12-80

Tankard, M. E., & Paluck, E. L. (2016). Norm perception as a vehicle for social change. *Social Issues and Policy Review, 10*(1), 181–211. doi:10.1111/sipr.12022

Ward-Horner, J., & Sturmey, P. (2012). Component analysis of behavior skills training in functional analysis. *Behavioral Interventions, 27*(2), 75–92. doi:10.1002/bin.1339

Whitehead, D. (2009). Reconciling the differences between health promotion in nursing and "general" health promotion. *International Journal of Nursing Studies.* doi:10.1016/j.ijnurstu.2008.12.014

Young, H. P. (2015). The evolution of social norms. *Annual Review of Economics, 7,* 359–387. doi:10.1146/annurev-economics-080614-115322

Recommended Readings

Glanz, K., Rimer, B. K., & Viswanath, K. (2014). *Health behavior: Theory, research, and practice.* doi:10.7326/0003-4819-116-4-350_1. Also see: https://www.med.upenn.edu/hbhe4/index.shtml

Page, R. M., & Page, T. S. (2015). *Promoting Health and emotional well-being in your classroom* (6th ed.). Sudbury, MA: Jones and Bartlett.

Online Resources

https://www.cdc.gov/healthyyouth/hecat—Health Education Curriculum Analysis Tool (HECAT) can be used to help select or develop appropriate and effective health education curricula, enhance existing curricula, and improve the delivery of health education.

https://www.cdc.gov/healthyschools/sher/characteristics—Providing more information on the characteristics of an effective health education curriculum.

https://www.cdc.gov/healthyschools/wscc—The Whole School, Whole Community, Whole Child, or WSCC model, is CDC's framework for addressing health in schools.

https://www.shapeamerica.org—Providing programs, resources and advocacy that support an inclusive, active, kinder, and healthier school culture.

II

21ST CENTURY SCHOOL HEALTHY PRACTICE

THE ROLE OF THE SCHOOL NURSE IN BUILDING HEALTHY COMMUNITIES

MARIA TORCHIA LOGRIPPO

LEARNING OBJECTIVES

- Compare the past, present, and future (2020 to 2030) of school nursing as it relates to school nurses' role in building healthy communities.
- Identify strategies to raise awareness of the strengths and also potential health and social inequities that exist within the community.
- Recognize collective interventions engaging strategic community partners designed to support healthier students and healthier families, healthier work environments and healthier communities.
- Describe and discuss the role of the school nurse for health promotion policy development that supports a culture of health and targets building a healthier community.

Introduction

As a trusted professional whose value is placed on honest, caring qualities, school nurses are well positioned to be drivers for collective interventions that promote health and health equity that goes beyond the confines of the classroom or school environment. With trust and a caring quality, school nurses are effective agents for change, especially for those communities with individuals who are most at risk for poorer health outcomes. School nurses must tackle and manage population health as they strive to deliver culturally competent nursing care while acknowledging the social determinants of health and health disparities that exist. With the emphasis on self-management of chronic illness and disease prevention, school nurses are key players in building healthier communities. The collaboration with strategic community partners and diverse stakeholders helps to bridge gaps and address best practices for individuals and populations within the community.

Strategic partnerships provide school nurses the tools and resources to deal with the challenges in their communities and can ensure the success of a healthier and more vibrant school community. This chapter provides a basic framework for school nurses to be leaders and champions for change to improve health and health equity within and across the communities they serve.

■ Tapping School Nurses as Change Agents in Communities to Address Health Goals

A school community's reach is far and wide. Students, faculty, administration, and staff make up the community within the confides of the school building. Parents, caregivers, and families play pivotal roles in the educational process to support a productive learning environment beyond the classroom. In addition, there are collaborative partnerships with public entities and private agencies whose contributions can promote a sense of community within the educational system. The potential for resources and collaboration across this community should equate to positive outcomes for learning. However, there remains strong influences on social needs and overall health of the community that can impede the process to learn (McGill, 2016; Robert Wood Johnson Foundation, 2016; Virginia Commonwealth University Center on Society and Health, 2015). Every day in schools across the country, "school nurses are embracing their roots as change leaders who improve the health of children, families, and communities" (Bergren, 2017), advocating for health and health equity. More than ever before, their leadership is critical to driving change needed for a healthier community.

Although much attention is paid to health and health promotion in the media and on the nation's agenda, health inequities exist and account for poorer health in communities. Erin D. Maughan, PhD, RN, PHNA-BC, FNASN, FAAN, Director of Research at the National Association of School Nurses (NASN), stresses that "being on the frontline of care, school nurses must make focused efforts to target and address health inequities as well as advocate for structural/macro-level changes needed" (Maughan, 2019). School nurses are acutely aware of the influences on health like one's zip code, the home environment, or family incomes. They see it daily: "School nurses know where their students and families live and the social stressors that impede them from getting proper healthcare or meet basic needs such as food" says Maughan. The World Health Organization's (WHO) definition of health equity "implies that ideally everyone should have a fair opportunity to attain their full health potential and that no one should be disadvantaged from achieving this potential" (WHO, 2019). Access to healthcare, community resources, and a fair share in utilization of services would certainly help to ensure equity in health. So what can a school nurse do to support health equity and reduce the health disparities that do exist?

In 1998, President Clinton challenged the nation to move to action and make eliminating racial and ethnic health disparities a national priority. David Satcher, MD, PhD, who served as surgeon general under President Clinton acknowledges that in order to eliminate health disparities, "we need leaders who care enough, know enough, do enough, and will persist until the job is done" (American Psychiatric Association, 2014). In January 2000 with the launch of the Department of Health and Human Services (DHHS) *Healthy People 2010*, the national agenda was set, aimed at delivering comprehensive health promotion and disease prevention with two overarching goals—increase the quality of healthy living and eliminate health disparities. On November 22, 2000, the National Center on Minority Health and Health Disparities (NCMHD) of the National Institutes of Health was established by the passage of the Minority Health and Health Disparities Research and Education Act of 2000, Public Law 106-525, which supported the expansion of programs to address a more highly qualified workforce and to provide funding for research. In 2005, the WHO Director-General established the Commission on Social Determinants of Health (CSDH) to address health inequity globally (CSDH, 2008) (Figure 4.1). Further objectives for the national agenda around eliminating health disparities are outlined in *Healthy People 2020*, which introduced the integration of reliable data and tools for action. This integration of data is vital to understanding population health and the considerations needed for effective planning and implementation of interventions to promote health and health equity. The Institute of Medicine (IOM) released its report *Unequal Treatment: Confronting Racial and Ethnic Disparities in Health Care* in 2002, which details an extensive study by experts on disparities research and offers

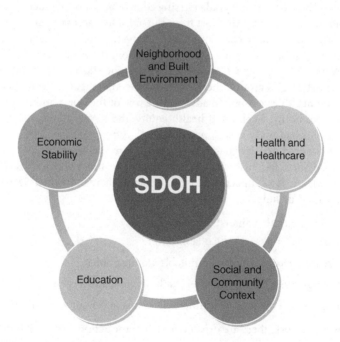

FIGURE 4.1 Healthy People 2020 Social Determinants of Health.

SDOH, social determinants of health.
SOURCE: HealthyPeople.gov.

recommendations addressing the need for increased awareness and education, policy interventions, health systems changes, and data/research. In 2006 at the National Leadership Summit for Eliminating Racial and Ethnic Disparities, the DHHS Office of Minority Health (OMH) put forth recommendations for best practices to eliminate disparities which would require a more systems-oriented approach directed at cross-sector collaboration and partnerships at the community level, this led to the formation of the *National Partnership for Action* (Office for Minority Health, 2018).

▪ Strategies for Community Engagement to Build a Culture of Health

As the nation's focus turns to health disparities, emphasis is placed on the profession of nursing as having great potential to develop leaders and advocates for promoting health and health equity. The Committee on the Robert Wood Johnson Foundation (RWJF) initiative on the Future of Nursing at the IOM began its work in 2008 outlining a plan for nurses to be critical players in advancing health and meeting the nation's health goals. With its release in 2010, the IOM's *Future of Nursing: Leading Change, Advancing Health* outlines recommendations on key areas to ensure a highly qualified nursing workforce ready to care for a complex, ever-changing and diverse population (IOM, 2011). These key areas include nursing education, scope of practice, leadership capacity, and data. A concerted effort from nurse leaders across a variety of national organizations and statewide coalitions provide targeted action plans to achieve IOM recommendations. Backed by the AARP Foundation, the AARP, and the RWJF, the *Future of Nursing: Campaign for Action*, coordinates the efforts of these organizations to implement strategies around the IOM recommendations that strengthen nursing and support a healthier nation. To advance the role of the nurse and to build on the momentum promoting health and health equity, the RWJF, along with the RAND corporation and national experts, put forth a *Culture of Health Action Framework* that supports a common language and vision where "(e)veryone has access to the care they need and a fair, just opportunity to make healthier choices" (RWJF, 2019). The framework aims to connect health to the places where individuals learn, live and play. Action areas include:

- ▪ Making Health a Shared Value
- ▪ Fostering Cross-Sector Collaboration
- ▪ Creating Healthier, More Equitable Communities
- ▪ Strengthening Integration of Health Services and Systems
- ▪ Improving Population Health, Well-Being, and Equity (RWJF, 2019)

For this framework, there are drivers in each of the action areas that indicate what is needed to make significant changes and the measures for progress (Chandra et al., 2017). Additional resources are available on the RWJF's Culture of Health website that can link users to valuable tools to help identify areas of improvements to advance health and health equity. Examples of such tools include County Health

Rankings and Roadmaps, AARP Livability Index©, and Build Healthy Places Network's MeasureUp©.

The next sections of this chapter provide examples of ways to deliver on these areas and to demonstrate the many ways school nurses are making a difference in the communities they serve. A consensus study from the *National Academy of Medicine's Future of Nursing 2020–2030* (2019) stresses that nurses are and will continue to play important roles in this vision for promoting a culture that supports healthier communities.

Focus on Upstream Interventions

Taking action to eliminate health disparities begins by understanding the social determinants of health within a community and to identify strategies that can promote upstream interventions (Bharmal, Pitkin, Felician, & Weden, 2015). To continue to drive change, the DHHS's subsequent initiative *Healthy People 2020* put understanding social determinants of health (SDOH) at the forefront. SDOH refers to "conditions in the environments in which people are born, live, learn, work, play, worship, and age that affect a wide range of health, functioning, and quality-of-life outcomes and risks" (U.S. Department of Health and Human Services [DHHS], 2019). See Figure 4.1 for the framework that depicts the five key areas in *Healthy People 2020* around SDOH. "Health starts in our homes, schools, workplaces, neighborhoods, and communities" with school nurses having a vital role in achieving the goal of creating "social and physical environments that promote good health for all" (DHHS, 2019). The roles and responsibilities of the school nurse cross several of these key areas. For example, school nurses understand the issues of safe housing, transportation to and from school, and the availability of community resources like after-school recreational activities that are critical to better health outcomes. When performing assessments like vision screening, the school nurse informs students and families on important health information. If there are any deficits or concerns, the school nurse advocates for access to needed care or additional services. However, what happens when there is limited access or unavailable resources to address a student's deficits or healthcare concerns? When it comes to social needs, where can the school nurse turn for solutions?

As a professional who relies on building trusting relationships, the school nurse gains a unique perspective and understanding of the community's needs. When the school nurse is aware of the SDOH, the next step to impact health for individuals and populations is taking action. Factors associated with the SDOH can be referred to as upstream, midstream, or downstream. Upstream determinants are the "features of the social environment, such as socioeconomic status and discrimination, that influence individual behavior, disease, and health status" (Gehlert et al., 2008). Upstream interventions occur at a macro level to influence the broader community, including "policy approaches that can affect large populations through regulation, increased access, or economic incentives" (Brownson, Seiler, & Eyler, 2010). Midstream determinants are associated with intermediate factors like health behaviors, and downstream determinants occur at the micro level—an example would be an individual's genetic predisposition. Global efforts are underway that promote public health interventions that require moving past midstream and focusing on upstream interventions. Castrucci and Auerbach (2019) depict individual and community impact gained from strategies involving upstream, midstream, and downstream interventions when considering the social determinants and social needs. In this model, the school nurse's responsibility in reporting communicable diseases would not end at teaching the school community health promotion strategies or providing community resources. Instead, the school nurse at the community-level is making changes through policy initiatives and legislative action such as immunization requirements that address factors associated with the spread of the diseases. This upstream community-level intervention does not happen overnight and cannot happen in isolation. As Director of Research for NASN, Maughan indicates that the data and stories support school nurses as strong advocates for policy changes (Maughan, 2019). She stresses that school nurses are aware of students' needs for appropriate housing in safe areas and housing free of asthma triggers. With data, school nurses can move to action and be the catalyst for building healthier communities.

With the primary goal to keep school children healthy, school nurses are critical stakeholders in community initiatives that address the full array of upstream, midstream, and downstream determinants. Upstream interventions aimed at the population rather than individual can have a great impact on the health and well-being of the community. Therefore, growing the body of healthcare and education research around interventions that support best practices can result in effective policy development and implementation.

▌ Engaging Strategic Community Partners and Diverse Stakeholders

To grow and develop intervention work in the community, school nurses can begin by tapping their ability as effective communicators on health education. There is great value having school nurses with a collective voice who can articulate the social needs and health concerns to the broader community, including key stakeholders. Stakeholders in the community can range from large hospitals and health systems to small, local businesses. Through the Affordable Care Act (ACA), nonprofit organizations, like many of the hospitals throughout the United States, receive tax exemption and have community benefit requirements. The purpose of the tax status is to acknowledge having the benefit of the organization in the community (James, 2016). These benefits are good opportunities for collaboration with school districts in raising awareness and addressing health and health needs of the community. In 2017, a Community Health Initiative by Nantucket Cottage Hospital provided grant funding of $762,000 to improve access to care, housing, and behavioral health (McGuire, 2017). The initiative also focuses on women's and children's needs by offering community programs and educational resources like *Sustainable Nantucket*'s Farm to School Nutrition Program (Sustainable Nantucket, 2019). This program links schools and local farmers to afford healthier meals in cafeterias, create school gardens, and support agricultural, health, and nutritional education.

Health systems also recognize the investment in community to address social determinants of health to prevent costly admissions. Major priorities for health systems that seek to build community initiatives involve making the connection between access to education and improved health. Whether it is keeping chronically ill children in school by advocating for the right medication or supporting health education for students to inform about immunizations, the school nurse serves as an important member of the healthcare team. The school nurse is a valued professional needed at the table during the planning of programs that impact the community. Nurses see hundreds of students, communicate with students' family members, coordinate care with healthcare providers in the community, and are entrusted to set practice guidelines according to standards set by the local and state government agencies. As a trusted nurse leader and advocate, the school nurse can identify what can work to meet the community's needs and what strategies are most effective to gain buy-in from the community members.

Building rapport and a strong relationship with the local health department office helps to ensure access to valuable services in the community as well as access to reliable health information. Public health services provide pertinent resources and health information to promote and protect health for individuals and populations. Working with members of the public health department can provide valuable resources in human capital and opportunities to engage in partnerships with key stakeholders in the community like the mayor, town administrators, local chamber of commerce, and faith-based organizations. Additionally, making connections with non-profit organizations like *Action for Healthy Kids* and *Healthy Kids, Healthy Future* offers tools and resources as well as a network of dedicated volunteers and partners ready for community engagement.

For ways to explore further public health engagement, the Centers for Disease Control and Prevention's Health Impact in 5 Years (HI-5) initiative offers cost-effective, evidence-driven, community-wide approaches geared toward public health interventions and designed to produce results within 5 years. For school communities, HI-5 (CDC, 2018) highlights school-based programs to increase physical activity, prevent violence, and ensure safe routes to school. Identifying programs that are backed by evidence and seek to engage the team of diverse stakeholders can help to support diverse needs of the community and can be a real win–win for all. Examples are provided by the CDC's website that discusses programmatic features, success stories, tools, and frameworks for school nurses to utilize as they consider the types of programs and the feasibility of these program in their community.

Pediatricians, advanced practice registered nurses (APRNs), and primary care providers are extremely valuable partners for community initiatives. In a policy statement made in 2016 by the American Academy of Pediatrics (AAP) Council on School Health, pediatricians acknowledge the dynamic role of the school nurse for community nursing and public health. In this statement, the Council calls for a minimum of at least one full-time registered nurse in every school. Breena Welch Holmes, MD, FAAP, who leads the work of the Council stresses that "(p)ediatricians who work closely with school nurses will serve all of their patients better" (AAP Council on School Health, 2016). On school health service teams, the school nurse functions as the lead in coordinating care across disciplines. The nurse collaborates with all members of the interprofessional team of physicians, health aides, school counselors, school psychologists, case managers, and social workers. Whether an entire health team or one provider, there is added value of such partnerships to drive change and promote health.

■ Collective School-Based, Population Health Interventions

At the National Academies of Sciences, Engineering, and Medicine's (NASEM) Roundtable on Population Health Improvement in June 2018, national experts came together to share stories and population-based interventions that link health and education. Megan Collins of the Wilmer Eye Institute at the Johns Hopkins University shared how their community is addressing gaps in care and barriers to securing eyeglasses for students who fail vision screening. In the *Vision for Baltimore* Initiative, a collaborative bringing together Baltimore City Health Department, the Johns Hopkins University, the Baltimore City Public School System, Vision to Learn, and Warby Parker, vision care and access to eyeglasses happens at the school level. In Alameda County, California, the Health Care Services Agency along with others from education, business, and philanthropy organizations came together to develop school health initiatives around the physical, social, and emotional needs of the students and their families. Strategic partnerships along with this system-integrated approach allow much needed access to care and services like trauma-informed care through school-based health centers (SBHCs).

There is a great deal of benefit when engaging academic partners as evidenced by the *Vision for Baltimore* project (NASEM, 2019). Schools of nursing seek opportunities for students to gain knowledge, skills, and attitudes in caring for individuals and populations in the community, often looking to school nurses for practicum hours and clinical experiences. In return, school nurses can also gain valuable resources through these academic partnerships to advance their goals in analyzing data, grant proposals, and disseminating current research that supports upstream intervention work. One example of an academic community partnership (ACP) at Vanderbilt University in Tennessee connects nursing faculty to the elementary school community in a large, urban school district. This ACP provides a school-based asthma management program (McClure et al., 2018). School nurses can leverage resources through collaborative partnerships with nursing programs and universities to deliver population-based interventions.

Linking health and education does present some challenges in the attempt to connect these two systems together. Examples of obstacles are access to data and costs/financing (Sharfstein & Santamaria, 2018). As stated earlier, school nurses rely on strong communication to achieve positive health outcomes. Electronic health records (EHRs) offer real-time data to support coordination of care and reduce duplication of services (HealthIT.gov, 2019). For school nurses, valuable communication with primary care providers and the healthcare team can occur using an EHR. In 2019, the National Association of School Nurses (NASN) released a position statement to stress the need for appropriate software platforms to allow school nurses to utilize EHRs that meet Health Information Portability and Accountability Act (HIPAA) and Family Rights Educational Privacy Act (FERPA) standards of confidentiality. With increased emphasis on EHRs, there is also an imperative to provide research on best practices to exchange, integrate, share, and retrieve private, secure patient information across these disciplines (Reeves et al., 2016). The access to EHR is a valuable tool for the school nurse to deliver high quality, timely, and safe practice.

As mentioned earlier, strategic partnerships and a systems approach can lead to improvements in access to care and service. To implement a SBHC model, for example, there are costs associated with startup and the operation. SBHCs require collaboration with strategic partners and a well-constructed planning process. Considerations for potential partnerships for the establishment of a SBHC include a local healthcare organization like a community health center or federally qualified health center (FQHC), hospital/health system or a local department of health. The mission of the SBHC—he intent to treat all students—can come at a big price tag. Therefore, proper planning must be undertaken by both systems to fully examine reimbursement and insurance practices, population data on insured versus uninsured, billing operations, and what can be deemed a billable visit.

Additional care coordination practices include services in SBHC linking to the medical home or other healthcare providers. Care coordination requires deliberate actions taken by the nurse to organize care for physical, psychological, and social needs as well as to share information among all members of the healthcare team "to achieve safer and more effective care...patient's needs and preferences are known ahead of time and communicated at the right time to the right people" (Agency for Healthcare Research and Quality [AHRQ], 2018). In this way, the healthcare team has the tools to deliver more efficient care that meets an individual's needs and can go beyond just medical care. The goal of care coordination then shifts from the individual to address population health management that is targeted and effective. School nurses are critical in their role to convey to the team the social needs and social determinants that can improve population health.

As agents for change, school nurses develop and implement appropriate health promotion programs for the community's benefit with the hope of influencing policy and making the move upstream. School nurses see firsthand how policy can drive change and prevent serious adverse events. Their leadership to establish life-saving policies for allergy and asthma prevention gives parents and families some comfort in knowing that the school is a safe place to learn. The CDC's National Asthma Control Program (NACP) funds 25 states and territories to promote evidence-based asthma programs designed to support asthma-friendly schools (AFSs). Through AFSs, collaborative practices across disciplines support the school nurse in ensuring that there is a safe and supportive environment for children to learn. With training and attention to population health management, school nurses reduce gaps in care and allow for timely, coordinated services and the promotion of self-management techniques. Beyond the immediate school team, school nurses are coordinating care for integrated primary care and behavioral health services that support student-centric counseling and social services.

▓ Health Promotion Policy Development

To begin the policy process, school nurses must understand how to move past the interventions at the individual level to develop effective interventions for improving population health. "At the policy development and implementation level, school nurses provide system-level leadership and act as change agents, promoting education and healthcare reform" (NASN, 2016). School nurses work with other professionals to develop the appropriate policy and procedures related to school health services. The call to action for building healthier communities puts the role of the school nurse at the community level to lead and advocate for policy beyond the immediate local school policies and procedures.

School nurses can begin working upstream by collaborating with district wide school personnel to develop policies to promote healthy work environments. The input and advocacy for policy development that ensures a healthy work environment within school systems can benefit school administrators, faculty, and staff. Beisser, Peters, and Thacker (2014) examined work-life balance, health, and nutritional status of school principals. Their findings suggest that principals need support in modeling wellness and dealing with stress (Beisser et al., 2014). With a school nurse as a valued member of the team, school nurses can lead healthy work environment initiatives to include healthy eating and weight loss programs as well as stress management programs. Nurses should help administrators to expand the health team or school safety committee to include physical and occupational therapists, nutritionists, and trained mindfulness facilitators to ensure that all can reap the benefit of a safer, healthier school community.

To deliver on broader community level policy development, there are a variety of resources and supports for the school nurse. Figure 4.2 represents the CDC's domains for the policy process specifically outlined for public health practitioners. The policy process involves steps from identifying the problem to translating a policy into action with two overarching domains that include (a) stakeholder engagement and education and (b) evaluation (CDC, 2015). A toolkit designed for public health practice by the Northeast Wisconsin Education and Practice (NEWLEAP) regional learning collaborative of the LEAP Project offers the basics from identifying a problem to evaluating the outcomes (NEWLEAP, 2010). Through funding from the CDC, the American Nurses Association (ASA), and NASN, the Enhancing School Health Services through Training, Education, Assistance, Mentorship, and Support (TEAMS) project provides online resources for policy development designed for the school nurse leader (AAP, n.d.). Additional supports from the ANA and NASN along with statewide chapters of professional nursing organizations can offer guidance and support to further the policy process (see Figure 4.2).

While developing policy seems like an arduous task, school nurses can champion policies and strategies aimed at health equity right in their own communities. In 2015 with the passing of the Every Student Succeeds Act (ESSA), emphasis is placed on access to quality education and cross-sector collaboration to facilitate supportive learning opportunities (Healthyschoolscampaign.org, 2020). Health in All Policies (HiAP) puts health considerations into all policies in every sector to stress that many

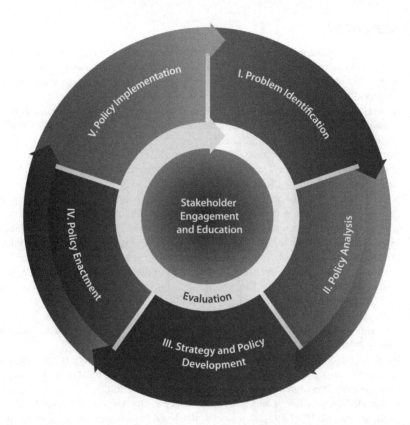

FIGURE 4.2 Centers for Disease Control and Prevention policy process.

factors impact health (CDC, 2016; WHO, 2014). An example of HiAP is advocating for energy efficiency in buildings across the district to reduce harmful pollutants. Whether at the local, state, or national level, it is important for the school nurse to stay abreast of legislation and have an advocacy role in policy making that can influence the health of the community.

With the complexity of health issues impacting children on the rise, community leaders are challenged with just what to do and who to turn to for solutions. Seeking counsel of the school nurse is a smart beginning point. Clearly, school nurses know the issues plaguing the children and young adults in their communities; they understand the real health concerns and struggles of individuals dealing with substance abuse, sexually transmitted diseases, mental and behavioral health disorders. "School nurses are the eyes and ears of public health," remarks Maughan as she stresses the role of the school nurse in identifying the factors that might attribute to barriers in optimizing health and health equity (Maughan, 2019). To end, it is a call to action for school nurses to be leaders and advocates for building healthier communities and a healthier nation.

References

Agency for Healthcare Research and Quality. (2018). *Care coordination.* Rockville, MD: Author. Retrieved from https://www.ahrq.gov/ncepcr/care/coordination.html

American Academy of Pediatrics, Council on School Health. (2016). Role of the school nurse in providing school health services. *Pediatrics, 137*(6):e20160852.

American Academy of Pediatrics. (n.d.). *TEAMS school health services policy development guidance.* Retrieved from https://schoolhealthteams.aap.org/uploads/ckeditor/files/aap%20policy%20guide%20FINAL.pdf

American Psychiatric Association. (2014). *Opening Session of APA's 2014 Institute on Psychiatric Services.* San Francisco, CA: Author. Retrieved from https://psychnews.psychiatryonline.org/doi/full/10.1176/appi.pn.2014.12a4

Beisser, S., Peters, R., & Thacker, V. (2014). Balancing passion and priorities: An investigation of health and wellness practices of secondary school principals. *National Association of Secondary School Principals Bulletin, 98*(3), 237–255. doi:10.1177/0192636514549886

Bergren, M. (2017). School nursing and population health: Past, present, and future. *Online Journal of Issues in Nursing, 22*(3), 1–6. doi:10.3912/OJIN.Vol22No03Man03

Bharmal, N., Pitkin, K. D., Felician, M., & Weden, M. (2015). *Understanding the upstream social determinants of health.* Santa Monica, CA: RAND Corporation. Retrieved from https://www.rand.org/pubs/working_papers/WR1096.html

Brownson, R., Seiler, R., & Eyler, A. (2010). Measuring the impact of public health policies. *Preventing Chronic Disease, 7*(4), A77. Retrieved from http://www.cdc.gov/pcd/issues/2010/jul/09_0249.htm

Castrucci, B., & Auerbach, J. (2019). Meeting individual social needs falls short of addressing social determinants of health. *Health Affairs Blog.* Retrieved from https://www.healthaffairs.org/do/10.1377/hblog20190115.234942/full/

Centers for Disease Control and Prevention, Office of the Associate Director for Policy and Strategy. (2015). *CDC policy process.* Retrieved from https://www.cdc.gov/policy/analysis/process/index.html

Centers for Disease Control and Prevention, Office of the Associate Director for Policy and Strategy. (2016). *Health in all policies.* Retrieved from https://www.cdc.gov/policy/hiap/index.html

Centers for Disease Control and Prevention, Office of the Associate Director for Policy and Strategy. (2018). *Health impact in 5 years.* Retrieved from https://www.cdc.gov/policy/hst/hi5/index.html

Chandra, A., Acosta, J., Carman, K. G., Dubowitz, T., Leviton, L., Martin, L. T., ... Plough, A. L. (2017). Building a national culture of health: Background, action framework, measures, and next steps. *Rand Health Quarterly, 6*(2), 3.

Commission on Social Determinants of Health. (2008). *CSDH final report: Closing the gap in a generation: Health equity through action on the Social Determinants of Health.* Geneva, Switzerland: World Health Organization.

Gehlert, S., Sohmer, D., Sacks, T., Mininger, C., McClintock, M., & Olopade, O. (2008). Targeting health disparities: A model linking upstream determinants to downstream interventions. *Health Affairs (Project Hope), 27*(2), 339–349. doi:10.1377/hlthaff.27.2.339

HealthIT.gov. (2019). *What is an electronic health record?* Retrieved from https://www.healthit.gov/faq/what-electronic-health-record-ehr

Healthy Schools Campaign. (2020). *School nurse leadership.* Chicago, IL: Author. Retrieved from https://healthyschoolscampaign.org/policy/national-policy/

Institute of Medicine. (2002). *Disparities in health care: Methods for studying the effects of race, ethnicity, and SES on access, use, and quality of health care*. Washington, DC: The National Academies Press.

Institute of Medicine. (2011). *The future of nursing: Leading change, advancing health*. Washington, DC: The National Academies Press.

James, J. (2016). Nonprofit hospitals' community benefit requirements. *Health Affairs, Health Policy Brief*. doi:10.1377/hpb20160225.954803

Maughan, E. D. (2019, October 23). *Email communication*.

McClure, N., Seibert, M., Johnson, T., Kannenberg, L., Brown, T., & Lutenbacher, M. (2018). Improving asthma management in the elementary school setting: An education and self-management pilot project. *Journal of Pediatric Nursing, 42*, 16–20. doi:10.1016/j.pedn.2018.06.001

McGill, N. (2016). Education attainment linked to health throughout lifespan: Exploring social determinants of health. *The Nation's Health, 46*(6), 1–19.

McGuire, S. (2017). NCH awards $762,000 to local nonprofits to address the island's most pressing health issues. *Nantucket College Hospital*. Retrieved from http://nantuckethospital.org/nch-awards-762000-to-local-nonprofits-to-address-the-islands-most-pressing-health-issues/

National Academies of Sciences, Engineering, and Medicine. (2019). *School success: An opportunity for population health. Proceedings of a Workshop in Brief*. Washington, DC: The National Academies Press.

National Academy of Medicine. (2019). *The future of nursing 2020-2030*. Washington, DC: The National Academies Press.

National Association of School Nurses. (2016). *The role of the 21st century school nurse (position statement)*. Silver Spring, MD: Author.

National Association of School Nurses. (2019). *Electronic health records: An essential tool for school nurses to keep students healthy*. Retrieved from https://www.nasn.org/advocacy/professional-practice-documents/position-statements/ps-electronic-health-records

National Institutes of Health. (2010). *History on minority health and health disparities*. Retrieved from https://www.nimhd.nih.gov/about/overview/history/

Northeast Wisconsin Education and Practice. (2010). *Shaping public health nursing practice: A policy development toolkit*. Retrieved from https://dpi.wi.gov/sites/default/files/imce/sspw/pdf/snpolicytoolkit.pdf

Office of Minority Health. (2018). *About the NPA*. Retrieved from https://minorityhealth.hhs.gov/npa/templates/browse.aspx?lvl=1&lvlid=11

Reeves, K. W., Taylor, Y., Tapp, H., Ludden, T., Shade, L. E., Burton, B., … Dulin, M. (2016). Evaluation of a pilot asthma care program for electronic communication between school health and a healthcare system's electronic medical record. *Applied Clinical Informatics, 7*(4), 969–982. doi:10.4338/ACI-2016-02-RA-0022

Robert Wood Johnson Foundation. (2016). *Commission to build a healthier America*. Retrieved from http://www.commissiononhealth.org/

Robert Wood Johnson Foundation. (2019). *Building a culture of health*. Retrieved from https://www.rwjf.org/en/cultureofhealth.html

Sharfstein, J., & Santamaria, R. (2018). Enabling school success to improve community health. *Journal of America Medical Association, 320*(11), 1096. doi:10.1001/jama.2018.12567

Sustainable Nantucket. (2019). *Sustainable nantucket: Cultivating a healthy nantucket*. Retrieved from https://www.sustainablenantucket.org/category/farm-to-school-community-agriculture/

U.S. Department of Health and Human Services, Office of Disease Prevention and Health Promotion. (n.d.). *Healthy people 2010.* Retrieved from https://www.cdc.gov/nchs/ healthy_people/hp2010.htm

U.S. Department of Health and Human Services, Office of Disease Prevention and Health Promotion. (n.d.). *Healthy people 2020.* Retrieved from https://www.healthypeople.gov/

Virginia Commonwealth University Center on Society and Health. (2015). *Why education matters to health: Exploring the causes.* Retrieved from https://societyhealth.vcu.edu/ work/the-projects/why-education-matters-to-health-exploring-the-causes.html

World Health Organization. (2014). *Health in all policies.* Retrieved from https://www.who .int/social_determinants/publications/health-policies-manual/key-messages-en.pdf

World Health Organization. (2019). *Health equity.* Retrieved from https://www.who.int/ topics/health_equity/en/

Online Resources

Action for Healthy Kids Campaign. Retrieved from https://www.actionforhealthykids .org/#

Health in All Policies. Retrieved from https://www.who.int/healthpromotion/framework forcountryaction/en/

Healthy Kids, Healthy Future. Retrieved from https://healthykidshealthyfuture.org/

Northeast Wisconsin Education and Practice (NEWLEAP). (2010). *Shaping public health nursing practice: A policy development toolkit.* Retrieved from https://dpi.wi.gov/sites/ default/files/imce/sspw/pdf/snpolicytoolkit.pdf

Robert Wood Johnson foundation Culture of Health Action Framework. Retrieved from https://www.rwjf.org/en/cultureofhealth.html

Sustainable Nantucket. Retrieved from https://www.sustainablenantucket.org/category/ farm-to-school-community-agriculture

TEAMS School Health Services Policy Development Guidance. Retrieved from https:// schoolhealthteams.aap.org/uploads/ckeditor/files/aap%20policy%20guide%20FINAL.pdf

The Future of Nursing: Campaign for Action. Retrieved from https://campaignforaction.org/

U.S. Department of Health and Human Services, Office of Minority Health. Retrieved from https://minorityhealth.hhs.gov

Further Readings

CDC. (n.d.). *CDC's health impact in 5 years.* Retrieved from https://www.cdc.gov/policy/ hst/hi5/index.html

CDC. (n.d.). *CDC policy process.* Retrieved from https://www.cdc.gov/policy/analysis/ process/index.html

CDC. (n.d.). *CDC's social determinants of health.* Retrieved from https://www.cdc.gov/ socialdeterminants/index.htm

Healthy People. (2020). Retrieved from https://www.healthypeople.gov/

National Academies of Sciences, Engineering, and Medicine. (2011). *Institute of medicine's future of nursing: Leading change, advancing health report.* Retrieved from https://www .nap.edu/catalog/12956/the-future-of-nursing-leading-change-advancing-health

FRAMEWORK FOR THE 21ST CENTURY SCHOOL NURSE PRACTICE

LAURA T. JANNONE | ANNEMARIE J. DELLE DONNE

LEARNING OBJECTIVES

- Identify the five principles of the *Framework for 21st Century School Nursing Practice*
- Compare how school nursing has changed from the early days to the 21st century
- Incorporate the National Association of School Nurses's *Framework for 21st Century School Nursing Practice* into their practice.

▆ Introduction

The school health program is an important component of community and public health. Though the primary responsibility of the health of the school-aged child lies with their parents and guardians, schools have immeasurable potential for affecting the health of the child, their families, and the health of the community. The school environment has dramatically changed in the past century. In concert with these changes, the school nurse's role has also changed. School nurses are still expected to care for children in school but now our responsibilities go beyond the school playground into the community. To meet these increasing responsibilities, the National Association of School Nurses (NASN) has given us a framework: The *Framework for 21st Century School Nursing Practice* (NASN, 2016a) is aligned with the *Whole School, Whole Community, Whole Child* model (Centers for Disease Control and Prevention [CDC], 2015) that sets forth a collaborative, comprehensive approach to child care and wellness.

Armed with this new insight, the school nurse will be prepared to meet the challenges of the 21st century.

As discussed in Chapter 1, School Nursing: Early Beginnings and the Unfolding of a New Nursing Specialty, school nursing developed at the turn of the century to meet the overwhelming needs of school-age children at the time, which included malnourishment, and the needs of the immigrant population. Many of these issues still exist but there are new issues facing school-age children in the 21st century. To address these new issues the NASN developed the *Framework for 21st Century School Nursing Practice* in 2016 (NASN, 2016a; Exhibit 5.1).

EXHIBIT 5.1

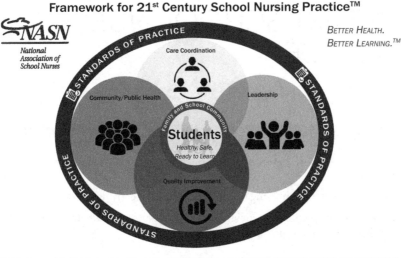

Framework for 21st Century School Nursing Practice™

NASN
National Association of School Nurses

BETTER HEALTH.
BETTER LEARNING.™

NASN's *Framework for 21st Century School Nursing Practice*™ (the *Framework*) provides structure and focus for the key principles and components of current day, evidence-based school nursing practice. It is aligned with the Whole School, Whole Community, Whole Child model that calls for a collaborative approach to learning and health (ASCD & CDC, 2014). Central to the *Framework* is student-centered nursing care that occurs within the context of the students' family and school community. Surrounding the students, family, and school community are the non-hierarchical, overlapping key principles of *Care Coordination, Leadership, Quality Improvement*, and *Community/Public Health*. These principles are surrounded by the fifth principle, *Standards of Practice*, which is foundational for evidence-based, clinically competent, quality care. School nurses daily use the skills outlined in the practice components of each principle to help students be healthy, safe, and ready to learn.

Standards of Practice	Care Coordination	Leadership	Quality Improvement	Community/Public Health
• Clinical Competence	• Case Management	• Advocacy	• Continuous Quality Improvement	• Access to Care
• Clinical Guidelines	• Chronic Disease Management	• Change Agents	• Documentation/Data Collection	• Cultural Competency
• Code of Ethics	• Collaborative Communication	• Education Reform	• Evaluation	• Disease Prevention
• Critical Thinking	• Direct Care	• Funding and Reimbursement	• Meaningful Health/ Academic Outcomes	• Environmental Health
• Evidence-based Practice	• Education	• Healthcare Reform	• Performance Appraisal	• Health Education
• NASN Position Statements	• Interdisciplinary Teams	• Lifelong Learner	• Research	• Health Equity
• Nurse Practice Acts	• Motivational Interviewing/ Counseling	• Models of Practice	• Uniform Data Set	• Healthy People 2020
• Scope and Standards of Practice	• Nursing Delegation	• Technology		• Health Promotion
	• Student Care Plans	• Policy Development and Implementation		• Outreach
	• Student-centered Care	• Professionalism		• Population-based Care
	• Student Self-empowerment	• Systems-level Leadership		• Risk Reduction
	• Transition Planning			• Screenings/Referral/ Follow-up
				• Social Determinants of Health
				• Surveillance

ASCD & CDC. (2014). *Whole school whole community whole child: A collaborative approach to learning and health.* Retrieved from http://www.ascd.org/ASCD/pdf/siteASCD/publications/wholechild/wscc-a-collaborative-approach.pdf

SOURCE: Courtesy of the National Association of School Nurses. (2015). *Immunizations* (Position Statement). Silver Spring, MD: Author. © National Association of School Nurses.

In this chapter, the reader will be able to identify and understand the five Principles of the 21st Century Framework including:

- Standards of Practice
- Care Coordination
- Leadership
- Quality Improvement
- Community/Public Health

Armed with this new insight, the school nurse will be prepared to meet the challenges of the 21st century.

21st Century Framework Standards of Practice: Overview and Background on Development

The *Framework for 21st Century School Nursing Practice (Framework)* provides guidance for evidence-based school nursing practice. Public health nursing focuses on population health; community/public health is the foundation school nursing is based on. The *Framework* was based upon the Whole School, Whole Community, Whole Child (WSCC) Model. This model was developed by the Association of Supervision and Curriculum Development (ASCD) in collaboration with the Centers for Disease Control and Prevention (CDC) in 2015 (Figure 5.1).

This model guides both educators and health professionals to include the student as an active participant in improving both their health and learning. Communities, including the school community and the outside community, collaborate in the coordination of policy development that supports new health and education processes and practices to improve student learning. School age children and adolescents are at the center of the WSCC model. This ensures that the model's focus is on keeping youth healthy, safe, engaged, supported, and challenged—outcomes that schools, teachers, health professionals, families, and communities value. In this model community strengths can boost the role of the school in addressing child health and learning needs, but can also be a reflection of areas of concern and needs in the community. The WSCC model provides the integration of education and health (CDC, 2015).

Looking back at the history of models of school nursing practice, there were other models that guided school nursing practice prior to the WSCC model. They included the Coordinated School Health Model (CSHP), written by Allensworth and Kolbe in 1987, which expanded other models which included only three important components of school health to eight components. These components included health instruction, health services, and also a healthful environment. Their newest model, CHSP, which was supported by the CDC Division of Adolescent and School Health, includes eight components: comprehensive health, physical education, school health services, school nutrition services, health promotion for staff, school counseling,

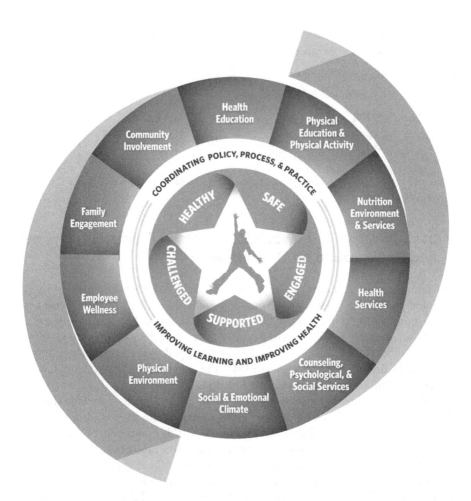

FIGURE 5.1 The Whole School, Whole Community, Whole Child (WSCC) model.

SOURCE: Centers for Disease Control and Prevention. (2014). *Whole school, whole community, whole child (WSCC)*. Retrieved from https://www.cdc.gov/healthyschools/wscc/

both psychological and social services, health school environment, and family and community involvement in the school (CDC, 2014).

   In 2000, responding to the CSHP model, the CDC developed and published an assessment tool called the School Health Index (SHI) to assist CSHP teams in program planning for individual schools. They developed both elementary and middle school/high school versions of this tool. It is both a self-assessment and planning tool that school personnel teams can use to identify the strengths and weaknesses of their health programs and policies, develop an action plan to improve them, and involve teachers, students, parents, and community members in promoting health behaviors and thereby improving health status. Both the CSHP and SHI were successful in assisting states, districts, and schools throughout the United States to establish policies and practices to support both healthy choices and lifestyles. Because of the complexities of school nursing in recent years due to complicated healthcare needs and other factors such as poverty and the interactions of education, health, and health equity, a newer more collaborative model which drew from a wider range of stakeholders in school health and education was developed (CDC, 2014).

The *Framework for 21st Century School Nursing Practice* (NASN, 2016a) explains essential principles of school nursing practice and is aligned with the WSCC model (ASCD & CDC, 2014). The WSCC model "calls for a greater collaboration across the community, across the school, and across sectors to meet the needs and reach the potential of each child" (CDC, 2014).

The NASN recognized the need for a framework because there was a lack of guidance, theory, or standard in school nursing practice. The NASN realized they needed more evidence to increase focus on prevention, and they knew there were increased numbers of medically fragile complex students in our schools. They developed the framework based on the review of the literature and the NASN Board of Directors' input and feedback from practicing school nurses through on-line surveys and conference feedback (NASN, 2016b). Once it was written and finalized, it was approved by the NASN Board of Directors—the NASN knew that school nurses advance the well-being, academic success and lifelong achievement and health of students. School nursing is a dynamic profession that changes with current needs. School nurses are leaders in school health and they use critical thinking, which includes the nursing process. The *Framework* focuses on the school community, which includes the student, family, staff, and the broader community.

The five principles of the *Framework* include Standards of Practice, Care Coordination, Leadership, Quality improvement, and Community and Public Health (NASN, 2016b). The principles are not hierarchical; each is an equally important part of school nursing practice.

Standards of Practice

The practice components of the Standards of Practice include *clinical competence, clinical guidelines, code of ethics, critical thinking, evidence-based practice (EBP), NASN Position Statements, Nurse Practice Acts,* and *Scope and Standard of Practice.* Tools that support competence and EBP include position statements and clinical guidelines along with peer reviewed journals for school nursing. The Institute of Medicine (IOM; now the National Academy of Medicine) defines clinical practice guidelines as "statements that include recommendations intended to optimize patient care that are informed by a systemic review of evidence and an assessment of the benefits and harms of alternatives care options (IOM, 2011, pp. 25–26). *Clinical Guidelines* enable the school nurse to translate research evidence into their practice. Some states have clinical guidelines published by their Department of Education (DOE) or Department of Health (DOH) or by their School Nurse Professional Organizations. NASN's position statements are evidence-based practice and include the history and political and scientific facets of topics that are relevant to school nursing, school health services, and children's health care (NASN, 2016b).

School nurses must also follow their *Nurse Practice Acts* in the state in which they practice; your State Board of Nursing usually publishes these.

Care Coordination Within the School and Community

The practice components of the Principle of Care Coordination include case management, chronic disease management, collaborative communication, direct care, education, interdisciplinary teams, motivational interviewing and counseling, nursing delegation, student care plans, student-centered care, student self-empowerment and transition planning. These are activities school nurses perform on a daily basis. The school nurse intervenes with actual and potential health problems, including first aid, emergency care and assessment, and planning for the management of chronic conditions. We know that when there is a school nurse, students are less likely to use an emergency department, and are more likely to visit an appropriate healthcare provider if they have a medical referral from a school nurse. Students are less likely to miss school due to an illness and the achievement gap for chronic conditions can be reduced (Lewallen, Hunt, Potts-Datema, Zaza, & Giles, 2015). Some partnerships provide dental and vision services along with pediatric specialty care.

Leadership

School nurses and school districts can partner with community healthcare providers to connect low-income students to health care. The leadership component is a standard of the school nurse practice (American Nurses Association [ANA] & NASN, 2017). The italicized words in the following are practice components of leadership: The ability to change, continuously learn and to adapt to changes are key leadership qualities in the complex role of the school nurse. School nurses can be *change agents* because they are often the only health professional in their school community. School nurses can *advocate* for their students and for education reform by working with others on the interdisciplinary team to promote healthy behaviors and healthy environments; they can also work with legislators to influence policy related to education and *healthcare reform*. Other practice components of the Principle of Leadership in the NASN's *Framework for the 21st Century* are *funding and reimbursement, lifelong learners, models of practice, technology, policy development and implementation, professionalism,* and *systems-level leadership.* Nurses' professionalism is recognized every year in public ranking which states that nurses are honest and ethical; professionalism is an integral part of school nurse leadership. To keep up with the changes in healthcare and education, school nurses must be lifelong learners and adopt technology to support both their research and their practice

▦ Quality Improvement

Continuous quality improvement can be accomplished in several ways; the components are *documentation/data collection, evaluation, meaningful health/academic outcomes, performance appraisal, and research. Uniform data sets* are an important component of Quality Improvement Data. What does it mean to you? Do you think of numbers, statistics, and charts? Do you consider it to be something other individuals are required to deal with, and you as a nurse don't need to be concerned? Does it overwhelm you? It can evoke different reactions from different people. Many school nurses think they have little involvement with data, yet they are in a unique position to collect it, analyze it, and incorporate it in their practice.

The NASN (2016c) has embarked on a new data initiative called *The National School Health Data Set: Every Student Counts! (Every Student Counts!)*. The *Every Student Counts!* data initiative includes developing a national school health data set that will influence local, state, and national student health policy, and identifies best practices in school health (NASN, 2017). It will also support the use of data to determine policies that will meet the needs of students, increase the use of evidence-based school nursing practice, and ultimately improve student health outcomes. The goals of *Every Student Counts!* will be realized by using a three-pronged approach and include (a) building school nurses' capacity for data collection, aggregation, and reporting; (b) further refining of the uniform data set; and (c) strengthening the national and state data collection infrastructure (NASN, 2017).

NASN will support school nurses by developing educational webinars, tool kits, templates, podcasts, and conference breakouts (Maughan, Johnson, & Bergren, 2017). These and other resources will improve the school nurse's ability to understand and use the data and be able to help show Evidence Based Practice for why we need school nurses. These resources are available on NASN's website in the area of *Every Student Counts!:* www.nasn.org/research/everystudentcounts

▦ Community/Public Health

Another one of the five principles of the framework, the principle of community/public health, is part of the school nursing's role. School nursing practice is built on the tenets of public health as school nurses provide health promotion and levels of prevention, a component of the framework (e.g., primary, secondary, and tertiary). Examples of primary prevention include health education and promotion of immunization compliance. *Screenings, referrals, and follow-up care* are perhaps the most common examples of secondary prevention, where health concerns are detected and treated in their early stages and where behaviors can be modified and symptoms treated before the health concern becomes more serious. The third tier of prevention, tertiary prevention, involves treating the existing disease and developing strategies to help improve the condition. Often the school nurse is the only *access to care* the student has and plays a vital role in *disease prevention*. The school nurse has the ability to reach children/adolescents slipping through the cracks of the healthcare system and at highest risk for poor health and potentially health-threatening behaviors. Other components of community/public heath are *health equity, population-based care,* and *risk reduction.*

School nurses are involved in wellness promotion, preventive services, and *health education:* access and/or referrals to the medical home or private health care provider, and support connecting school staff, students, families, community, and health providers to promote the healthcare of students in a health and safe school environment Because school attendance is required in the United States, schools represent our best opportunity to reach many children and adolescents in need of proper health care.

If you are member of the NASN you have access to VSP Sight for Students®: https://www.nasn.org/nasn/membership/current-members/vsp-sight-for-students

School nurses must be aware of the *social determinants of health.* Factors such as income, housing, transportation, access to health care, employment, social support, education/literacy, physical environment, neighborhood safety, and other elements can influence health outcomes (Office of Disease Prevention and Health Promotion, 2019). The *practice component of cultural competency* helps build trust and furthers communication between the school nurse, students, and their families.

School nurses must be cognizant of these factors and others, such as the environment and how it influences the health of their students and their families. Children are especially vulnerable to environmental effects from air and water pollution, food safety, chemical, biological risks, and psychological influences (NASN, 2018). School nurses are in a position to monitor environmental conditions in the school setting, as well as the community, and act as change agents to advocate for safer surroundings to promote health and learning, thereby maintaining *environmental health.*

According to the World Health Organization (WHO, n.d.), public health surveillance is the continuous, systematic collection, analysis, and interpretation of health-related data needed for the planning, implementation, and evaluation of public health practice. Such surveillance can:

- Serve as an early warning system for impending public health emergencies;
- Document the impact of an intervention, or track progress toward specified goals; and
- Monitor and clarify the epidemiology of health problems, to allow priorities to be set and to inform public health policy and strategies.

Whether they realize it or not, school nurses play an essential role in surveillance. Noting the number and type of injuries may result in changes to or maintenance of playground or gym equipment. Attendance records are often monitored and the incidence of certain diseases, such as influenza-like illness (ILI) is reported to health departments. Trends in illnesses during the school day, such as gastrointestinal illness, may need further investigation to determine the cause (e.g., food/water-borne contamination or bacterial or viral causes). The school nurse is poised to identify those at risk, provide education, and make referrals for treatment.

School nursing has deep roots in community and public health. Moved by the plight of poor immigrant families on New York City's Lower East Side, Lillian Wald moved into their neighborhood in 1893 to provide nursing care and establish public health nursing (Bergren, 2017). The Henry Street Settlement was established in 1895, focusing on child health and public health nursing. During this time, school health dealt primarily with health inspectors screening and excluding children with contagious diseases from school. Students were sent home and instructed to see a physician. Families often lacked the financial resources and knowledge to address the health concerns identified at the screening and their children remained untreated and excluded from school.

Lillian Wald assigned Lina Rogers, a nurse from the Henry Street Settlement, to promote hygiene and preventive health measures to 10,000 children in four New York City schools. This 1-month experiment resulted in a 50% reduction in school absenteeism and dramatically increased the health of these children by decreasing treatable illnesses and preventing others (Hanink, 2019). The New York experiment was repeated in other large cities, such as Los Angeles, Philadelphia, and Boston, with similar results (Bergren, 2017). In 1908, Jane Addams, the founder of Hull House Settlement in Chicago, home of the Chicago Visiting Nurse Association, observed that physicians were focused on excluding students with communicable diseases from school, whereas the visiting nurse was able to have the well child return (Bergren, 2017).

As described in the first chapter, in the early years of the 20th century school nurses were often public health nurses and had a significant presence in the community. School nurses would render treatments as directed by protocols and would consult with healthcare providers (physicians or dispensaries) as needed. School nurses saw students at school as well as in their homes, and health education was an essential part of the role they played in disease prevention and health promotion. The role of the school nurse was not limited to the school year and the summer months had many health promoting initiatives, such as instruction on hygiene and sanitation. This approach "represented the most efficient means of reaching the greatest needy populations" (Apple, 2017).

Fast forward to present day school nursing, where the focus remains on preventing illness and promoting health. In addition to caring for increasing numbers of students with chronic and often life-threatening conditions, the school nurse has responsibilities directly related to public health. Schools were often settings for transmission of what are now vaccine preventable diseases (VPDs), such as measles, mumps, rubella, polio, pertussis, and varicella. Vaccines are among the 10 greatest public health achievements in the United States (CDC, 2011) and requiring children to be immunized according to the Advisory Committee on Immunization Practices (ACIP) has drastically reduced the number of VPDs. All 50 states have instituted mandatory vaccine requirements for school enrollment; all states permit medical exemptions, 45 states allow religious exemptions, and 15 states allow philosophical exemptions (National Conference of State Legislatures, 2019). The NASN (2015) support school nurses in their public health role in promoting immunizations. School nurses are compelled to maintain accurate immunization records and enforce state mandatory immunization requirements. The school nurse must recognize which children are at increased risk of contracting or transmitting

VPDs, whether due to a compromised immune system, or suboptimal immunization status (Davis, Varni, Barry, Frankowski, & Harder, 2016). The school nurse should not only have medical knowledge, but should have formal training in health education and understanding the health needs of all children and adolescents in pre-K through 12th grade.

Healthy People 2020 represents national health priorities that school nurses are in a position to incorporate into their health programs and services, in both their schools and communities, through school health programs. School nurses are in a key position to work with others in the community in *health promotion* activities such as health fairs, and other *outreach* programs that identify students at risk for *poor access to care*. The school nurse can assist students and their families in finding appropriate healthcare, financial resources, food, and shelter (NASN, 2016b).

In conclusion school nursing has increased in complexity since the early days of Lina Rogers. The specialty of school nursing practice must continue to grow to meet the demands of our population in the 21st century. The NASN *Framework for the 21st Century School Nursing Practice* incorporates principles and concepts from previously used frameworks, theories, and models to provide a comprehensive overview of school nursing practice that incorporates the needs of today's student population. NASN's *Framework for 21st Century School Nursing Practice* can be found at https://www.nasn.org/nasn/nasn-resources/professional topics/framework

■ References

Allensworth, D., & Kolbe, L. (1987). The comprehensive health program: Exploring an expanding concept. *Journal of School Health, 57*(10), 409–412. doi: 10.1111/j1746 -1561.1987.tb03183.x

American Nurses Association. (2017). *Public health nursing.* Retrieved from https://www .nursingworld.org/practice-policy/workforce/public-health-nursing/

American Nurses Association & National Association of Nurses. (2017). *School nursing: Scopes and standards of practice: School nursing* (3rd ed.). Silver Spring, MD: Author.

Apple, R. D. (2017). School health is community health: School nursing in the early twentieth century in the USA. *History of Education Review, 46*(2), 136–149. doi: 10.1108/ HER-01-2016-0001

Association of Supervision and Curriculum Development & Centers for Disease Control and Prevention. (2014). *Whole school, whole community, whole child. A collaborative approach to learning and health.* Retrieved on from http://www.ascd.org/ASCD/pdf/ siteASCD/publications/wholechild/wscc-a-collaborative-approach.pdf

Bergren, M. D. (2017). School nursing and population health: Past, present, and future. *Online Journal of Issues in Nursing, 22*(3), 3. doi: 10.3912/OJIN.Vol22No03Man03

Centers for Disease Control and Prevention. (2011). Ten great public health achievements-United States, 2001-2010. *Journal of the American Medical Association, 306*(1), 36–38. Retrieved from https://jamanetwork.com

Centers for Disease Control and Prevention. (2014). *Whole school, whole community, whole child (WSCC).* Retrieved from https://www.cdc.gov/healthyschools/wscc/

Centers for Disease Control and Prevention. (2015). *Components of the whole school, whole community, whole child (WSCC)*. Retrieved from https://www.cdc.gov/healthyschools/wscc/components.htm

Davis, W. S., Varni, S. E., Barry, S. E., Frankowski, B. L., & Harder, V. S. (2016). Increasing immunization compliance by reducing provisional admittance. *Journal of School Nursing, 32*(4), 246–257. doi: 10.1177/1059840515622528

Hanink, E. (2019). Lina Rogers, the first school nurse. *Working Nurse*. Retrieved from http://www.workingnurse.com/articles/Lina-Rogers-the-First-School-Nurse

Institute of Medicine Committee on Standards for Developing Trustworthy Clinical Practice Guidelines. (2011). *Clinical practice guidelines we can trust*. Washington, DC: National Academies Press. Retrieved from https://www.ncbi.nlm.nih.gov/books/NBK209539?

Lewallen, T. C., Hunt, H., Potts-Datema, W., Zaza, S., & Giles, W. (2015). The whole school, whole community, whole child model: A new approach for improving educational attainment and health development of students. *Journal of School Health, 85,* 729–739. doi: 10.1111/josh.12310

Maughan, E. D., Johnson, K. H., & Bergren, M. D. (2018). Introducing NASN's new data initiative: National school health data set: Every student counts! Make this YOUR year of data. *NASN School Nurse, 33*(5), 291–294. doi:10.1177/1942602X18791572

National Association of School Nurses. (2015). *Immunizations* (Position Statement). Silver Spring, MD: Author.

National Association of School Nurses. (2016a). Framework for the 21st century school nursing practice. *NASN School Nurse, 31*(1), 45–53. doi: 10.1177/1942602X15618644

National Association of School Nurses. (2016b). *The role of the 21st century school nurse* (Position Statement). Silver Spring, MD: Author.

National Association of School Nurses. (2016c). *National School Health Data Set: Every Student Counts*. Silver Spring, MD: Author.

National Association of School Nurses. (2017). *Whole school, whole community, whole child: Implications for 21st century school nurses* (Position Statement). Silver Spring, MD: Author. Retrieved from https://www.nasn.org/nasn/advocacy/professional-practice-documents/position-statements/ps-wscc

National Association of School Nurses. (2020). VSP Sight for Students. Retrieved from https://www.nasn.org/nasn/membership/current-members/vsp-sight-for-students

National Association of School Nurses. (n.d.). *Professional practice documents*. Retrieved from https://www.nasn.org/ /advocacy/professional-practice-documents

National Conference of State Legislatures. (2019). *States with religious and philosophical exemptions from school immunization requirements*. Retrieved from http://www.ncsl.org/research/health/school-immunization-exemption-state-laws.aspx

Office of Disease Prevention and Health Promotion. (2019). *Healthy People 2020: Social determinants of health*. Retrieved from https://www.healthypeople.gov/2020/topics-objectives/topic/social-determinants-of-health

World Health Organization. (n.d.). *Public health surveillance*. Retrieved from https://www.who.int/topics/public_health_surveillance/en/

INTERDISCIPLINARY PRACTICES AND THE NEW SCHOOL ENVIRONMENT

MATT BOLTON

LEARNING OBJECTIVES

- Discuss the role of the school nurse as a member of an interdisciplinary team.
- Identify two ways an effective school nurse coordinates care for student health inside and outside of the school.
- Describe how a school nurse contributes to a culture of health and wellness in a school.
- Name two effective communication strategies to establish rapport with varies school stakeholders.
- Evaluate the role of the school nurse in providing educational services to students.

■ Introduction

Growing up as the son of a practicing school nurse and district-level school administrator, dinner table conversations typically focused on daily life in a school setting. My mother would often share accounts of her day in the school health office, which included the details surrounding scraped knees, fevers, height and weight screenings, and even the occasional four-letter word ... lice. While I recall these dinner conversations in vivid detail, I have no recollection of this school nurse sharing the intricacies of her role in the broader school community. I do not recall her offering her sentiments on evaluation criteria or mandatory student growth objectives. I do not remember hearing her thoughts on being an integral member of her school's Section 504, Child Study, or Intervention Services teams. I certainly do not remember her discussing strategies for garnering commitment from faculty member delegates to administer epinephrine or glucagon injections.

The role of the school nurse has changed dramatically during the past 30 years. The 21st century school nurse is tasked with responsibilities that permeate the entire school community. This chapter details the many challenges, tasks, and roles that require the school nurse to be an active member, if not curator, of an interdisciplinary team within the school setting.

Cultivating Relationships and Building Trust

After 3 long days of screening the heights and weights of over 800 middle school students Martha heads back to the health office, organizes her notes, and examines the data she collected about her students. For the most part, her students generally fell within the acceptable range for body mass index guidelines; however, her meticulously kept records kept bringing her back to three students whose measurements feel well outside of acceptable guidelines. The state and board of education in which Martha is employed has well-established laws and policies that guide her work as a school nurse. In this instance, those laws and policies dictate that Martha is required to notify the parents of the three students whose health screening results deviated from the normal distribution. Martha's school district has a standard form, which is mailed to the parents of all students to inform them of their child's screening results. Martha believes that it is important to go beyond the minimum expectation of mailing a form letter, especially when the subject of the discussion is as personal as height or weight.

Her first phone call is to Emily's mother. The results of Emily's height and weight screening revealed that her weight was well beyond the established norm. Having been a certified school nurse for more than 15 years, Martha knows two things for certain about the phone call she's about to make: (a) Emily's obesity puts her at risk for serious health problems such as diabetes, high blood pressure, and heart disease. This is something that Emily's parents need to be aware of, and should be provided with the resources to properly address it. (b) The subject of a child's height and weight, particularly when those results fall beyond established norms, can be a very delicate and challenging conversation to have with a parent. Martha has had this conversation with parents before and knows that by being empathetic, understanding, resourceful, and factual, she can effectively communicate the importance of her message.

Thankfully, Martha has a secret weapon in her difficult conversation arsenal … established trust within the school community. Martha's difficult conversations with parents don't always go as planned, but the vast majority of her more challenging messages are well received by parents because she has done a tremendous amount of work prior to build trust with parents, teachers, administrators, and colleagues. As the school nurse in a large suburban middle school she has an extremely busy job, but she designates time to be a visible presence in the school. She greets parents with a reassuring smile; she sends a weekly email communication that promotes healthy habits; when teaching health classes, she makes positive phone calls home to celebrate student successes; and when students visit the health office they are greeted by someone who listens and never dismisses their concerns. The genial attitude that frames Martha's work has very little to do with the difficult phone call she is about to make, and yet … it has everything to do with the ultimate outcome of that phone call. As a result of the trust that this school nurse has established within her school community, parents are more disposed to accept difficult news.

Emily's mother and father confirm with Martha that they are aware of Emily's recent weight gain that began over the summer months. Emily's mother at first responds with apprehension about the information Martha provides, then shares, "She began putting on weight over the summer as a result of a new medication she is taking." Martha was unaware that Emily was taking any medication. Emily's mom continues, "Emily was experiencing some concerning thoughts and was generally depressed after the last school year. Her doctor put her on an antidepressant, which has result in her gaining some weight." Martha thanks Emily's mother for sharing this important information and also informs her of the resources that are available from both the school's counseling department and the greater community to help Emily with her depression. Martha adds that it could also be helpful for Emily's mother to communicate Emily's experience with her teachers so that they can alert her to any changes in Emily's mood or behaviors in school. At the conclusion of their conversation, Emily's mother is grateful to Martha for making the phone call and makes an appointment to meet with the school counselor to discuss some of the challenges that Emily has been experiencing.

In addition to working to establish trust with parents in the school community, the effective school nurse builds trust and rapport with their teacher colleagues. School nurses do not work in isolation. They are an integral part of an educational system. The educational system, regardless of location, generally holds a few fundamental objectives that pertain to keeping students safe and healthy, and provide students with a fair, equitable, and high quality education so that they can find success in college and career (Every Student Succeeds Act, 2015). A quality education system requires the collaborative efforts of many key stakeholders within a school community. School nurses are expected to work in conjunction with teachers, administrators, nurse colleagues, secretaries, paraprofessionals, school psychologists, learning consultants, behaviorists, lunchroom supervisors, and just about everyone else who is employed within a school.

The demands currently placed on the school nurse are extensive and include responsibilities associated with student instruction, clinical health care, emergency response to critical incidents, planning and intervention teams, record retention, culture and climate improvement, and faculty training, just to name a few. Each one of these responsibilities requires the school nurse to interact effectively and often garner support and buy-in from other members within the school.

Val is a school nurse in a small elementary school. She is required to teach health classes to students in third, fourth, and fifth grades multiple times each year. In order to do so, she must carefully coordinate her schedule to ensure that those teachers are able to accommodate her teaching time in their classroom. Val must also communicate her teaching schedule to her principal and the two main office secretaries so that they are aware that she will be away from the health office while teaching. Val has already emailed each of the teachers and asked them to provide her with times that they could meet to schedule her lesson and discuss its content. Prior to meeting with the teachers, Val confers with her principal to review her lessons and discuss her approach to scheduling time in an already jam-packed elementary school classroom. Her principal reminds her that the teachers really struggle with interruptions to their daily routines, but would more than likely be grateful for some additional planning time while she is teaching her lessons.

During Val's meeting with the teachers, she reminds them that because she possesses an instructional certificate, they can leave the room to accomplish some much needed work while she teaches her health lessons. Val's collaborative and thoughtful approach to the teacher's work load is appreciated and the teachers welcome her into their classrooms.

This anecdote about a school nurse whose work is made far less complicated as a result of the trust she has established within her school community reinforces the important role relationship building and community outreach play in an effective interdisciplinary approach to school nursing. Through their pleasant communication style, high visibility, and investment in relationship building with all school stakeholder groups, Val and Martha are effective collaborators. Ultimately, the trust they have developed enables them to find more successes than obstacles in their professional work.

Coordinated Care

Three years ago my wife, Lisa, was diagnosed with breast cancer. After the initial diagnosis, Lisa and I planned for upcoming surgeries, recovery, and treatment by meeting with breast surgeons, plastic surgeons, oncologists, and therapists. We were inundated with information at a time when it was challenging to think rationally. While each member of Lisa's medical team was absolutely amazing, the person that was invaluable to us throughout the process was Lisa's nurse navigator, Carol. Carol was the person charged with coordinating the care Lisa received. She assisted in scheduling appointments, contacting doctor's to receive updates, advocating for Lisa's care, and generally ensured that all parties were working collaboratively on behalf of their patient.

School nurses do not work in isolation. They are an integral part of a larger educational community that services students with wide ranges in social, emotional, cognitive, psychological, and medical needs. Working with students with chronic conditions whose various needs are accommodated for within a public school setting is becoming more commonplace. "The number of students in the United States who suffer from one or more chronic illnesses has dramatically increased in the past four decades, doubling from 12.8% in 1994 to 26.6% in 2006" (Van Cleave, Gortmaker, & Perrin, 2010).

The school nurse often serves as the primary point of contact, or case manager, for students with chronic illnesses who often require Individualized Health Plans and other possible institutional supports such as an Individual Education Plan (IEP) or Section 504. While working in this capacity, the school nurse is not only responsible for assessing students' daily health and administering medications, but also for organizing, planning, communicating, and evaluating students' long-term care and daily management of care plans.

As the primary coordinator of care for students with chronic health issues, the school nurse is the student's school based communicator, collaborator, and medical advocate. The nurse will regularly share communication between the student's physician, Section 504 and IEP teams, school counselor, and teachers. The nurse participates in a constant loop of supporting the medical needs of the chronically ill student; communicating necessary interventions to the various teams of teachers, family, and support personnel; and gathering feedback to continuously monitor the impact of both the student's illness and provided interventions on their educational experience. Moreover, while serving as the student's medical case manager and coordinator of care, the school nurse is positioned in an optimal role to develop rapport, engage in communication, and receive feedback directly from the student. The role the school nurse plays to support a medically fragile quarter of the school population is critical. Without the school nurse to coordinate resources and services on behalf of chronically ill students, the consequences are well researched and quite stark. Forty-five percent of students with chronic illness report falling behind academically. "Fifty-eight percent of students with a chronic illness routinely miss school with 10% missing more than 25% of the school year" (Thies, 1999).

Core Team Member

The school nurse is often a standing member of the many student support, instructional intervention, crisis, and pre-referral teams in the school. The nurse's in-depth knowledge of the large groups of students, as well as clinical background in assessing student learning, social, emotional, behavioral, and health needs, positions them as an essential part of the school's support, referral, and intervention teams. The following outlines the various school level teams, requirements, and responsibilities of the 21st century school nurse.

Section 504 Team

Section 504 of the Rehabilitation Act of 1973 prohibits discrimination against students with disabilities. This law requires that all students receive a free and appropriate public education (FAPE; U.S. Department of Education, 2010). Section 504 requires that those students who have been diagnosed with some form of mental or physical disability that substantially limits a major life function be identified through evaluative measures and be provided with a plan of accommodations/services designed to meet their individual needs. Major life functions can range from hearing, learning, and attending to walking, bending, and using the bathroom. A 504 team is made up of those school personnel who are knowledgeable about the student and the nature of their disability. When health related issues rise to the level of substantially limiting a major life function of a student, the nurse will be invited to be an essential member of that school's 504 team. The role of the school nurse on the 504 team can be to conduct the initial evaluation and referral to the team, as in the case of a student identified with vision difficulty through the student's annual vision screening. The nurse can also serve as an integral part of the accommodations within the developed 504 plan. For example, a student recently diagnosed with type 1 diabetes may require the nurse to monitor blood sugar levels throughout the day and administer insulin as part of a second grader's 504 plan.

Child Study Team

The Individuals with Disabilities Education Improvement Act of 2004 requires that schools districts work to identify, locate, and evaluate all students with disabilities. This Child Find mandate also requires that school districts work to develop a practical method for identifying which children are receiving special education services and which students are not (Wright & Wright, 2006). The child study team is a multi-disciplinary group of school professionals who possess an expertise in conducting the necessary evaluations to properly identify those students in need of special services. The school nurse serves as a critical connection between the educational community and the healthcare community in schools. The school nurse is often an essential member of the Child Study Team in that they are able to both conduct necessary health assessments and provide professional insight into the potential impact any existing or chronic health conditions can have on learning outcomes (Galemore & Sheetz, 2015).

Pre-Referral and Intervention Teams

In the current context of American education, the process of identifying and intervening in the educational life of students who are making minimal academic, social, or behavioral progress begins promptly as students begin school. School districts are often required by law, administrative code, or best practices, to develop a team of educational professionals to create intervention plans for students prior to referral for a Child Study Team evaluation. These teams hold a variety of names such as: intervention and referral services team, pre-referral team, learner assistance team, and response to intervention team.

The school nurse often plays an integral role on pre-referral teams. The nurse's in-depth understanding of large groups of students and knowledge of health and family histories of students can be critical to the overall function of these teams. The school nurse's function on an intervention team can include the following functions:

- Serving as a case manager for individual students, maintaining requests for assistance, progress, and performance reports
- Coordinating the services of community-based social and health provider agencies and other community resources
- Providing support, guidance, and professional development to school staff who are working with a student with a health-related intervention plan
- Reviewing and assessing the effectiveness of the designed intervention plan

■ Fostering a Culture of Health and Wellness

Patty is in her third year as the school nurse of a large elementary school. Prior to entering school nursing, she had a long and rewarding career as a critical care nurse at a local hospital. Every 2 weeks, Patty takes part in a full day of meetings where she discusses students, collected data, and the outcomes of implemented strategies as part of her school's intervention team. During one early October meeting, Patty addresses the group on a trend she has observed in the health office. Patty reports that in the past 2 weeks she has needed to contact the families of multiple students regarding complaints of toothaches. From a cursory examination, Patty can see (and smell) that large numbers of students are not practicing proper dental hygiene. She also reports that parents in her community either do not have the resources or awareness to access quality dental care. Patty asks the intervention team and her principal for their thoughts. After a few days of research and a phone call to the community board of health, Patty has an idea and a few leads. Patty was referred to a local dentist who is the parent of a former student. He was thrilled with Patty's proposal to come to the school to provide the students with a short assembly about the importance of dental hygiene. In addition to speaking with the students, the visiting dentist provided Patty with a list of resources for a sliding fee scale and free dental clinics in the community to share with parents.

The previous example highlights the significant role the school nurse plays in bridging the gap between the academic and health care fields, initiating school-wide programs, and promoting a culture of health and wellness throughout the school. Examples of where school nurses foster a culture of health and wellness throughout a school highlight their leadership, collaboration, and communication skills. Creating a culture that blends the values of student academic performance as well as health and wellness is accomplished through strategically implemented programs as well as sustained, ongoing, and contextually embedded education.

In order to successfully implement an initiative across a school, the effective school nurse must have collected data regarding a felt need. Typically, the evidence that supports the need for a grade-level or school-wide initiative is not solely directed toward the school's health office. This evidence, and the concerns regarding a health, wellness, or safety issue, are communicated to the school nurse, principal, teachers, central office administrators, community agencies, and school counselors. Think for moment about the current health and wellness issues facing 21st-century students: stress, anxiety, vaping, drug abuse, obesity, cell phone regulation, and bullying. These issues significantly hinder students' ability to access their education and drastically impact the overall health and wellness of the student body. These issues impact large groups of students and must be addressed through a systemic school-wide approach. The school nurse does not work in isolation to address these issues; they are part of a much larger team of educators and community stakeholders. The Centers for Disease Control and Prevention's (CDC) *Whole School, Whole Community, Whole Child Model* (CDC, 2019) proposes an approach to health and wellness that includes the following components:

- Physical education and physical activity
- Nutrition and environment services

- Health education
- Social and emotional school climate
- Physical environment
- Health services
- Counseling psychological and social services
- Employee wellness
- Community involvement
- Family engagement

Health and wellness initiatives often encompass areas and competencies that fall beyond the scope of the school nurse, but require the nurse's influence and expertise to coordinate. As the bridge between the educational and health care communities, the school nurse is perfectly positioned to organize the interdisciplinary efforts to address the challenging health and wellness topics that impact students. The vast majority of issues facing 21st-century students are not solely home/parent problems, nor are they solely school/educator problems. The issues facing the 21st-century student occupy the space in between the home and the school. They are problems that must be addressed collaboratively by both parents and educators.

School nurses use a variety of formats and approaches to move the culture of the school toward health and wellness. The primary objective of implemented initiatives is to educate students and parents through communicating information and strategies regarding healthy habits and trending issues. For example, take a walk through the vast majority of middle and high schools at the current time and you will see, hear, and feel the influence school nurses have in creating a culture of health and wellness. You will see flyers for parent programs about the opioid crisis. You will pass by bulletin board displays informing students about the dangers of vaping. You will hear announcements about upcoming anti-bullying, peer leadership, and social emotional learning programs.

While school nurses use a variety of tools, in conjunction with a viable health education curriculum, to collaboratively create a school-wide culture of health and wellness, the most often used and most effective are being a sustained, visible, and inclusive of all school stakeholders. The following are a few examples of strategies used by school nurses to promote a culture of health and wellness.

Displays

Visual displays are an important aspect of promoting a healthy climate and culture. Figure 6.1 depicts a bulletin board created by the school nurses of Edison Intermediate School in Westfield, New Jersey, as part of a district-wide initiative in social emotional learning.

Programs

School-wide programs serve as an often utilized method for the school nurse to demonstrate leadership within the school, integrate community resources in the

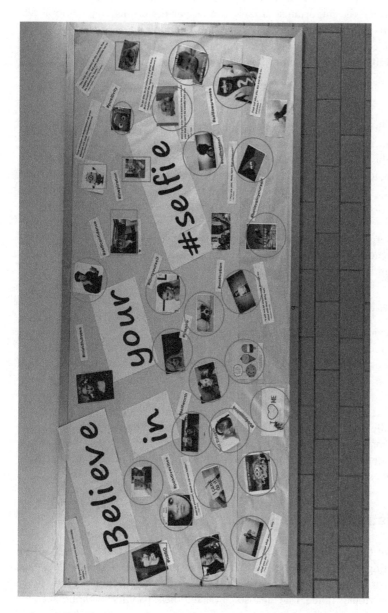

FIGURE 6.1 Example of visual display: Bulletin board presenting a social emotional learning initiative.

school day, and collaborate with teachers and administrators to strategically impact student health and wellness. Programs can vary in scope and in length. Some programs address a specific need that has been identified, such as a walking club during recess to promote the importance of daily exercise at the elementary school level. The school nurse can also play a critical role in health and wellness programs that are broader, more comprehensive, and involve numerous school stakeholders such as a school-wide initiative in social emotional learning.

Events

Another way that the school nurse can effectively collaborate with teachers, administrators, and community agencies to further a culture of health and wellness is through working collaboratively to plan, organize, and facilitate school events designed to address trending topics affecting the health of students. School-wide events can include students, such as having all students wear a specific color of clothing to recognize the importance of an issue (blue for anti-bullying; Stomp Out Bullying, 2019), red to bring awareness to heart disease in women (Gored for Women, 2019), or teal to promote food allergy awareness (Food Allergy & Anaphylaxis Connection Team, 2019). Other events can include the planning of a guest speaker to address a key health topic for students and parents.

Communication

As noted previously, regular communication from the school health office to all school stakeholders is one of the most effective methods for the school nurse to use to establish trust, build confidence, and share important information. A weekly or bi-weekly newsletter from the health office can serve as an important tool for both parents and educators. Often, through their network of connections with community agencies and their affiliation with professional organizations, the school nurse is aware of trending health issues affecting students well before the general public. Sharing this information in a sustained, concise, digestible, and constructive manner not only builds public trust in the school nurse, but also fosters conversations between schools, families, and children.

Administrator–Nurse Rapport

Emily was not the only student who Martha mailed height and weight referrals to after conducting her assessments. Martha also sent referrals to two other students whose height or weight fell beyond established guidelines and required parental notification. As previously noted, Martha also contacted these parents by phone to communicate that a letter with sensitive information was on its way to the house. Two days after mailing her notifications, William's parents arrive at the school at 8:00 a.m. sharp and demand a meeting with the school principal. The principal can immediately see that William's parents are livid as he greets them. They proceed to tell the principal how extremely angry they are to receive what they believe to be an inappropriate letter regarding a practice that violated the rights of privacy of their child. They demand to know why the school nurse thinks that she should not only measure, but also make judgments about their son's weight. William's parents want an explanation immediately or they have vowed to contact the superintendent of schools as they drive to their attorney's office.

Thankfully, Martha not only possesses sound nursing judgment, she also has an excellent rapport with her school principal. The rapport that exists between Martha and her principal was established over time and is grounded in mutual respect and constant communication. Prior to notifying parents about screenings that fell beyond established guidelines, Martha informed her principal that she would be sending out the letters. She respected the students' privacy rights and did not believe that each student's identity needed to be shared with her principal. She was also able to inform her principal that when contacted by phone about the referral, William's parents were both surprised and not happy about the news. Martha's proactive communication with her principal allowed him to prepare for what can be contentious information for a parent. As a result of Martha's communication prior to notifying parents, her principal had the time to prepare himself for the possibility of this parent concern and was able to provide William's parents with copies of the district policy that mandated the screenings as well as background about the importance of the information that results from the screenings.

The school nurse and principal must develop and maintain a professional rapport. Both the school nurse and principal must regularly collaborate throughout the day as they respond to critical issues, plan to properly address the needs of students, parents, and teachers, and ensure that the school is operating in compliance with local and state health codes and requirements. The rapport between the school nurse and principal takes many forms and depends greatly on the personalities, backgrounds, length of time working together, leadership style, and established routines and procedures within the school. While multiple variables exist that will dictate the nature and type of relationship between the school nurse and principal, non-negotiables must exist regarding the school nurse's role and function within the school, communication between both parties, and supervision and evaluation methods.

Chain of Command

Throughout this chapter multiple vignettes have been offered to demonstrate the importance of various school nursing functions within an interdisciplinary environment. Each of these examples places heavy emphasis on the importance of communication. In some instances the school nurse is communicating as a function of their role while serving on a school-based team; in other examples the school nurse is communicating with parents and teachers to collaboratively plan instructional endeavors. Each scenario presents an opportunity for the school nurse to communicate with their principal. Many of the scenarios offered are examples of where the nurse is required, as a result of the chain of command, to report to her principal.

Schools districts, and the schools therein, function as part of a bureaucratic hierarchy. School and district hierarchies allow for school districts to organize work flow, management, reporting, and information sharing to ensure that the district is working in an efficient manner. The basic elements of this hierarchy involve a board of elected citizens that govern the development and implementation of policies. The board of education relies on a chief school administrator or superintendent to implement the board's vision and lead the district's schools through the management of policy and program implementation. The superintendent in turn relies on a school principal to ensure that the daily operations and district's program of studies is facilitated effectively at the school level. The school principal relies on the teachers, school nurses, counselors, and support personnel who work directly with students to provide daily instruction, support, counseling, coaching, and caring for their general welfare. Each of the distinct positions within a school district bureaucracy requires formal mandatory reporting obligations and informal communication responsibilities.

When to Report

School nurse's typically report directly to the school principal or another school administrator such as an assistant principal. In some spaces, school nurses also report to a supervisor, director, or coordinator of nurses. These positions can be formal administrative positions or stipend positions assigned to a nurse in the district who has demonstrated organizational and leadership abilities. Knowing what to report and to whom are critical responsibilities of the school nurse, and tasks that can be made much less burdensome when a positive and professional rapport exists between the principal and school nurse.

- An elementary school nurse identifies the fifth student that morning in two classes with active nits in their hair.
- A high school physics teacher escorts a sophomore to the health office because the student fell asleep in his class and he believes he smells marijuana emanating from his jacket.
- A middle school nurse just returned from an excellent workshop offered by the community board of health about anti-vaping education. She is has big ideas about changes she would like to make to the district's outdated curriculum.
- At the height of cold and flu season, an elementary school nurse sends home her sixth student of the day, all with similar symptoms of fever, chills, and nausea.

Which of these scenarios requires a report to the school principal? Which of these scenarios would the effective school nurse not only report to their principal, but also to the district coordinator of school nurses? Which of these scenarios requires immediate administrative support and intervention, and which do not?

Each of the above scenarios presents an opportunity for a school nurse to report to their principal. Communicating about an accident, incident, or problem are situations where reporting procedures are often required and guided by state law or district policy. These reports must be made as soon as possible and be communicated and documented thoroughly. Reports regarding ideas and trends are also occasions when communication between supervisor and nurse can occur. These are often less pressing issues that can be discussed over time. Regardless of the issue being communicated to a principal or other supervisor, all reports should be guided by a sound understanding of school law, school board policy, and sound nursing judgment.

Nurse Evaluation

The beginning of the school year is always a hectic time for the effective school nurse. Days are filled with the receipt and cataloging of student medications, verification of required medical forms and immunization records, facilitation of training for faculty and staff in communicable diseases, epinephrine auto-injectors, and glucagon, and sharing important medical information about hundreds of students with scores of teachers. Hectic would be an understated way of describing the month of September in the life of a school nurse.

In the middle of the craziness of September, a principal was approached by one of his school nurses with a question about a recent email that the principal sent earlier in the day. The email reminded all teaching faculty about deadlines for required information as part of the teacher evaluation system. Teachers were reminded of the requirement to submit beginning of the year rubric self-assessments, two professional development goals, and two student growth objectives to the principal by the end of the week. The nurse, who had established open lines of communication with the principal during their 7 years of working together, asked the principal why the school nurses had to submit professional development goals and student growth objectives like the classroom teachers. The principal could see that the nurse was communicating from a place of exhaustion, so the principal took a moment and then responded. The principal offered, that with less than 50% of the country's public schools employing a full-time school nurse, as well as school nurse positions being cut and outsourced more frequently than ever (Camera, 2016), it is critical that that school nurses do every single thing they can to viewed as a full-time, critical, and professional component of the school faculty. One of the best ways to achieve this professional recognition is to be evaluated in the same manner as every other teacher in the school.

School nurse observations and evaluations are most typically conducted by a school principal or assistant principal. Evaluations of the school nurse conducted solely by non-nursing personnel create a juxtaposition for both the school nurse as well as the administrator. The school administrator can offer substantive feedback on classroom teaching, communication skills, collaboration with faculty, planning, and other professional responsibilities. However, the school administrator does not possess the background experience or capacity to offer evaluative feedback on the nurse's clinical delivery of nursing service. The National Association of School Nurses (NASN, 2018) recommends that evaluations of school nurses be conducted by both registered school nurses as well as non-nurse school administrators.

The supervision and evaluation of school nurses is most effectively conducted when it is grounded in a systemic evaluation framework that is informed by standards of practice such as provided by a state or national school nurse association. Established evaluation models of teachers such as Charlotte Danielson's *Framework for Teaching* (2014) and Kim Marshall's Evaluation Model (2013) have been effectively modified to include evaluative indicators and domains specific to the school nurse. While each evaluation model contains idiosyncratic processes, each encourages self-assessment, observations conducted by a supervisor or principal, and a mid-year or final summary evaluation. When the evaluation process is conducted thoughtfully and with fidelity, it is can be mutually beneficial in promoting a positive rapport between the principal and school nurse.

References

Camera, L. (2016, March 23). Many school district don't have enough school nurses. *US News and World Report*. Retrieved from https://www.usnews.com/news/articles/2016-03-23/the-school-nurse-scourge

Centers for Disease Control and Prevention. (2019, May 29). *Whole School, Whole Community, Whole Child (WSCC)*. Retrieved from https://www.cdc.gov/healthyschools/wscc/index.htm

Cleave, J. V., Gortmaker, S. L., & Perrin, J. M. (2010). Dynamics of obesity and chronic health conditions among children and youth. *JAMA, 303*(7), 623. doi: 10.1001/jama.2010.104

Danielson, C. (2015). *The framework for teaching: evaluation instrument*. Moorabbin, Australia: Hawker Brownlow Education.

Food Allergy & Anaphylaxis Connection Team. (2019). Retrieved from https://www.foodallergyawareness.org/

Galemore, C. A., & Sheetz, A. H. (2015). IEP, IHP, and Section 504 primer for new school nurses. *NASN School Nurse, 30*(2), 85–88. doi: 10.1177/1942602x14565462

Gored for Women. (2019). Retrieved from https://www.goredforwomen.org/

Marshall, K. (2013). *Rethinking teacher supervision and evaluation: how to work smart, build collaboration, and close the achievement gap*. San Francisco, CA: Jossey-Bass.

National Association of School Nurses. (2018). *Supervision and evaluation of the school nurse* (Position Statement). Silver Spring, MD: Author.

Stomp Out Bullying. (2019). Retrieved from https://www.stompoutbullying.org/

Thies, K. M. (1999). Identifying the educational implications of chronic illness in school children. *Journal of School Health, 69*(10), 392–397. doi: 10.1111/j.1746-1561.1999.tb06354.x

U.S. Department of Education. (n.d.). *The Every Student Succeeds Act (ESSA): A new education law*. Retrieved from www.ed.gov/essa?src=rn

U.S. Department of Education, Office for Civil Rights. (2010). *Free appropriate education for students with disabilities: Requirements under Section 504 of the Rehabilitation Act of 1973*. Retrieved from https://www2.ed.gov/about/offices/list/ocr/docs/edlite-FAPE504.html

Wright, P. W. D., & Wright, P. D. (2006). *Wrightslaw: Special education law*. Hartfield, VA: Harbor House Law Press.

Further Readings

American Academy of Pediatrics. (2008). Role of the school nurse in providing school health services. *Pediatrics, 121*(5), 1052–1056. doi:10.1542/peds.2008-0382

New Jersey Department of Education. (n.d.). *Intervention and referral services*. Retrieved from https://www.state.nj.us/education/students/safety/behavior/irs/

Sampson, C. H., & Galemore, C. A. (2012). What every school nurse needs to know about Section 504 eligibility. *NASN School Nurse, 27*(2), 88–93. doi: 10.1177/1942602x12437879

THE SCHOOL NURSE, HEALTH OFFICE, AND THERAPEUTIC INTERVENTIONS

JANICE LOSCHIAVO

LEARNING OBJECTIVES

- Define school nursing
- Identify the key provision of the Tenth Amendment to the United States Constitution.
- Describe the various functions of the school nurse
- List 10 components of an individual health folder
- Explain two reasons why accurate documentation is essential.

▓ Introduction

The health office is a vital part of the school community. Always busy, many accurately refer to it as the "heart of the school." School nurses would readily agree. In command of this office is the school nurse who, hopefully, will demonstrate the utmost professionalism, sincere concern, and unconditional acceptance toward all who pass through the door. Many will make this office their first stop when entering the building. Therefore, the atmosphere should always be warm and welcoming.

The daily activities in this office will vary. It is almost impossible to plan specific tasks as priorities will come into play. Best to imagine the day as a bucket containing several pounds of uncooked rice. Each rice morsel represents a task to be completed, within the bucket, your time. As the day progresses people come and occupy space in the bucket. By the end of the day, there is no room left and the people overflow with their many needs unmet.

A better scenario is to start the day by putting people in your bucket, gradually adding the rice (tasks), which now will fill in the open spaces. In other words, put the children *first* in your day. The tasks can wait.

In this chapter you will learn the academic requirements and essential attributes the school nurse must possess, the practical aspects of setting-up a health office, as well as the many required tasks that are to be accomplished. Once properly prepared with the appropriate tools available, the school nurse can utilize acquired skills to assess students through the nursing process, monitor physical assessments, document health information, deal with areas of concern, and effectively run the school health office.

Educational Preparation for the School Nurse

In 1791, the Tenth Amendment to the United States Constitution was passed. This Amendment was intended to keep power in the hands of the people, not the federal government. Therefore, unless specifically granted to the central government, exclusive rights on the remaining issues are given to the individual states. This covers all aspects of education, including school nurse preparation. Therefore, educational preparation for the school nurse will vary from state to state. Some states will require a bachelor's degree in addition to specific courses relevant to school nursing. Others may require little or no advanced training.

The National Association of School Nurses (NASN) recommends that every school-aged child have access to a fully qualified school nurse. For some children, the nurse will be the only health professional seen on a regular basis. Therefore, the school nurse should possess, at minimum, a baccalaureate degree in nursing from an accredited college or university, and should be licensed as a registered, professional nurse through a board of nursing or equivalent body, as required by the state in which the nurse practices.

These requirements constitute minimal preparation needed to practice at the entry level of school nursing (American Nurses Association [ANA] & NASN, 2016). Additionally, NASN supports state school nurse certification and endorses national certification of school nurses through the National Board for Certification of School Nurses (NBCSN; NASN, 2016).

Considering the varied role of the school nurse, comprehensive educational preparation is crucial. The school nurse must develop skills in many areas since this nurse may also serve as a:

- Pediatric nurse
- Health educator
- Community health nurse
- Social worker
- Office manager
- Nurse administrator

- Mother figure
- Health counselor
- Psychologist
- Emergency department nurse
- Mediator
- Advisor
- Child study
- Intervention/referral team member
- Crisis management team member
- Section 504 team member

Attributes of a School Nurse

Parents have no choice. They must leave their children daily for at least 6 hours and, for many students, the school day is even longer. While they are apart, parents rely on school personnel to meet their child's physical and emotional needs so learning can take place. The school nurse serves as the bridge between the home and school. Teachers change each year or each semester but the school nurse is a constant presence in that child's school experience (Loschiavo, 2019, p. 16).

Any new school nurse can quickly become overwhelmed with the prospect of working independently and might even question if they made the right career choice. Recognize that fate will sometimes place you in situations much larger than you can completely understand. Be alert to these challenges and receptive to the influences placed before you. Each incident will create a better you: more confident, more capable. To do the job well and best manage the stress level, certain qualities are essential. These attributes represent the pillars of our profession. If you feel that you personally lack these qualities, work to develop them. They include:

- *Professional Pride*

According to the 2019 Gallop poll, nurses were voted the profession most trusted, for the 18th consecutive year. This honor should bring tremendous pride. No other profession can make this claim (Brennan, 2019).

- *Communication Skills*

We communicate verbally and nonverbally. How well you speak and write is a direct reflection on you.

- *Listening Skills*

Learn to be an active listener. Display attentive body language which simply means paying attention to the speaker. Students and staff will then feel valued and understood.

■ *Curiosity*

Unless you remain interested and are curious about people, you will find school nursing is not challenging. Much of what we do is repetitious. If you limit your day to rendering first aid, doing screenings, checking immunizations, and completing paperwork, boredom and monotony will define your role.

■ *Sense of Humor*

So often our work is upsetting and we must seek ways to find fun in the day. Do not take every situation seriously. Look for opportunities to laugh and give joy to others.

■ *Flexibility*

Today, more than ever, we must adapt to the ever-changing student, parent, and lifestyles. Change is hard for many. Sometimes we resist change simply because it is new. Be willing to bend and look for the new, right way.

■ *Interpersonal Skills*

Good interpersonal skills will allow the school nurse to interact positively and effectively with all; students, parents, teachers, and administrators.

■ *Trustworthiness*

You cannot demand trust. Trust must be earned. Trust will come when you act with integrity and never mislead or lie. Do not display favoritism toward students or teachers.

■ *Decision-Making Skills*

When it comes to the health and well-being of students, you make the decisions. Do not be swayed by those not qualified to do so.

■ *Respect*

Before you can respect others, you must respect yourself. Only then you can respect others' right to be different.

■ *With-It-Ness*

Remain focused and engaged throughout the school day. Stay in the moment and you will prevent small problems from becoming big ones.

■ *Self-Confidence*

Confidence shapes the foundation of your endurance. It will help improve the way people see you (Loschiavo, 2019a).

■ The School Health Office

Most school nurses would agree that the nurse's office should be titled *The School Health Office*. This allows the assumption that we are dealing with a healthy, school environment. This office is open the entire school day and is where students can get help from a knowledgeable, caring health professional. For some staff, students, and families, this is the extent of their health service availability.

Location

The School Health Office is usually located near the front entrance, just steps away from the principal and main office. Since you are so visible, many visitors will stop in to say hello and frequently you will have unwanted interruptions in your work. If there are children present, explain to the visitor that you cannot stop to talk at that point. If they insist they need to speak with you, unless it is urgent, give them an appropriate time later in the day/week when you can speak with them. The size of the health office should be reflective of the number, age, and health needs of the student body. Older buildings were originally designed this way but with the addition of so many new support staff, frequently the office is moved to other areas. If this is the situation, consider the following requirements for every health office in every school regardless of enrollment size:

- Locked cabinet for medicine
- Central location, ground level
- Doors wide enough to accommodate a stretcher or wheel chair
- Area spacious enough so there can be separation for the ill and well child
- Place where children can shelter-in-place if necessary
- Office work area
- Rest station with at least one cot
- Bathroom with window or exhaust system and doorway wide enough for a wheelchair
- Consider not having a lock for the bathroom door; if a student becomes ill, you need to enter quickly
- Private conference place
- Storage area for Go-Kit
- Bathroom sink and, if possible, a second, clean sink with an eyewash station outside of the bathroom
- Air conditioner and proper ventilation

Equipment

The School Health Office should be equipped much as other offices in the building (Box 7.1). A separate copy machine or fax is not necessary as long as the nurse can locate these services quickly so an ill child is not left unattended and private documents are not accessible to other school personnel. In addition to the standard equipment seen in most offices, the school nurse will need specialized equipment relevant to nursing and the need for document privacy (Box 7.2).

BOX 7.1

HEALTH OFFICE EQUIPMENT

Phone—land line and cell

Desk

Computer

Several chairs

Copy machine

Refrigerator with lock

Examining light

Chair with wheels

Appropriate software

Fax machine

File cabinets with locks

BOX 7.2

NURSING EQUIPMENT IN THE HEALTH OFFICE

Thermometers

Nebulizer—mask and tubing

Sphygmomanometer with child, adult, and obese cuffs

Wheelchair

Glucometer

Eye wash station

Masks (paper and CPR)

Emesis basins

Vision testing equipment

Peak-flow meter

Bandages/gauze in assorted sizes

Ice packs

(continued)

Gloves—sterile and unsterile

Tooth preservation kits

Tissues

Go-Kit

Oxygen

Pulse Ox

Stethoscope

Privacy screen

Flash lights

Otoscope

Scoliometer

Automated external defibrillator—child and adult pads

Leg and arm splints

Topical antiseptics

Cotton balls

Lotion

Hand wipes

Paper/medication cups

Forceps/nail clipper

The Nursing Process

Throughout the school day, students will come and go with various complaints/issues to be addressed. In order to deal effectively with each adult or child who seeks you out, the Nursing Process must be enacted. The Nursing Process is designed for all nurse specialties. It is considered the essential core of practice needed to deliver comprehensive care and the one procedure which unites all nurses. Developed by Ida Jean Orlando in 1958, it is still useful for nursing care today.

Definition of the Nursing Process

The Nursing Process is a sequential, systematic guide to patient-centered care. Fundamental principles of critical thinking, client-centered approaches to care, goal-oriented procedures, evidence-based practice recommendations, and strong nursing intuition are employed. The five sequential steps include assessment, diagnosis, planning, implementation, and evaluation.

▓ Components of the Nursing Process

The Nursing Process involves five, sequential components or steps: assessment, diagnosis, planning, implementation and evaluation (ANA, n.d.) This process in enacted for each child for every visit to your office (ANA, n.d.). Make it clear to all teachers that no child should be denied permission to see you. Nor should they have to explain the reason they are requesting to come to the school health office. If visits become excessive you will work with the child, teacher, and parent so excessive class time is not missed. Be mindful that it may not actually be a stomach or headache but something that drew the child to you. You will need to discover what the actual problem is.

Assessment

The first step in the process is for the nurse to gather as much information as possible. This includes physiological data as well as psychological information. The school nurse should question the student about the nature of the complaint. Vital signs can be taken while the nurse notes the student's demeanor and body language. Relevant questions might be:

- ▪ Were you ill before coming to school?
- ▪ Describe how you feel?
- ▪ On a scale of 1 to 10, how much pain are you experiencing?
- ▪ When did you eat/drink/go to the bathroom last?
- ▪ What were you doing in class before asking to see me?
- ▪ How did you sleep last night?
- ▪ Is there anything upsetting you?

Diagnosis

After gathering the required information, the school nurse can make an educated guess as to the nature of the problem and formulate a Nursing Diagnosis. Keep in mind that there may be several, possible, concurrent problems. A child might be struggling in class, be a bully victim, and actually be acutely ill with the flu. No possibility should be overlooked.

Outcomes/Planning

With the information gained from the assessment and the formulated Nursing Diagnosis, the nurse develops a plan to help the child. This might include providing:

- Bathroom access
- Snacks
- Opportunity to rest a while
- Return to class and check on later
- Exclusion from school
- Opportunity to talk with you
- Refer for counseling
- You-do-not-have-to-be-sick-to-visit-me talk, assuring the child that if they need to stop in periodically it is okay. They should just tell you they need to talk and are not ill and come when they are not missing valuable class time.
- Call parent to conference and/or to come pick up child
- Call 911 if warranted

Implementation

Once you have considered the options, make your decision and implement the plan as you deem best at that moment. Keep in mind to always err on the side of caution. If you have to think about calling 911, make the call.

Evaluation

Now the school nurse must evaluate whether the plan was effective. Were your goals met? Ask yourself if you assessed the situation correctly. Should you have done anything differently? Are modifications needed? Is a follow-up home call warranted (Toney-Butler & Thayer, 2019)?

Example of the Nursing Process With Poor Outcome

An eighth grade boy enters the health office at 9 a.m. complaining of an upset stomach. This student is one you see repeatedly for various minor issues. You ask him the routine questions, when he ate last, does he need the bathroom, was he ill during the night or before school. Nothing appears significant.

His temperature is normal but his color is poor and he appears out of sorts. You question if anything is bothering him and remind him he can just come and talk. He shares that his parents are talking about getting a divorce. You spend a few minutes reassuring him that although his parents may not love each other anymore, they still love him. He is comforted and you tell him to return to class.

The next morning you note he is absent and call home. His mother tells you that he was hospitalized during the night with acute appendicitis. She asks you if he saw you the day before and asks why she was not notified?

This scenario would have had a better outcome if the nurse had checked the student's abdomen for tenderness. Even if no symptoms presented at that time, she should have checked on the student later in the day. Was he still uncomfortable? Did he eat lunch? Was he looking better?

The final phase, evaluation, is so important. The nurse went with what appeared most obvious, emotional distress caused by issues at home. This may have been true but along with that was an underlying illness. Even if the child does not return to see you, check on them later in the day. If the child is still exhibiting symptoms, it will be apparent. A phone call home is always appreciated, even if it is to say you are not sure if a problem is developing.

▨ Assessments

It has long been established that to learn a child must be healthy and happy in the school environment. An ill, sad child simply cannot be properly educated nor can they fully participate in the various enrichment programs now offered in the school setting. Today we refer to physical examinations as assessments since we consider subjective as well as objective information. We look at all body systems as well as emotional wellness. Whenever possible, these assessments should be provided by the child's primary care physician at regular health supervision visits and should be performed as recommended in the Guidelines for Health Supervision, Third Edition, from the American Academy of Pediatrics (AAP, 2018). Additional visits may be necessary if circumstances suggest variations from normal (AAP, 2018). This exam should include (AAP, 2018):

- ▪ Health history (pregnancy/birth trauma, injuries, surgeries, congenital defects)
- ▪ Comprehensive appraisal (blood pressure, temperature, abdominal masses, dental caries)
- ▪ Growth and development assessment (height, weight, Tanner scale)
- ▪ Body systems check (pulse, lung sounds, abdominal mass check)
- ▪ Blood work as appropriate for age
- ▪ Child's and family's mental health evaluation (teen depression survey)
- ▪ Immunization appropriate to age recommendations
- ▪ Health education on nutrition and exercise
- ▪ Evaluation for athletic participation (permission for contact sports, previous traumatic brain injury [TBI])
- ▪ Specific recommendations as health needs require

The exams may be conducted by a licensed physician or advanced practice nurse. If the child is under 18 years of age, parental input is needed. The AAP also recommends that each comprehensive, periodic health assessment visit beginning at 3 years of age should include attention to school health issues. Can the child attend? Does the child easily separate from the parent?

A number of states also require examinations and/or assessments when the student is participating in interscholastic sports, following a traumatic brain injury, prior to beginning work, if suspected of being under the influence of alcohol or a controlled substance, or undergoing Child Study Team evaluation. These assessments will undoubtedly contain additional, specific tests/information relevant to the nature of the required assessment.

Depression Screening

The AAP now recommends that adolescents 10 to 21 years of age be screened for depression by their primary care clinicians. This recommendation is in response to the report by Dr. Zuckerbrot that cites that 50% of adolescents with depression are diagnosed before they reach adulthood and as many as two in three depressed teens do not get any help or care (Zuckerbrot et al., 2018).

▪ Documentation

The school nurse is the one person totally responsible for maintaining health records for students. School nurses face decisions every day regarding health information: how much should be written in files, where they should be stored, and who should be permitted to see these files knowing that unauthorized personnel should not have access to a student's private data.

Record-keeping tasks are endless and time-consuming. They keep school nurses from spending needed time with students. We grudgingly do it, and far too frequently, we omit valuable information. Each school district has some variation as to the documentation required by the school nurse. In general, all schools will require the nurse to keep a record of emergency information for students and staff, a daily log of health office visits, and a comprehensive, individual health folder for every student (Loschiavo, 2019, pp. 97–106).

▪ Emergency Information

The first priority the school nurse must tend to is to annually secure emergency information for every student and staff member. This information should be secure yet available for quick access. Do not discard previous year's information as you may have to reconfirm information. Each card or computerized form should include the student's name, both parents' names and contact information or that of the legal guardian, address, and physician' name and phone number.

Included also should be a list of at least two, previously informed family members or friends who would be willing to pick up the child in the event you cannot reach the parent. Keep in mind that you should not release a child to anyone not listed unless the parent gives written or verbal permission. This includes a person who might answer the home phone. The child must be able to identify the person and be comfortable with them. When calling a parent at work, do not discuss the child's health with anyone other than the parent. This emergency card can also be used to update any health information and give consent for information to be shared. Consider adding a note asking for health updates and have the parent initial if they do *not* wish information to be shared. Make sure the parent or guardian signs the card.

Daily Log

One of the first commandments we learned as we prepared to be nurses was: *If it was not documented it was not done*. This is especially true in school nursing since no one comes in to relieve you at the end the day. What you have not written, no one else will.

The school nurse must document all student visits to the health office either electronically or in hard copy. Ideally, entries should be made immediately. However, the health office is a busy place, and this is often not possible. The following procedure may help you keep track of numerous visits. If age-appropriate, have students enter their names and time of arrival on a clip board or laptop. No other information is needed since this information is confidential. The very young students should bring a note from the teacher containing the time and any classroom observations or information the teacher may have received from the parent.

Assess each child according to the Nursing Process, document your findings, and retain these records for each student according to district policy. If there was another student involved in the injury, or if there is potential for complications, complete an Accident Report. Notify parents and administration as needed. It will help diffuse a potentially libelous situation. Document your actions carefully on the student's log. Include parental conversations, student assessment notes, your follow-up efforts, and the outcome.

Individual Health Folders

The student's health folder is a compilation of a number of essential documents. The folder can be maintained electronically or in hard-copy format. It should contain, at minimum, a permanent, cumulative form that covers the entire school tenure. Each form should include the child's name, birth date, parents'/guardian's names, addresses, phone numbers, screening data, immunizations, growth and development statistics, disease history, hearing, vision, dental, blood pressure, scoliosis, height and weight screenings. Include tuberculosis testing results and a section for nurse's notes. The nurse's notes should contain a record of when the child enrolled and when/if they transferred out, along with any significant health issue not included elsewhere on the form. The folder should also house registration health information, previous school records, the student log sheet, medication record, copies of accident reports, referral notes, physical assessments reports, parental notes, and your personal notes not included in the permanent record.

The school nurse is responsible for gathering and maintaining an updated health record for each student. Any deficiencies noted should be followed up according to state/district policies. Add the written permission from the parent(s) to share confidential health information with teachers and other personnel whom you deem appropriate.

Administrative Reports

The school nurse is responsible for a number of reports throughout the school year. Not all reports are required by every school, district, or state. Check with your administration and school nurse colleagues to see what is relevant for you and the date on which any reports are due. The school nurse must also write and keep secure a number of documents to guide their practice. Again, these documents will vary from state to state and district to district but basically are essential references for all school nurses. Some of the more commonly requested reports are described in the following sections.

Accident or Incident Reports

An accident or incident report is a written statement by an eyewitness, which is obtained and provided as part of the legal record as close to the time of the event as possible. The person who actually witnesses an incident should provide the firsthand information. If no adult observed an incident firsthand, the nurse should document in the form, for example, "Mrs. Smith stated that Robert fell, hitting his head." Include only factual information. Reference the accident on the student's log sheet as you would for any health office visit. Be alert for incidents that could have been prevented and inform administration if further investigation is needed.

Daily, Weekly, Monthly, and Annual Reports

These reports are made upon request and help justify how you are spending your time. Prepare a checklist of the number of health office visits, exclusions, medications given, phone conferences, screenings performed, deficiency notices sent out, classes taught, and so on. This is an excellent way to communicate with your administrator and keep a record of statistics.

Section 504 Accommodation Plan

Students with 504 Accommodation Plans have difficulty with one or more activities of daily living. There are children who require accommodations during the school day so that maximum learning can take place. Be aware of these children, know the extent of the required accommodations, and ensure that the accommodations are implemented.

Tuberculosis Report

Most states require some type of report so they can follow up on the incidence and prevalence of tuberculosis. This is how they evaluate the need for testing in particular areas. Standardized forms asking for the number of students and staff tested and the results are usually sent by the state and must be completed by the school nurse.

Immunization Status Report

Once you have completed checking all your students' immunizations, you must file an annual report with the state. It includes information on the number of students with provisional admission as well as those with medical, philosophical, and religious exemptions.

School Nurse Resources

Since almost all school nurses work independently, it is essential that physician-directed, clear, concise information and orders be readily available. Every health office should contain an accessible reference area for the substitute school nurse. Various documents needed for best practice:

- *Substitute Nurse Folder:* This folder should contain basic information such as location of keys for medications, how to access phone lines, emergency egress plans, and directions for shelter-in-place. The student alert list should be included as well as a list of students who receive daily and emergency medications. Add where and how the medications should be charted.
- *School Nurse Manual:* The manual should contain copies of newsletters generated from your office as well as any notice sent out.
- *Standing Orders:* These orders are written by the school nurse and contain directions for the routine care of students. These include when the child should be excluded, what topical medications can be given, and so on. Every school district should have a Medical Director or School Physician who must review and sign the orders annually.
- *Nursing Service Plan:* Some states require an annual quality assurance report. Part of this report asks school nurses to identify those students needing specialized nursing care. It is designed to make sure students with medical needs are cared for adequately.
- *Policy and Procedure Manuals:* The state sets forth policies and procedure for implementation of various mandates for each district. A copy of the Policies and Procedures should be available.

◼ Special Considerations for the School Nurse

Technology

As soon as we learn one program, a new one is developed. Learning the new world of technology takes time, patience, and a willingness to humble yourself and ask for help, often from someone half your age. Most health offices today have some computerized charting and the nurse will therefore have some technology background. However, when we forward records, we do not know if what we send will be compatible with the receiving district. Often, work has to be transferred into hard copies, doubling the amount of work. Be open to finding the new, better way. The very definition of a professional is a person with a growing body of knowledge. If a new student entered your school with a condition you never heard of, you would research it so you could best do your job. Technology is no different. Work at it and you will be successful.

Lack of Health Office Coverage

Sad stories of school nurses who could not take a needed day off abound. Once you do find a willing substitute, she is hired for her own school. Consider recruiting from your parent base. As long as you feel you can trust their discretion, ask administration if you can have a mother who is a registered nurse work for the small pay just to be close to her young children. Work to increase the substitute pay for nurses. A nurse has a license to protect and should be compensated at a higher rate than a substitute teacher. You might also try recruiting from a local university with a bachelor program for nurses. Offer to allow nurses to work just a few hours. If they can split the shift, more might be available.

Infection Control

So many nurses work in less than ideal conditions. As previously mentioned, school health offices frequently have been relocated to less desirable locations in the building to make room for the increasing number of special service personnel. Insist that your office be accessible to children, ground level, and meets the required specifications for safety. The room must be large enough for you to be able to separate the ill from the well child, have a bathroom, sink, a resting place, and an area to shelter in place if necessary

Conflict With Personal Beliefs and District/State Mandates

The school nurse must deal with everyone they come in contact with respect and compassion. Regardless of how you might personally feel about transgender students, same-sex marriages, and other sensitive issues, you must remain nondiscriminatory. If you cannot deal objectively, seek professional help or another profession.

Non-Nursing Assignments

It is not uncommon for school nurses to be assigned to cover the office secretary for lunch, do the attendance, cover a late-arriving or early departure teacher's class, have hall duty, tend to school bus arrivals/departures, and other nonnursing tasks. Usually, the nurse is very willing to help and, for administrators, represents the path of least resistance. In most instances the rationale is that there is no one else to do the task. This is not your problem. It is important for administration to distinguish what no other person can do or what no other person wants to do. Tactfully explain that you have responsibilities that no one else can do and must tend to these first.

Frequent Flyers

If you have spent more than a day in the school health office you realize that there are students that must see you every day. They will present with a variety of complaints that must be addressed immediately. You patiently tend to them while trying to deal with the many others who truly need immediate care. These children do have a reason for seeing you; it is just not the one they share with you. There might be unrest at home, or the student might be new and not have found a comfortable place yet. Perhaps they are being bullied or marginalized because of another issue. Sometimes, if the teacher is absent, the young student will want to be with you. If the work presented is too difficult and the teacher not attentive to the child's needs, they will seek you out. Many children just have a need to move about and sitting in one room for prolonged periods is just too difficult. One remedy might be to have a you-do-not-have-to-be-sick-to-visit-me talk. Advise them that they do not have to have a physical symptom. It is okay just to say they need a time out or want to talk. Consider allowing this child to see you daily at a predetermined time when they are not missing class and it is not your busiest time.

Work with the student, parent and teacher to try and resolve whatever the underlying issue is. Eventually, the student will find a comfortable place outside your office. You will then have time to welcome the next frequent flyer.

■ References

American Academy of Pediatrics. (2018). Physical examination. *Bright Futures*. Retrieved from https://brightfutures.aap.org

American Nurses Association. (n.d.). *The nursing process*. Retrieved from nursingworld .org

Brenan, M. (2018). Nurses again outpace other professions for honesty, ethics. *Gallup Poll*. Retrieved from https://news.gallup.com/poll/245597/nurses-again-outpace-professions -honesty-ethics.aspx

Loschiavo, J. (2019a). *Fast facts for the school nurse* (3rd ed., p. 16). New York, NY: Springer Publishing Company.

Loschiavo, J. (2019b). *Fast facts for the school nurse* (3rd ed., pp. 97–106). New York, NY: Springer Publishing Company.

National Association of School Nurses. (2016). *Position statement education, licensure and certification*. Retrieved from https://nasn.org

Nursing Process. (2019). *Purpose of NursingProcess.org*. Retrieved from nursingprocess.org

Toney-Butler, T. J., & Thayer, J. M. (2019). *Nursing process*. Treasure Island, FL: StatPearls Publishing. Retrieved from https://www.ncbi.nlm.hih.gov

Zuckerbrot, R., Cheung, A., Jensen, P. S., Stein, R. E. K., Laraque, D., & GLAD-PC Steering Group. (2018). Guidelines for adolescent depression. *Pediatrics, 120*(5), e1299. doi:10.1542/peds.2017-4081

▨ Further Reading

National Center for Constitutional Studies. (n.d.). *The Bill of Rights Amendments 1-10*. Retrieved from https://nccs.net/blogs/americas-founding-documents/bill-of-rights-amendments-1-10

THE DEVELOPING CHILD AND CHALLENGES TO LEARNING

HUGH BASES

▓ Introduction

Today's educational environment has dramatically changed. Schools are now barrier free, guided by many more federal regulations, and include a growing number of special needs students. In addition, the child of today attends school, or some type of formal institution, at a much earlier age, for a longer school day and, often, an extended school year.

Yesterday's child was kept at home until 5 years of age. The gifted child had few enrichment experiences offered and, isolated, the special needs child remained unidentified. Early intervention was not an option. Fortunately, children with special needs have now been brought into the light sooner so problems can be addressed, a treatment plan formulated, and progress monitored by professional personnel. This places enormous responsibility on school personnel. We, the educators, who work within the school walls, are given the challenge of meeting the individual needs of students with unique learning profiles.

Therefore, it is essential that all those involved in education today add to their knowledge base by understanding the basic function of the brain and the impact of neurodevelopmental variation on a child's ability to obtain school-related skills. This valuable information is helpful in recognizing the various stages of a child's maturation and can highlight potential problems. The information contained in this chapter will enable the reader to identify the child in need of services, deal with the different issues affecting the child's behavior, establish the nurse's role in educating parents about their child's educational rights, and support the teacher who may or may not be adequately prepared to deal with the special needs child in a mainstream classroom setting.

Scope of the Chapter

Success or failure in school relies upon a multitude of factors impacting the life of a developing child. Each child has a unique set of neurodevelopmental strengths and weaknesses that impact school performance. In addition, each individual child is raised in unique home/learning environments that may promote or hinder learning skills. It is this variability of inherent neurological functioning, layered on the milieu in which the child is raised, which impacts the acquisition of school-related skills. As Mel Levine eloquently summarized in the textbook *Developmental and Behavioral Pediatrics*:

> variation of function that represents a weakness is considered a dysfunction. If the dysfunction interferes with application of a skill, that becomes a disability. If the skill set impaired by the disability is relevant to productivity and the acquisition of reasonable gratification then the disability can be considered a handicap. (Carey, 2009, p. 535)

As a result, about 10% of school-aged children are receiving some sort of special education services because they are having difficulty with school performance (Parker, Zuckerman, & Augustyn, 2005). Therefore, this chapter begins with a review of basic functions of neurons, neuroanatomy, and the lobes of the brain. Variation in neurological functioning as a result of either medical, genetic, or environmental factors are discussed. Particular detail is spent studying specific types of disorders that impact a developing child's ability to successfully learn in a general education classroom setting. Federal law that supports the needs of children with diverse learning profiles is discussed. Medical conditions which may contribute to learning disorders is reviewed, including reading disorders, attention deficits, intellectual disabilities, language disorders, autism, and sensory impairments.

Basic Neuroanatomy

An adult human brain contains an estimated 100 billion neurons (Bahra, Nagamatsu, & Liu-Ambrose, 2016). Neurons are the basic cell types that allow for neurological processing and output of neurological phenomenon to occur. All neurons have a similar structure. A neuron consists of a cell body (soma), an axon, and dendrites (branchlike structures that communicate with other neurons and axons (Figure 8.1). The cell body houses the nucleus of the neuron. This area contains DNA material which directs the neuron to perform its particular function. Initiation and processing of neurological phenomena occur through electrical impulses. The speed at which a neuron is able to transmit electrical impulses is dependent on the amount of myelin

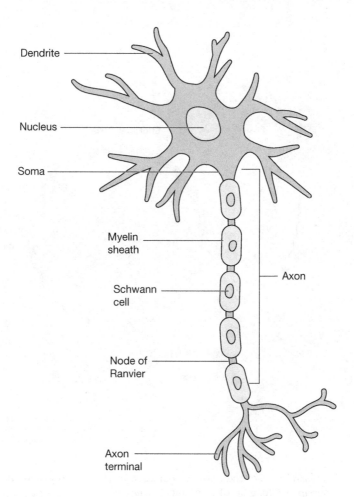

FIGURE 8.1 A neuron.

SOURCE: Reproduced from Myrick, K. M., & Karosas, L. M. (2020). *Advanced health assessment and differential diagnosis: Essentials for practice.* New York, NY: Springer Publishing Company.

covering the axon. As more myelin is produced, the faster and more complex the neurological processing will be. Myelination, the process by which myelin is produced and covers the axon, begins in infancy and progresses to completion by age 25 years. Myelination starts at the baby's head and progresses, sequentially to the toes. Therefore, a baby will be able to lift their head before they can sit up unsupported or crawl.

After an electrical impulse stimulates a neuron, chemicals called neurotransmitters are released from the neuron into the space between them (Figure 8.2). This space is called the synaptic cleft. The neurotransmitters cross the space and bind to receptors on the receiving neuron. This has an effect upon the neuron on the opposite side (post-synaptic neuron). This can effect the neuron by either exciting or inhibit-

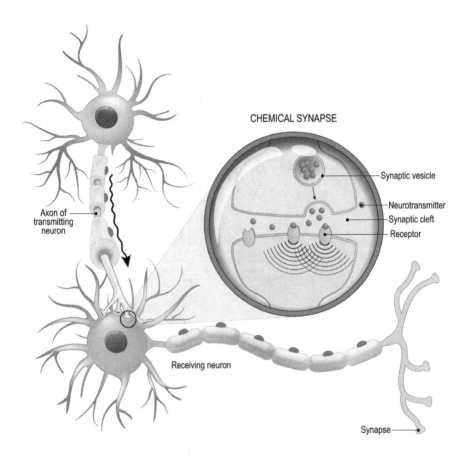

CHEMICAL SYNAPSE

Axon of
transmitting
neuron

Synaptic vesicle

Neurotransmitter

Synaptic cleft

Receptor

Receiving neuron

Synapse

FIGURE 8.2 Transmission of the nerve signal between two neurons with axon and synapse. Close-up of a chemical synapse.

SOURCE: Designua/Shutterstock.com.

ing the neuron's function. The neurotransmitters are then metabolized and degraded or recycled back to the pre-synaptic side.

Glutamate is the most common excitatory neurotransmitter in the brain. It is formed from glutamine.

Gamma-aminobutyric acid (GABA) is the main inhibitory neurotransmitter in the brain and spinal cord. GABA is formed from glutamate. Medications such as benzodiazepines (Ativan, valium, etc.) increase GABA functioning, causing relaxation. Barbiturates used for anesthesia and treatment of epilepsy also bind to these receptors. **Acetylcholine** is a neurotransmitter that exists where the neuron interacts with muscle. This is called the neuromuscular junction. It is also found in several areas of the brain and is involved in cognition and motor control. Once released, acetylcholine is inactivated by an enzyme called acetylcholinesterase.

Epinephrine and norepinephrine are involved in the autonomic nervous system's fight-or-flight response. Epinephrine increases attention and concentration and norepinephrine affects arousal.

Dopamine is involved in the coordination of voluntary movement and is also implicated in motivation, reward, and reinforcement. **Serotonin** regulates mood, sleep, appetite, and pain. Many antidepressant drugs work by blocking the reuptake of serotonin and are called selective serotonin reuptake inhibitors (SSRIs). Problems with functioning of serotonin has been implicated in depression, bipolar disorder, and anxiety (Barha et al., 2016).

Brain Structure

The central nervous system consists of two types of neurological tissue: gray matter and white matter. Gray matter is composed mostly of the cell bodies, dendrites, and synapses, whereas white matter is composed of the axons and the myelin.

The central nervous system is also composed of two major systems. The somatic motor system regulates skeletal muscles and the autonomic nervous system regulates functions in the body's internal organs. The autonomic nervous system is further divided into the sympathetic and parasympathetic systems. The sympathetic nervous system is involved in the fight-or-flight response and the parasympathetic nervous system is involved in rest and digestive functions. The sympathetic nervous system starts in the spinal cord; the parasympathetic nervous system starts in the sacral region of the spinal cord and the medulla.

The **cerebral cortex** is the outermost layer of the brain. It is divided into two halves or hemispheres and that are connected to each other by a structure called the corpus callosum. This structure is made up of about 300 million axons and is around 10 cm long. It ensures that both sides of the brain communicate and send signals to each other. Sensory, motor, and cognitive information is constantly being transferred between hemispheres via the corpus callosum. If the corpus callosum is severed, or if a child is born without this structure, the brain's hemispheres are not able to communicate properly. This can result in a loss of many functions such as changes to visual perception, speech, and memory. Surgical severing of the corpus callosum may be required for patients who have intractable seizures. It prevents seizure activity from spreading across the brain.

The brain has also been divided into four lobes: frontal, parietal, temporal, and occipital (Figure 8.3).

The **frontal lobe** is where executive functioning takes place. This is the set of higher neurocognitive processes by which people make decisions. It is where information is collected and analyzed in the brain. This portion of the brain helps provide timely pauses and inhibitions in order to make appropriate decisions. Patients with attention deficit hyperactivity disorder often have difficulties because of weaknesses in this area.

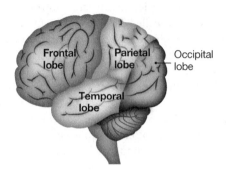

FIGURE 8.3 Anatomical illustration of lobes of the brain.

SOURCE: Reproduced from Gawlik, K. S., Melnyk, B. M., & Teall, A. M. (2020). *Evidence-based physical examination: Best practices for health and well-being assessment.* New York, NY: Springer Publishing Company.

The **parietal lobe** is located behind the frontal lobe. It is responsible for integrating sensory information including touch, temperature, pain, and pressure. The primary motor cortex is an area in the parietal lobe that is highly connected to motor output for planning, initiating, and directing sequences of movements. The motor system responds to sensory system information by generating movements and other behaviors. Movement is controlled ultimately by muscles that receive nerve input by the brainstem and spinal cord.

The **temporal lobe** is the area of the brain that is responsible for processing sensory information. This area is important for hearing, recognition of language, and creating memories. Auditory information is received by the ears and processed in this portion of the brain. This portion of the brain also contains a structure called the hippocampus, which is responsible for memory, learning, and emotions.

The **occipital lobe** is at the back of the brain and is the major visual processing center. The primary visual cortex receives information from the eyes and allows for interpretation of visual information including depth perception, distance, and location (University of Queensland, n.d.).

The Limbic System

Within the deeper portions of the brain, a specialized system of neurons, called the limbic system, plays a central role required for survival including memory, reproduction, and nutrition. Two structures within the limbic system are responsible for memory and emotion. The **hippocampus** is a cluster of neurons responsible for cataloging and forming long-term memories. It has connections between the frontal and temporal lobes and integrates information from sensory inputs. The **amygdala** plays a central role in emotional responses, including feelings like pleasure, fear, anxiety, and anger. It plays a role in forming new memories (Figure 8.4).

The Hindbrain

The **hindbrain** is located at the lower part of the brain. It is made up of three main parts: The brainstem (pons, and medulla oblongata) and cerebellum (Figure 8.5). The brainstem connects the brain to the spinal cord. It is responsible for driving a person's heartbeat and respiratory effort.

Pons

The **pons** connects the brainstem to the cerebral cortex. It coordinates signals that travel between the hemispheres and the spinal cord.

Medulla Oblongata

The **medulla oblongata** is the lowest part of the hindbrain. It controls involuntary, autonomic functioning such as heart rate, blood pressure, and respiratory effort. It also controls many involuntary reflexes used in swallowing and sneezing.

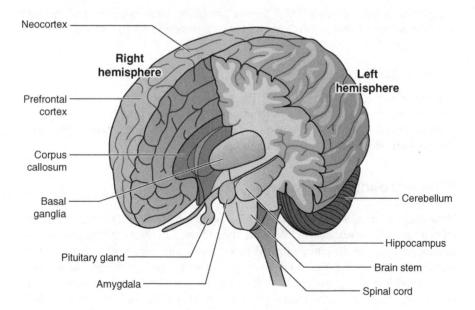

FIGURE 8.4 Anatomical illustration of the limbic system.

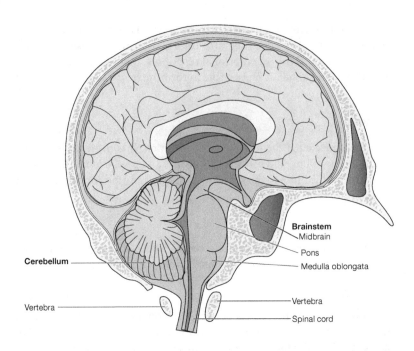

FIGURE 8.5 The hindbrain: The brainstem (pons and medulla oblongata) and cerebellum.

SOURCE: Reproduced from Myrick, K. M., & Karosas, L. M. (2020). *Advanced health assessment and differential diagnosis: Essentials for practice*. New York, NY: Springer Publishing Company.

Cerebellum

The cerebellum is located behind the pons. It has special neurons called Purkinje cells, which can process many signals at once. This then allows the cerebellum to provide smooth, coordinated voluntary muscle movement. It also takes input from the inner ear which helps with balance and posture.

▉ Background History

Neurological functioning is the foundation upon which students develop school-related skills. However, many children do not advance in their development, based upon differences in their neurological functioning. This may lead to poor performance and the development of a learning disability. Prior to changes in the law, children with learning and medical disorders were not provided with any educational support. In 1975, the federal government passed the All Handicapped Children Act (PL 94-142) and updated it over the ensuing years as the Individuals with Disabilities Education Act, No Child Left Behind, and the IDEA Improvement Act of 2004. These federal laws provided that public schools must offer free, appropriate public education (FAPE) to students with disabilities. Any person between 3 and 21 years of age who is suspected of having a disability is entitled to a comprehensive, multidisciplinary evaluation, and if eligible, to an individualized learning plan (IEP) and to monitoring over time showing that adequate progress is being achieved. Part C of the law includes the educational services provided to children from birth to 3 years in a program called Early Intervention Program (EIP; Benitez & Carugno, 2019).

Therefore, children who have educational special needs are entitled by law to receive services and accommodations that will help them perform to the best of their abilities and reach their academic potential. Special education is the process by which students with special needs are educated. This type of educational structure supports their educational differences and integrates them into mainstream settings as much as possible.

Common Terms Used in Special Education

Individuals with Disabilities Education Act (IDEA): This is a federal law that requires public schools to provide students, if eligible, with special education services. It covers students starting at age 3 and provides services up to age 21.

Free Appropriate Public Education (FAPE): Students with special needs have a right to a free and appropriate public education.

Individualized Education Program (IEP): This is a legal document that identifies a student's educational needs, develops goals and objectives, and outlines related services to be offered.

General Education: This is a regular educational program that does not provide any special accommodations or modifications.

Response to Intervention (RTI): This is the school district's initial intervention to give support to a student who is struggling. It allows educators to monitor a student's progress before pursuing a formal psychoeducational evaluation and development of an IEP.

504 Modifications/Accommodations: This is named from Section 504 of the Rehabilitation Act of 1973. This is a civil rights law that prohibits discrimination on the basis of disability. It allows for modifications or accommodations to the curriculum based on a medical diagnosis.

Accommodations: Changes to classroom or homework that provide students with an opportunity for academic success. This is usually based upon a medical or academic disability. It may include extra time for assignments or exams, preferential seating, or taking tests in a quiet place.

Related Services: Extra services that help students achieve academic success. This may include counseling, occupational therapy, physical therapy, or speech/language therapy.

Early Intervention Program (EIP): Services provided to children from birth to 3 years old who either have developmental delay or who are at risk for delay. It does not provide a diagnosis, but rather assesses whether or not a child qualifies for services.

Committee for Preschool Special Education (CPSE): Educational services provided to children 3 to 5 years old with educational needs.

Committee for Special Education (CSE): Educational services for children 5 to 18 or 21 (Benitez & Carugno, 2019).

Definition of Learning Disability: A disability based upon a discrepancy between a person's overall intellectual ability and actual academic achievement.

■ Evaluation Process

In a developing child, integrated complex neurological functioning is required for the successful acquisition of school-related skills. Lack of progress in developing these skills may come as a result of a child's intrinsic neurological status (neurological/medical conditions) as well as environmental factors. The combination of these factors can influence, affect, and interfere with a child's school performance.

When neurodevelopmental dysfunction is overtly disruptive of learning, these problems are often referred to as learning disabilities. Approximately, 10% of school-aged children receive special education and other services. Learning disabilities impact approximately 3 million children in the United States (Rimrodt & Lipkin, 2011). The Individuals with Disabilities Act defines it as a "disorder in one or more of the basic psychological processes involved in understanding or in using language, spoken or written, that may manifest itself in an imperfect ability to listen, read, spell, or do mathematical calculations" (U.S. Congress Senate Committee on Labor and Human Resources, 1997). When there is a discrepancy between a student's overall intellectual ability and academic achievement, a learning disability may be diagnosed. A student's intellectual potential and academic achievement are typically reported as standard scores (SS), with 100 being an average score with a 15-point standard deviation. Therefore, when comparing intellectual potential and actual academic achievement, scores should be within range of each other. When there is more than a 12 to 15 point discrepancy between potential and achievement, a learning disability may be diagnosed.

Signs of a learning disability may present themselves in pre-school. Children with speech/language disorders may later on have difficulties with comprehension of language-based instruction. Phonological processing used in the development of speech may lead to problems with word reading or decoding. Preschoolers who avoid reading activities should be suspect of a later learning disability. Difficulty with recognition and drawing of shapes may manifest itself later as problems with letter recognition or writing. Lack of recognition of letters of the alphabet or inability to associate sounds associated with letters is a red flag. Parents often report that their child cannot retain the information that has been taught to them. They often will say "it is as if he has never seen it before," even though it was reviewed recently. The process of evaluating a child's learning profile begins with identifying that a student is struggling in school. There has to be exposure to formal learning instruction before an assessment is considered. This is usually noticed when a child is in kindergarten. Schools are required by law to identify students who are struggling in their academic development. Once a student is identified, the parent must consent to an evaluation. With the re-authorization of IDEA in 2004, school districts were allowed to provide additional support for struggling students before establishing a diagnosis through psychological and educational testing (Psycho-Ed eval). This process was called response to intervention (RTI). This typically involves providing extra assistance to a child. The child's progress is monitored for a period of time. If the child continues to struggle, a multidisciplinary team evaluation is completed. This usually consists of measuring intellectual ability, learning profile, and other evaluations depending on the needs of the student. Once this is completed, a decision is made as to whether or not the student is eligible for an IEP (Rimrodt & Lipkin, 2011). This is a legal document created by the school district. It documents the student's current levels of performance, sets out goals and objectives to be achieved in the area of need, and provides for related services (speech therapy or occupational therapy, etc.). The IEP is updated yearly and full re-evaluation occurs every 3 years (triennial). Educational services may include placement in a collaborative environment. This is usually a regular classroom with an additional special education teacher. Students needing more support may be placed in a self-contained, smaller class setting. Sometimes, student's needs are beyond the capacity of the district and a specialized out-of-district school placement may be indicated.

If a student has a medical condition that interferes with the "free and appropriate education," accommodations and modifications of the school program may be offered. Section 504 of the Rehabilitation Act of 1973 and the Americans with Disabilities Act of 1990 (ADA) allow for these accommodations to occur. For example, a student with attention deficit hyperactivity disorder (ADHD) may be allowed to have preferential seating or extended time on tests. The law protects students against discrimination and "reasonable accommodations" must be provided.

There are genetic and neuroanatomic bases for learning disabilities. Family and twin studies show that 50% of learning problems can be accounted for by heritable factors. Genetic linkage analysis suggests various chromosome locations for learning disability. Environmental influences have a larger impact in children with lower IQs (Fletcher & Grigorenko, 2017).

The most common form of learning disability is a reading disability or dyslexia. This accounts for 80% of learning disorders. Estimates of prevalence are 5% to 10% of the general pediatric population. It is far more common in boys than girls (Rimrodt & Lipkin, 2011). Students with this disability have difficulty with phonemic awareness. They take a long time to recognize letters of the alphabet. Once they recognize letters, they have difficulty linking the sounds associated with those letters. Dyslexia has little to do with reversing letters or numbers. As a result, students with dyslexia develop a large sight word vocabulary or they guess at words because they start with a letter with which they are familiar. When shown an unfamiliar word or a "pseudoword," they can't decode it. Reading disabilities are best remediated using a multi-sensory approach to reading instruction. One common approach is Orton-Gillingham remediation. The student may require daily remediation as part of their general education plan. Parents should be reminded that their children are not "lazy." They are trying but it can be a frustrating and exhausting process for them. By the time the child gets home from school, they may be mentally and emotionally exhausted. This will make homework an even more challenging experience for the family.

Accommodations and modifications will be provided for any other comorbid condition. The prognosis for children with learning disabilities can vary. Affected children have a higher incidence of poor academic performance and dropping out of high school.

Other Barriers to Learning

Attention Deficit Hyperactivity disorder

ADHD is the most common neurodevelopmental disorder among children. In the United States, approximately 5.4 million children between 6 and 17 years of age receive an ADHD diagnosis (Feldman & Reiff, 2014). The prevalence of ADHD varies depending on the criteria used to diagnose the condition. An accepted estimate is between 4% and 6% of American school children have ADHD. The disorder has been found worldwide, with rates ranging from 3% to 18%. Prevalence of ADHD is higher in children from homes with low socioeconomic status. It is not clear whether this represents a true increase or is the result of an environment with fewer resources to ameliorate the challenging behaviors. It is more common in boys than girls (Parker et al., 2005).

There are three patterns of behavior that lead to a diagnosis. Children can be inattentive, hyperactive/impulsive, or a combination of both. The ratio of the disorder in boys versus girls is estimated to be about 4:1 to 6:1. However, this ratio may be overestimated since many girls are not referred for evaluation since they are often inattentive and don't attract the same attention boys do. Boys typically have more externalizing behaviors that get noticed in a classroom. Girls tend to be more inattentive and often do not receive the same attention as children who can be more disruptive to the classroom (Parker et al., 2005). Therefore, the actual ratio may be as low as 2:1. Boys commonly meet criteria for ADHD, combined type, whereas girls often meet criteria for ADHD, inattentive type. This is commonly called ADD.

ADHD has a genetic component. Family, twin, and adoption studies show heritability to be estimated at 76%. Multiple genes have been found in the dopamine and serotonin pathways which may be implicated in the pathogenesis of ADHD (Faraone & Mick, 2010). From clinical experience, parents often report that their child "reminds" them of some other family member.

The diagnosis is made by taking a thorough history about the symptoms from parents and caregivers. Additional information is collected from teachers. Diagnostic criteria require at least six of nine symptoms, as defined by the Diagnostic and Statistical Manual of Medntal Disorders, Fifth Edition (DSM-5; American Psychiatric

Association [APA], 2013., in the domains of an inattention and hyperactivity/impulsivity, to be rated as being in the "significant range." Symptoms must be present before age 12 and the diagnosis can be made in people who have a diagnosis of autism as well as other developmental disorders. Symptoms must also occur in two different areas of a child's life (school and home). Therefore, data are collected from teachers and parents. Scores are interpreted in conjunction with other relevant information about the child's birth, medical, family, and school history. A physical and neurological examination is indicated as well. Once this has been completed, appropriate educational support can be provided. It is important to rule out medical problems which can appear as ADHD symptoms. This should include ruling out a seizure disorder, sleep problems, and thyroid disease. Emotional problems from physical and/or sexual abuse may appear to have similar symptoms. ADHD is associated with genetic conditions such as autism, fragile X syndrome, and Tourette's syndrome (Wolraich et al., 2011).

A large percentage of children with ADHD have comorbid conditions; 20% to 60% may have a specific learning or language disorder. Up to 10% of children may have intellectual disability. Thirty percent to 60% may have oppositional defiant disorder and up to 50% may have conduct disorder. Five percent to 30% may have tic disorders (Parker et al., 2005).

Medications are commonly used to control symptoms. First-line treatment of ADHD is use of stimulant medications. Commonly use medications in this category are methylphenidate products (e.g., Concerta, ritalin, Focalin), and a mixture of amphetamine salts (Adderall or Adderall XR). Behavioral therapy is an important component. In 1999, the longest follow-up study of children with ADHD was published. It followed children with ADHD for 14 months. The multimodal treatment of ADHD study (MTA) compared the use of medication, intensive behavioral therapy, and the combination of medical and behavioral therapy and community-based care in children diagnosed with ADHD. Medication was better than behavioral therapy in decreasing the core symptoms of ADHD. The combination of medical and behavioral therapy was not significantly more effective than the medication alone. When compared to medication alone, combination therapy showed greater improvement in academic performance and reduction in conduct problems, higher levels of parental satisfaction, and the use of lower doses of medication. Combined therapy was also superior for treating children with low socioeconomic status and those with co-existing anxiety (Feldman & Reiff, 2014).

Stimulant medication is considered the first line treatment of ADHD. The onset of action is usually within an hour after taking it. The effect of the medication usually lasts for several hours, often wearing off by the end of the school day. Common side effects of stimulant medication is a slightly increased elevation of heart rate and blood pressure. This is often not clinically significant. Stimulants may also cause suppression of appetite. As a result of poor appetite, the velocity of height may slow, especially in children who take the medication for long periods of time. However, once the medication wears off, appetite returns to normal. Parents may choose to skip the dose on weekends or school holidays, since there is no need to taper the medication. It essentially "self-tapers." Catch up growth occurs after discontinuation of medication.

Rebound is a phenomenon where children feel irritable or moody as the medication is losing its effect. Therefore, teachers may notice some of the rebound effects toward the end of the school day. During this period of time when the medication is wearing off, children might feel irritable or "annoyed" by small problems. They may be easily frustrated or cry easily. This usually resolves within an hour or so. If the irritability occurs all throughout the day, the medication may not "agree" with the child and a different medication can be offered. In addition, if teachers notice rebound effects during the middle of the day, perhaps around lunchtime, then the dose of the medication may need to be adjusted. It is important for teachers and nurses to encourage students being treated with stimulant medication to eat some of their lunch during the school day. The role of the school nurse may be important in that sometimes children are required to take medication during the school day. Parents and teachers should communicate frequently so the effect and proper dosing of the medication can be monitored.

In 2008, the American Heart Association recommended electrocardiography prior to starting stimulant medication. However, follow-up studies found children taking stimulants were at no greater risk of unexpected cardiac death than children in the general population who were not taking stimulant medication. Therefore, if there is no family history of sudden cardiac death, syncope, or chest discomfort, and the child has a normal cardiac exam and blood pressure, no further cardiac workup is required prior to starting stimulant medication. Stimulants may cause vocal or motor tics in children with a family history of tics/Tourette's syndrome. This is considered a relative contraindication, not an absolute contraindication to starting stimulants.

Intellectual Disability

Intellectual disability is a term used to describe what was previously called "mental retardation." This is a lifelong condition based upon significant deficits in cognitive and adaptive abilities. Approximately 1% to 3% of the population exhibit intellectual disability. It is more commonly found in boys than girls with a 1.4:1.0 ratio. Based upon current population figures and using a 1% prevalence, there are more than 6 million children with intellectual disability in United States (Shea, 2012).

Students who have below-average intellectual functioning, accompanied by deficits in adaptive skills, with onset of symptoms before age 18 may qualify for this diagnosis. The degree of intellectual disability has been characterized as having an IQ score of less than 70. IQ scores are typically reported as SS with 100 being an average score and a 15 point standard deviation. Therefore, children with IQs below 70 are functioning two or more standard deviations below the mean. Adaptive functioning includes conceptual, social and practical skills of life. Information about adaptive functioning is obtained by the caregiver who reports how the child functions in language, social, motor, and daily living skills. The child is not required to do anything; rather, the caregiver reports how the child functions in these areas.

The clinical presentation can vary. Typically, children often present with delayed developmental milestones. Gross motor development is typically within normal limits.

The causes of intellectual disability are wide and varied. Often no specific ideology can be identified. **Prenatal** causes can be related to maternal infection, genetic abnormalities, exposure to toxins, congenital hypothyroidism, and inborn errors of metabolism. **Perinatal** causes can be related to birth complications such as hypoxia, or complications of prematurity, intracranial hemorrhage, or perinatal central nervous system infection. **Postnatal** causes can be related to an acquired brain injury, hemorrhage, infection, environmental deprivation, severe malnutrition, or exposure to toxins such as lead and mercury (Shea, 2012).

In determining an etiology, complete physical and neurological examination is important. This may give clues into genetic disorders. It is important to screen for vision and hearing in all children when they enter school as well. Metabolic testing and testing for seizures often is a low yield endeavor. Neuroimaging is rarely indicated unless there is some specific focal neurological finding. Family history is important especially if there are inherited forms of intellectual disability. The most common would be X-linked inheritance pattern, such as Fragile X syndrome.

Assessment of intellectual disability is often done as part of an individual educational plan. Intellectual testing such as the Wechsler Preschool and Primary Scale of Intelligence (WPPSI-IV) or the Wechsler Intelligence Scale for Children (WISC-V) are common tests used to determine intellectual abilities.

There is evidence that improved functional outcome is associated with inclusion of individuals with intellectual disabilities within the mainstream classroom. These are typically children who have mild symptoms. The vast majority of students with intellectual disabilities have intellectual functioning in the mild range. Expectations for outcomes vary according to level of intellectual disability. Students with mild intellectual functioning have good self-help skills, can read at an early-to-late elementary school level, may achieve independent living and employment but may need some support/supervision. Students with moderate intellectual disability may perform basic self-help skills, have early elementary reading/math skills, and will need support and supervision. Students with severe/profound intellectual disability will not be able to live independently, but may succeed in a sheltered work setting. Profound intellectual disability is associated with limited communications skills and caregiver dependency for self-help and daily living skills. The child will be dependent on others for all or most activities (Shea, 2012).

During times of transitions, especially as children age from preschool to elementary school and elementary school to middle and high school there can be some regression of their functioning. In addition, puberty is often a time of concern but most individuals negotiate this without any difficulty.

Language and Speech Disorders

The prevalence of languages disorders is about 2% to 3% in school-aged children; there may be no obvious underlying genetic or neurological disorder. The prevalence of speech disorder is about 3% to 6%. This assumes there are no underlying medical or genetic disorders. Speech and language disorders are more common in boys than girls and more common in children with a family history of speech/language, or reading disorders. Children with low socioeconomic standing are more likely to show delays in language development.

Language disorders may be features of deficits in neurological functioning such as cerebral palsy or motor disorders that inhibit the coordination of speech. Seizures may also be present. The seizure disorder, Landau-Kleffner is an acquired aphasia seizure disorder that may present with loss of language skills. Children with muscular disorder such as Duchenne's muscular dystrophy may show some early speech/language deficits (Feldman, 2005).

Significant language disorder should not be explained away as being the result of having been exposed to two languages or being the youngest of several children. Exposure to two languages may show some mild delay, but is often associated with mixing of the languages. In addition, the language development of boys is only a 1 to 2 months behind that of girls. Therefore, it is not appropriate to delay referral for a speech/language assessment based upon male gender or coming from a large and/or multi-lingual family. Children with language delay may have no specific findings on physical examination. Audiology examination is essential. However, the most common cause of mild to moderate hearing loss in children's is otitis media with effusion. Placement of pressure equalization to help reduce the incidence of hearing loss can improve language development.

Autistic Spectrum Disorders

Autistic spectrum disorders is a spectrum of neurodevelopmental disability that impacts the ability of a child to socialize. It is comprised of three main areas which affect a child's development: socialization, language, and an array of unusual behaviors. Results from the national survey of children's health 2011 to 2012 estimates parent-reported autistic spectrum disorders to be about 2% (Blumberg et al., 2013). The Centers for Disease Control and Prevention (CDC) and the Autism and Developmental Disabilities Monitoring Network estimates that the prevalence of autistic spectrum disorder is approximately 1 in every 88 children. Boys outnumber girls 4 to 1 which corresponds to an incidence of 1 in 54 for boys and 1 in 252 in girls (Christensen et al., 2016). Over the last 20 years, the incidence and prevalence of this disorder has increased dramatically. It is unclear whether or not this has come as a result of some environmental trigger or whether or not the diagnostic category allows for more variation and therefore more variability in the severity of symptoms. It has been well documented that vaccines are not implicated as a trigger to developing autistic spectrum disorders (Spencer, Pawlowski, & Thomas, 2017). Diagnostic substitution may also play a critical roll. Patients previously diagnosed with intellectual disability may be given a diagnosis of autism. In addition, subspecialists such as developmental–behavioral pediatricians have taken on a more prominent role in the management of children with developmental disorders. Therefore, children who have autism are more easily recognized. Finally, new and better screening instruments have been developed. The American Academy of Pediatrics has recommended using a screening instrument at pediatric well visits at 18 and 24 months of age. The combination of these factors are likely to contribute to the increasing numbers of cases that have been diagnosed.

Recent fraternal and identical twin studies revealed that genetic and environmental factors are likely to have an equal effect on determining the diagnosis with sibling risks at about 25% or above (Hallmayer et al., 2011).

Symptoms of autistic spectrum disorder are typically found when a parent becomes concerned about a child's language development. This typically occurs at 18 to 24 months of age. During this visit to the pediatrician, parents often bring their concerns that their child's language development is lagging behind other siblings or other children with whom the child plays. From an expressive language standpoint, the child may have only one or two words in their vocabulary. From a receptive language standpoint, the child may not be able to follow directions or identify body parts. The child may not consistently know how to wave "bye-bye" or point to pictures in books. However, the key determining factor of whether or not a child has autistic spectrum disorder has more to do with a lack of social development. Typically, children with autistic spectrum disorder tend to play by themselves. They are described as being "self-directed." They will not initiate play with other children or if other children initiate playing with them, they may not know how to reciprocate. Eye contact is characterized as being poor. In addition, they do not alert to their name when it is called. Another key factor is lack of joint attention behavior. This developmental skill is the ability to direct a parent's attention to something of interest. A typically developing child may point to a plane in the sky or to the moon. Children with autism often point to only things they need or can't reach (refrigerator/snacks) and lack or have reduced ability to point to things of mutual interest. They may have difficulty following a point. If a parent points to something of interest, the child should follow and look at the described item. Finally, there is a unique behavioral profile. Children with this diagnosis may be very rigid or play in ways that are repetitive in nature. They may only like to line up objects or take notice of objects that spin. Therefore, they may prefer to spin the wheels of cars/trains or notice fans. They like to do things in a repetitive fashion such as turning on and off light switches or opening and closing doors. Occasionally, they may have unusual motor movements such as flapping the hands or tensing up their arms. They may track or look at objects from the corner of their eye or roll toy cars close as eye level. This is known as self-stimulatory behavior. There may be associated sensory difficulties. Children with autistic spectrum disorder may seek out or avoid certain sensory input such as loud noises or textures. They have difficulty transitioning from one activity to the next. Changes in routine or unexpected outcomes are difficult for these children. They may refuse or tantrum when there is a change in the routine.

The *DSM-5* (APA, 2013) updated the diagnostic categories for autistism spectrum disorders in May 2013. The manual outlines three diagnostic categories including deficits in social communication and/or social interactions, and restricted and repetitive patterns of behavior, interests, or activities. Symptoms must be present in a child's development and cause clinically significant impairment in social, occupational, or other important areas of current functioning. The problems are not better accounted for by an intellectual disability or global developmental delay. Patients who have been previously been given a diagnosis of pervasive developmental disorder—not otherwise specified (PDD-NOS), and Asperger's syndrome should be given a diagnosis of autism spectrum sisorder (APA, 2013).

Screening for autistic spectrum disorders was recommended by the American Academy of Pediatrics in 2007. The most commonly used screening tool used by primary care pediatricians is the Modified Checklist for Autism in Toddlers (M-CHAT). It can be used in children from 16 to 30 months of age. It is a 23 item "yes/no" questionnaire (Robins, 2008).

Since the rise in prevalence of autistism spectrum disorders, there have been developed many different types of educational interventions that attempt to treat the core symptoms of autism. Applied behavior analysis (ABA) is a behavioral treatment designed to increase socialization and reciprocal interactions and decrease behaviors which are intrusive and nonfunctional. Research has shown that ABA results in improvements in communication and social relatedness, and decreases repetitive behaviors (Harrington & Allen, 2014).

Comorbid diagnoses such as anxiety and obsessive-compulsive disorders may exist. More than one third of children with autistism spectrum disorder have some type of obsession or compulsion that interferes with their socialization skills (Williams, 2010).

ADHD is another comorbid condition often associated with autistism spectrum disorder. Medical treatment of ADHD in children with autism can be effective; however, commonly used stimulant medication may have increased likelihood of adverse effects such as irritability.

Complementary and alternative medicine treatments have become popular over the last several years. Nutritional supplements or dietary changes, immunomodulation, metabolic therapies, detoxification, sensory integration therapy, and music therapies have not been shown to support or improve the outcomes of children with autistism spectrum disorder (Vohra et al., 2012).

Children with autistism spectrum disorder will have an IEP. Nursing care may include the administration of medication during the school day. In addition, the nursing office may be a safe haven for children who become overwhelmed by large classrooms or lunchrooms. Participation in social skills training is a key component to the educational plan. Often, they have related services of speech/language therapy, occupational therapy, and/or physical therapy. School personnel should be sensitive to children with autistism spectrum disorder need for predictability of the school program. Changes or unexpected outcomes are often difficult to tolerate.

A genetic component to autism spectrum disorders may be found in some cases. Common genetic disorders such as Fragile X syndrome and micro-deletions or duplications have been implicated as well. In the majority of cases, an identifiable genetic cause cannot be found.

Sensory Impairments

Hearing loss may have a significant impact upon development of academic skills. Students with hearing loss often have difficulty with phonemic awareness and therefore reading and reading comprehension becomes challenging to them. Hearing loss may, be a result of otitis media with effusion, cholesteatoma, or dislocation of the ossicular apparatus. Sensorineural hearing loss comes as a result of many genetic disorders, autosomal recessive, dominant and X-linked syndromes. Acquired hearing loss may be the result of prenatal factors such as maternal infection with rubella or cytomegalovirus or toxoplasmosis and syphilis, perinatal issues such as perinatal asphyxia or hyperbilirubinemia, or postnatal factors such as meningitis, encephalitis, ototoxins, injury, or tumor (Carey, 2009).

◼ Family Dysfunction

The stress of family dysfunction will have an impact upon a child's school performance. Parental separation, divorce, child abuse and neglect, or death of an immediate family member will have an effect upon their school performance. Changes or a decline in academic performance may be a due to a psychosocial issue impacting the child.

◼ Classroom Strategies for Common Behavioral Problems

Medical issues that are impacting the child's ability to learn often present with behavioral difficulties in the classroom. This may range from children who act out or become oppositional when required to do tasks that requires effort or a task the child finds difficult. It may manifest itself as a child who refuses to do work. Sometimes they make any little excuse to get up and avoid tasks. They may "take the long way back from the water fountain," or want to use the bathroom frequently, or complain of a medical ailment that allows them to go to the nurse's office. Behavioral problems may also manifest as a symptom of a learning problem since children who are quiet and nervous may be reluctant to ask for help. They may be embarrassed or do not want to bring attention to the fact that they are struggling.

One of the most important things a teacher can recognize in these situations is that the behaviors are often not volitional. They are driven by some underlying medical or learning issue that needs to be addressed. Therefore, it is important not to be punitive to a child struggling to learn. Teachers must recognize that all children have the desire to learn and please their teachers and parents, but that their unique challenges may preclude them from achieving this. It is important for teachers to try, at every turn during the day, to find something kind to say to a child. In addition, it is important for teachers to recognize how they feel about a particular child. Every teacher will not adore every student. Teachers may find some students challenging and feel annoyed or angry toward the student. Children are acutely aware of when a teacher does not like them or is frustrated by them. It is important for teachers and school staff to be aware of how a student makes them feel. They have an obligation to do their best to teach challenging students. The goal should be to help children feel successful in school.

Behavioral strategies that can be implemented in the classroom should be designed in order for the child to feel successful. Motivation to achieve a reward is often helpful in shaping behavior you want a student to achieve. Therefore, giving rewards, such as stickers or stars, should be easy to achieve. Children with learning challenges, ADHD, or other behavioral issues often have difficulty in achieving the goal of receiving, say, 10 stickers for the entire week. It is much more effective for a child to receive one or two stickers per day. If they can achieve that over the course of a day or even 2 days in a row, then the reward should be provided. This can be simple things as having some key role or responsibility in the classroom or being given extra time on a favorite activity. It is of no use to set the standards so high that it is essentially not achievable. In addition, it's important not to remove stickers for off-task or problematic behaviors. If a child achieved them, then they should get credit and the sticker should remain. In addition, being held back from recess time should not be a punishment for not completing work. Every child needs exercise. In addition, it is not useful for unfinished classwork to be sent home as extra homework. The National Education Association recommends 10 minutes of homework for each year a child is in school. Therefore, a first grader should receive about 10 minutes of homework, a second grader should receive about 20 minutes of homework, and so on (Vohra et al., 2012). Parents should be encouraged not to check their child's homework or "to go back and make it neat." Parents should inform teachers that they will not be checking it and to leave that for the teacher. In addition, if homework is taking too long to complete, then the parent should step in and stop after an allotted amount of time, relevant to the child's grade. If completion of homework becomes too stressful, tearful, or combative, parent should hire a high school student to sit with the child to complete it.

Other strategies that can help a struggling learner is for the teacher to plan in advance with the student that the student will not be called upon in class, unless the teacher is, say, standing right near the student's desk and the teacher knows that the student knows the answer. No student wants to be called upon if they feel that they cannot answer the question. Again, the idea is to create an environment where a student can feel successful.

Over the course of a child's elementary school career, teachers will change each year and school administrators are often far removed from the day-to-day classroom strategies. Therefore, school nurses can be a consistent presence and support in the child's life.

References

American Psychiatric Association. (2013). *Diagnostic and statistical manual of mental disorders* (5th ed.). Arlington, VA: American Psychiatric Publishing.

Barha, C. K., Nagamatsu, L. S., & Liu-Ambrose, T. (2016). Basics of neuroanatomy and neurophysiology. In M. J. Aminoff, F. Boller, & D. F. Swaab, (Eds.), *Handbook of clinical neurology* (*Vol. 138*, pp. 53–68). Philadelphia, PA: Elsevier.

Benitez A., & Carugno, P. (2019). *Special education.* Treasure Island, FL: StatPearls Publishing. Retrieved from https://www.ncbi.nlm.nih.gov/books/NBK499857/

Blumberg, S. J., Bramlett, M. D., Kogan, M. D., Schieve, L. A., Jones, J. R., & Lu, M. C. (2013). Changes in prevalence of parent-reported autism spectrum disorder in school-aged U.S. children: 2007 to 2011-2012. *National Health Statistics Report, 65*(65), 1–11. Retreived from www.ncbi.nlm.nih.gov/pubmed/24988818

Carey, W. (2009). *Developmental-behavioral pediatrics* (4th ed.). Philadelphia, PA: Saunders/Elsevier.

Christensen, D. L., Baio, J., Van Naarden, B. K., Bilder, D., Charles, J., Constantino, J. N. … Yeargin-Allsopp, M. (2016). Prevalence and characteristics of autism spectrum disorder among children aged 8 years—Autism and developmental disabilities monitoring network, 11 sites, United States, 2012. *MMWR. Surveillance Summaries, 65*(3), 1–23. doi:10.15585/mmwr.ss6503a1. (Erratum in: Morbidity and Mortality Weekly Report, *65*(15), 404.)

Faraone, S. V., & Mick, E. (2010). Molecular genetics of attention deficit hyperactivity disorder. *Psychiatric Clinics of North America, 33*(1), 159–180. doi:10.1016/j.psc.2009.12.004

Feldman, H. M. (2005). Evaluation and management of language and speech disorders in preschool children. *Pediatrics in Review, 26*(4), 131–142. doi:10.1542/pir.26-4-131

Feldman, H. M., & Reiff, M. I. (2014). Clinical practice. Attention deficit-hyperactivity disorder in children and adolescents. *New England Journal of Medicine, 370*(9), 838–846. doi:10.1056/NEJMcp1307215. (Erratum in 2015. *New England Journal of Medicine, 372*(2), 197.)

Fletcher, J. M., & Grigorenko, E. L. (2017). Neuropsychology of learning disabilities: The past and the future. *Journal of the International Neuropsychological Society, 23*(9/10), 930–940. doi:10.1017/S1355617717001084

Gawlik, K. S., Melnyk, B. M., & Teall, A. M. (2020). *Evidence-based physical examination: Best practices for health and well-being assessment.* New York, NY: Springer Publishing Company.

Hallmayer, J., Cleveland, S., Torres, A., Phillips, J., Cohen, B., Torigoe, T., … Risch, N. (2011). Genetic heritability and shared environmental factors among twin pairs with autism retrieved no results. *Archives of General Psychiatry, 68*(11), 1095–1102. doi:10.1001/archgenpsychiatry.2011.76

Harrington, J. W., & Allen, K. (2014). The clinician's guide to autism [Review]. *Pediatrics in Review, 35*(2), 62–78; quiz 78. doi:10.1542/pir.35-2-62. (Erratum in: *Pediatrics in Review, 35*(3), 113.)

Myrick, K. M., & Karosas, L. M. (2020). *Advanced health assessment and differential diagnosis: Essentials for practice.* New York, NY: Springer Publishing Company.

Parker, S., Zuckerman, B. S., & Augustyn, M. (2005). *Developmental and behavioral pediatrics: A handbook for primary care* (2nd ed.). Philadelphia, PA: Wolters Kluwer Health.

Rimrodt, S. L., & Lipkin, P. H. (2011). Learning disabilities and school failure. *Pediatrics in Review, 32*(8), 315–324. doi:10.1542/pir.32-8-315

Robins, D. L. (2008). Screening for autism spectrum disorders in primary care settings. *Autism, 12*(5), 537–556. doi:10.1177/1362361308094502

Shea, S. E. (2012). Intellectual disability (mental retardation). *Pediatrics in Review, 33*(3), 110–121; quiz 120-121. doi:10.1542/pir.33-3-110

Spencer, J. P., Trondsen Pawlowski, R. H., & Thomas, S. (2017). Vaccine adverse events: Separating myth from reality. *American Family Physician, 95*(12), 786–794. Retrieved from https://www.aafp.org/afp/

The University of Queensland. (n.d.). *Lobes of the brain.* Retrieved from https://qbi.uq.edu.au/brain/brain-anatomy/lobes-brain

U.S. Congress Senate. Committee on Labor and Human Resources. (1997). *Reauthorization of the Individuals with Disabilities Education Act: Hearing of the Committee on Labor and Human Resources, United States Senate, One Hundred Fifth Congress, First Session, January 29, 1997* (Report 105-1). Washington, DC: United States Government Printing Office.

Wolraich, M., Brown, L., Brown, R. T., DuPaul, G., Earls, M., Feldman, H. M., ... Visser, S.; Subcommittee on Attention-Deficit/Hyperactivity Disorder; Steering Committee on Quality Improvement and Management. (2011). ADHD: Clinical practice guideline for the diagnosis, evaluation, and treatment of attention-deficit/hyperactivity disorder in children and adolescents. *Pediatrics, 128*(5), 1007–1022. doi:10.1542/peds.2011-2654

Vohra, S., Surette, S., Mittra, D., Rosen, L. D., Gardiner, P., & Kemper, K. J. (2012). Pediatric integrative medicine: Pediatrics' newest Subspecialty? *BMC Pediatrics, 12*, 123. doi:10.1186/1471-2431-12-123

Williams, K., Brignell, A., Randall, M., Silove, N., & Hazell, P. (2010). Selective serotonin reuptake inhibitors for autistic spectrum disorders. *Cochrane Database of System Review, 8*(8), CD004677. doi:10.1002/14651858.CD004677.pub3

Further Readings

A 14-month randomized clinical trial of treatment strategies for attention-deficit/hyperactivity disorder. The MTA Cooperative Group. Multimodal Treatment Study of Children with ADHD. (1999). *Archives of General Psychiatry, 56*(12), 1073–1086. doi:10.1001/archpsyc.56.12.1073

ADDITUDE: ADHD Parenting. (2017, May). *"What Does That Mean?" Glossary of special education terms and acronyms*. Retrieved from https://www.additudemag.com.special -education-terms-acronyms-glossary

Austerman, J. (2015). *Cleveland Clinic Journal of Medicine, 82*(11, Suppl. 1), S2–S7. doi:10.3949/ccjm.82.s1.01

Carey, W. (2009). *Developmental-behavioral pediatrics* (4th ed.). Philadelphia, PA: Saunders/Elsevier.

Liu, X. L., Zahrt, D. M., & Simms, M. D. (2018). An interprofessional team approach to the differential diagnosis of children with language disorders. *Pediatric Clinics of North America, 65*(1), 73–90. doi:10.1016/j.pcl.2017.08.022

Protopapas, A., & Parrila, R. (2018). Is dyslexia a brain disorder? *Brain Sciences, 8*(4), 64. doi:10.3390/brainsci8040061

Shaywitz, S. E., & Shaywitz, B. A. (2003). Dyslexia (specific reading disability). *Pediatrics in Review, 24*, 147. doi:10.3390/brainsci8040061

Schulte, E. E. (2015). Learning disorders: How pediatricians can help. *Cleveland Clinic Journal of Medicine, 82*(11, Suppl. 1), S24–S28. doi:10.3949/ccjm.82.s1.05

Stein, J. (2018). What is developmental dyslexia? *Brain Sciences, 8*(2), 26. doi:10.3390/brainsci8020026

Stein, D. S., Blum, N. J., & Barbaresi, W. J. (2011). Developmental and behavioral disorders through the life span. *Pediatrics, 128*(2), 364–373. doi:10.1542/peds.2011-0266

The University of Queensland. (n.d.). *The brain*. Retrieved from https://qbi.uq.edu.au/brain/brain-anatomy

Voigt, R., Macias, M. M., & Myers, S. M. (Eds.). (2011). *AAP developmental and behavioral pediatrics*. Itasca, IL: American Academy of Pediatrics.

9

ACUTE CONDITIONS IN THE SCHOOL-AGED CHILD

LEWIS W. MARSHALL, JR.

LEARNING OBJECTIVES

- Classify acute conditions that require immediate intervention versus those that are non-life-threatening.
- Manage traumatic injuries in the school setting.
- Recognize the most common infectious conditions.

■ Introduction

Most illnesses and injuries that arise in schools are minor and can be cared for by the school nurse. The problem is easily addressed and the child can return to class.

If the issue is more serious, other actions should be considered. The school nurse must be prepared to address the problem quickly, without diagnostic tools or other medical personnel, and respond appropriately. This is when our past experiences and current knowledge will come into play. School nurses must be prepared for the inevitable emergencies that will present themselves. Utilizing the Nursing Process where the school nurse assesses, formulates a nursing diagnosis, develops a plan, implements the plan, and then evaluates the outcome, each child is systematically tended to according to the level of need.

The chapter is divided into four sections: Urgent, Life-Threatening Conditions; Common Infectious Diseases; Traumatic Injuries; and Common Complaints. Each section includes a description, causes, signs/symptoms, evaluation, first aid, and follow-up recommendations.

While not an exhaustive list of conditions, it should provide the school nurse with information that can be applied toward many presenting illnesses or injuries that occur during the school day. It is assumed that the school nurse has a physician-directed set of Standing Orders or guidelines and will carefully document all activity in the appropriate manner. What follows is a guide to provide additional background information as the school nurse tends to the unique needs of each student.

◾ Urgent and Potentially Life-Threatening Conditions

Children with any of the following conditions must have an Individualized Healthcare Plan:

Upper Airway Obstruction

Description: Any condition that causes upper airway obstruction (UAO) can be life-threatening. UAO is any blockage of the airway above the base of the neck. The universal sign for choking is hands on the throat.

Causes: Common causes of UAO include severe allergic reaction (anaphylaxis), foreign body ingestion, trauma, and infections. Students may present with cough, change in voice, or difficulty swallowing. Some of these infections can cause sudden life-threatening symptoms. Foreign bodies can be swallowed and may cause UAO.

Signs and Symptoms: Students may present with stridor (high pitched, crowing breathing sound) or abnormal, high-pitched, musical breathing sound. It is caused by a blockage or narrowing in the upper airways. It is more often heard during inspiration, frequently without the aid of a stethoscope. Symptoms may include: inability to talk, trouble breathing, turning blue, and loss of consciousness. In children, croup, a viral respiratory infection, has stridor as a symptom. When a child has swallowed a foreign object and it becomes lodged in the upper airways, stridor sounds can be heard.

Evaluation: Observe the child for good breathing, ability to speak, listen for stridor, grunting, or wheezing. Check the base of the neck for retractions, look for nasal flaring.

First Aid: Place the child in a position of comfort. Call 911. Do not force them to lie down. If the child becomes unconscious begin basic life support and CPR. If the student is in an environment where a foreign body is more likely such as toys and food consider intervention using the Heimlich maneuver (Mayo Clinic Staff, n.d.-a).

Follow-Up: No specific follow-up is required when the student returns to school. The school system should consider training cafeteria and other staff in first aid.

Diabetic Reaction—Hyper/Hypoglycemia

Description: Diabetes is an endocrine disorder involving insulin that results in alterations in blood glucose levels. Many students with diabetes will be identified early in life. In the school setting the risk to the student is elevated or decreased glucose levels. Both of these extremes can cause symptoms in many patients. In many diabetic patients the blood glucose level will vary and symptoms will vary as well.

Causes: Diabetes affects how your body uses glucose. In type 1 diabetes the body does not produce insulin and these students will require insulin injections either intermittently or through an insulin pump. It is also known as Juvenile or Insulin-Dependent Diabetes (Mayo Clinic Staff, n.d.-c). Type 2 diabetes is more common in adults but the incidence in children is increasing due to increased obesity in the school-aged groups. In type 2 diabetes the body makes insulin but cells are not as responsive to the insulin (Mayo Clinic Staff, n.d.-d; National Association of School Nurses [NASN], 2016b).

Signs and Symptoms: As glucose blood levels increase, students may begin to have increased thirst and hunger and increased urination. Other symptoms that may occur with hyperglycemia are blurred vision, tiredness, not participating in break/gym activities, and nausea. When a student with known diabetes is asking to go to the bathroom more frequently than normal, doesn't want to participate in gym, or complains of vision disturbance, notify the parents and suggest checking sugar level (Brutsaert, n.d.-a). Students with diabetes may also have low blood sugar. This may be due to medication, decreased food intake, or increased exercise. The symptoms that may occur include sweating, feeling shaky or having tremors, feeling lightheaded and hungry. If the blood sugar continues to go down other symptoms such as dizziness, confusion, slurred speech,and syncope may occur (Brutsaert, n.d.-b).

Evaluation: Initial nursing assessment should include vital signs, alertness, and orientation. If the student has their own glucose monitor, ask them to check their glucose level. You may also assist in testing using the student's monitor or insulin pump.

First Aid/Treatment: If the student has symptoms of low blood sugar and there is no ability to test, then provide the student with glucose. Glucose can be in the form of hard candy or if available oral glucose gel can be given as well. If there are any symptoms of high glucose level, contact the parent/guardian and recommend that the student be evaluated by the student's medical provider. If the student can check the glucose level and has permission to self-administer insulin, monitor the student during this process. If the student is symptomatic with high or low blood sugar level contact the parent/guardian to advise them to pick up the student. If the student is lethargic or confused call 911 first then notify the parent/guardian of the student's condition and the actions you have taken. If permitted by state regulations, Glucagon can be administered.

Follow-Up: No specific follow-up is needed and the student may return to normal school activities when symptoms have resolved.

Anaphylaxis

Description: Anaphylaxis is a potentially life-threatening allergic reaction. The onset is rapid and requires emergency management.

Causes: The most common causes of anaphylaxis are allergies to foods, insect bites, and medications.

Signs and Symptoms: Students will usually present with itching, urticarial welts, and possibly flushing or redness of the face. Students quickly develop itching or fullness in the throat, chest tightness or shortness of breath, and dizziness. Students may also have abdominal pain, diarrhea, wheezing, runny nose, and low blood pressure. Symptoms progress and the student will become unable to follow instructions eventually lose consciousness and go into arrest.

Evaluation: Evaluation and diagnosis is clinical. Check for exposure to known and unknown allergens such as food. If the student has been outdoors then consider bee sting or similar insect bite.

First Aid: Allow the student to remain in a position of comfort. Notify 911. If the student has known allergies and has an epinephrine auto-injector then administer or assist the student in administering the dose. If the school district has epinephrine auto-injectors on site then administer the appropriate one (pediatric or adult). Provide oxygen if available. All students with anaphylaxis should be transported to the closest emergency department due to the risk of recurrence of symptoms which can occur 3 to 4 hours after the initial symptoms have cleared (Tintinalli et al., 2016).

Follow-Up: An attempt should be made to determine the offending agent and the student should be prescribed epinephrine auto-injectors to carry at all times.

Drug Overdose

Description: Deaths from prescription opioids have increased exponentially. According to the Substance Abuse and Mental Health Services Administration's (SAMHSA) National Survey on Drug Use and Health in 2018, there were 4.2 million adolescents aged 12 to 17 in 2018 were past year illicit drug users (SAMHSA, 2018). This is potentially a huge issue for school nurses and school health systems.

Causes: The causes are multifactorial. Access and availability of prescription medications, cheap street drugs, and teen experimentation all can lead to substance use disorder and death.

Signs and Symptoms: Opioid or narcotic overdose symptoms are due in part to the area of the brain that regulates breathing. High doses and overdoses can cause respiratory depression. Three main symptoms are pinpoint pupils, loss of consciousness, and slow breathing rate.

Evaluation: When responding to a location with an unconscious student you should always keep overdose in mind. Assess the students level of alertness by calling their name or pinching the skin to see if there is purposeful movement. The student should try to move away from the painful stimuli or try to move your hand away. Check the respiratory status. Is the student breathing at a normal rate and effort (may need to consider other causes)? Is breathing slow and shallow (consider narcotic overdose)?

First Aid/Treatment: Call 911 for transport to the closest emergency department. Any student found unconscious with shallow breathing should be considered an overdose and treated with Naloxone. Naloxone is an opioid antagonist used to reverse the effects of opioids. It is potentially lifesaving and should be available in all schools in the intranasal form and staff trained in its use and administration. Naloxone is available as an injectable medication and for intranasal administration by spray. Both are effective. Intranasal is easy to administer. Naloxone has essentially no side effects and if given to a patient with another cause of unconsciousness will not have any adverse effect. Be prepared that someone with an opioid overdose that is reversed may be combative and have vomiting (NASN, 2015; World Health Organization [WHO], 2018).

Follow-Up: This is an opportunity to get help for the person who survived an opioid overdose. Many resources are available.

Status Epilepticus

Description: A seizure, also known as a convulsion, may begin with no warning or the student may get a feeling that they are going to have a seizure. Status epilepticus is defined as a seizure lasting more than 5 minutes or two or more seizures without a lucid interval.

Cause: Seizures are due to increased inappropriate neuronal activity in the brain.

Signs and Symptoms: Focal seizures can be with or without loss of consciousness. There are many types of generalized seizures. Absence seizures often occur in children. The child may stare into space, have subtle body movements, and have a loss of awareness. Other types include tonic or muscle tightening, atonic or drop seizures, clonic or jerking movements of the face or arms, myoclonic or jerking of the arms and legs and tonic–clonic also known as grand mal associated with loss of consciousness. A seizure lasting 5-minutes or longer is classified as status epilepticus and is a medical emergency (Clayton, 2019).

Evaluation: The student will be in obvious distress, have jerking movements of the arms and legs, and be unresponsive. Most seizures will stop spontaneously but those that last more than 5 minutes are potentially life-threatening.

First Aid: Call 911 to transport the student to the closest emergency department. Immediate action is required. Remove hazards from the student's immediate area. Prevent the patient from injuring themselves. Turn the patient on their side to help prevent aspiration in the event the patient vomits. Monitor the patient for respiratory distress.

Follow-Up: No specific follow-up is needed.

■ Common Infectious Diseases

Conjunctivitis/Eye Infections/Pink Eye

Description: Conjunctivitis is inflammation of the conjunctiva and is a cause of red eyes. It can be highly contagious but usually not serious.

Causes: Conjunctivitis is usually caused by viruses and will typically resolve on its own. Other causes include bacterial, fungal, parasitic, allergic, or chemical.

Signs and Symptoms: Symptoms include red eye, photophobia, feeling like there is sand in the eye, and tearing. Symptoms typically affect one eye and, within a few days, spreads to the other.

Evaluation: The nurse should wear gloves to prevent contamination. Check the student's eyes for redness, discharge, swelling of the eyelids. Viral conjunctivitis will last 1 to 3 weeks and resolve on its own. Bacterial conjunctivitis will most likely require antibiotic eye drops prescribed by the primary care provider. Older students may not need to be sent home. While in school they should wash their hands frequently, avoid sharing clothing, towels, and so on with other students. If there is any concern, send the student home and request a note from the provider to return to school.

First Aid: If the student wears contact lenses they should be removed. For symptomatic treatment, a cool or warm compress may be used on the affected eye. Avoid using the compress on the unaffected eye (Mayo Clinic Staff, 2019b).

Follow-Up: Once back in school the student should report to the nurse's office for clearance to return to class.

Ear Infection/Pain

Description: Ear infections will typically present as ear pain. The student may also have fever. Ear infections can be in the ear canal which is otitis externa or behind the ear drum which is otitis media.

Causes: Most ear infections are caused by bacteria and frequently follow an upper respiratory infection. Some common bacterial causes include *Streptococcus pneumonia*, *Haemophilus influenza*, and *Moraxella catarrhalis*.

Signs and Symptoms: Early symptoms may include an itchy ear and ear pain. Uncommon symptoms include drainage from the ear, hearing loss, ringing, and vertigo. The student may or may not have fever.

Evaluation: If the provider has been trained and is comfortable using an otoscope, the canal and tympanic membrane can be observed directly. If this is not the case, then base the diagnosis on the clinical symptoms.

First Aid Treatment: If permitted in the school's physician-signed standing orders, analgesia with acetaminophen or ibuprofen for pain would be appropriate. A warm moist compress may also be helpful. The student's parents should be informed and the student picked up and referred to the student's primary care provider (Tintinalli et al., 2016).

Follow-Up: As with other febrile illnesses, once the student has been fever free for 24 hours they may return to school. No documentation should be required.

Impetigo

Description: Impetigo is a highly contagious skin infection that affects children.

Causes: It is caused by exposure to the bacteria when coming in contact with an infected individual or items the individual has used including clothing, towels, and toys.

Signs and Symptoms: Classically impetigo presents with red sores that rupture and begin to ooze a yellow-brown liquid. The sores typically occur around the mouth but can spread to other areas of the body.

Evaluation: Most doctors diagnose impetigo by looking at the sores. Lab tests are not needed.

First Aid: Refer to family provider for treatment.

Follow-Up: The child should be kept at home until crusting has stopped or the student has been on antibiotics for 24 hours (Contra Costa Health Services, 2014; InformedHealth.org, 2006; Mayo Clinic Staff, 2019a).

Coxsackie

Description: Coxsackie virus commonly causes hand, foot and mouth disease (HFMD). This is common in children but can also affect adults.

Causes: The cause of this disease is the Coxsackie virus which is an RNA virus.

Signs and Symptoms: Like many viral illnesses patients may present with a fever, generalized weakness, rash, and sore throat. In this particular viral illness, the rash is blister-like and located on the palms and soles and in the mouth.

Evaluation: This condition is diagnosed clinically by a provider. No blood tests or tests of blister fluid are needed to make the diagnosis.

First Aid/Treatment: Prevention of the spread is key. Avoid contact with students with this condition. Particularly avoid contact with stool, saliva, and blister fluid. Wash hands frequently. Washing items in the classroom handled by a student with HFMD is helpful in preventing spread. There is no antiviral therapy available to treat this condition.

Follow-Up: Students should remain at home until the fever has resolved. If there are a large number of blisters the school may ask the child to be kept home until the blisters dry up. Students may return to school when they are feeling better and the fever has resolved. This may be 3 to 5 days. Exclusion from school is not beneficial because the student can shed virus when symptom-free and be in the stool for weeks (healthychildren.org, 2016).

Upper Respiratory Infection (URI or Common Cold)

Description: A URI is a common illness in children and adults. School children can get as many as eight colds a year, mostly in the fall and winter. Adults get a URI less frequently.

Causes: The most common cause of URIs are viruses. There are hundreds of viruses that can cause a URI in humans. The majority of URIs are caused by rhinoviruses. Cold viruses are transmitted through the air when a sick individual coughs or sneezes. They can also be transmitted by direct contact and through contact with toys and other objects touched by someone with a URI.

Signs and Symptoms: The common signs and symptoms of a URI are runny nose, scratchy throat, sore throat, tearing, cough, sneeze, aches and pains, fever, chills, and fatigue. These symptoms can present with many infections including influenza.

Evaluation: Review the child's symptoms and if there is the capability, take vital signs.

First Aid/Treatment: There is no specific treatment for URI. Treatment is symptomatic and can be accomplished with over-the-counter medications. If the child has a fever the parents should keep the child home until the child has been fever free for 24 hours (Johns Hopkins Medicine, 2019).

Follow-Up: No follow up is required.

Pediculosis Capitis (Head Lice)

Description: Lice (AKA "cooties") are insects that cause infestation of the scalp. There are over 12 million cases in the United States every year.

Causes: The cause of this condition is the infestation of wingless, six-legged insects that only live on scalp hair. Head lice is spread by direct contact or spread by contact with objects.

Signs and Symptoms: The classic symptom is intense itching, although some students may be asymptomatic. Some individuals with head lice can develop secondary bacterial infection particularly with *Staphylococcus aureus* or *Streptococcus pyogenes*.

Evaluation: In the student with itchy scalp consider the diagnosis of head lice. Findings are typically limited to the scalp. Definitive diagnosis is made by finding nits (eggs) or lice on the hair follicles.

First Aid/Treatment: No treatment is indicated while the child is in school. Students with head lice should remain in school and go home at the end of the day and receive treatment. Once treatment has begun they may return to classes (NASN, 2019). A physician/provider should be contacted for recommended treatment (American Family Physician, 2019).

Follow-Up: The school nurse should ensure that treatment has begun. A physician/provider note is not required. No-nit policies in schools should be discontinued because the transfer from one person to another is unlikely and misdiagnosis is common (Centers for Disease Control and Prevention [CDC], 2015).

Common Childhood Exanthem (Rashes)

Description/Cause: There are six common childhood exanthems named in order of the dates they were described: rubeola or measles (Figure 9.1), scarlet fever (Figure 9.2), rubella or German measles or 3-day measles (Figure 9.3), Ritter's disease or Staphylococcal scalded skin syndrome (Figure 9.4) Fifth's disease or erythema infectiosum (Figure 9.5), and roseola or exanthem subitem (Figure 9.6; Chamberlain, 2013).

Signs and Symptoms: Students may present with fever, runny nose, headache, sore throat, nausea, and diarrhea. Two to 5 days after the symptoms present the rashes may appear. In the school setting, we may see measles, Fifth's disease, and roseola.

Evaluation: Assess the child for cold symptoms, fever, chills, sore throat, and rash.

First Aid/Treatment: No specific first aid is required. If the student has a fever, follow district policy and exclude. Any undiagnosed rash must be evaluated by a physician.

Follow-Up: Most students will recover quickly but should have clearance from the primary care provider to return to school. In addition, for measles you should consider possible exposure of others and the incubation period which can be up to 21 days. Measles is a reportable disease. Check with the child's physician to make sure it has been reported. Vaccination status of those students who were potentially exposed should be evaluated to ensure they have immunity.

FIGURE 9.1 Measles (rubeola).

SOURCE: From Gawlik, K. S., Melnyk, B. M., & Teall, A. M. (2020). *Evidence-based physical examination: Best practices for health and well-being assessment.* New York, NY: Springer Publishing Company.

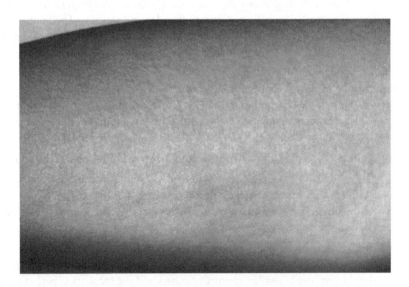

FIGURE 9.2 Scarlet fever.

SOURCE: From Gawlik, K. S., Melnyk, B. M., & Teall, A. M. (2020). *Evidence-based physical examination: Best practices for health and well-being assessment.* New York, NY: Springer Publishing Company.

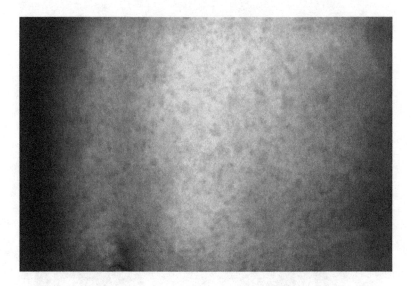

FIGURE 9.3 Rubella (German measles or 3-day measles).

SOURCE: From Gawlik, K. S., Melnyk, B. M., & Teall, A. M. (2020). *Evidence-based physical examination: Best practices for health and well-being assessment.* New York, NY: Springer Publishing Company.

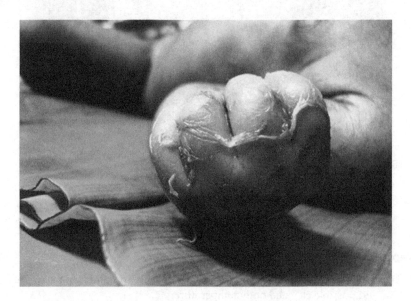

FIGURE 9.4 Ritter's disease (Staphylococcal scalded skin syndrome).

SOURCE: OpenStax Microbiology Publishers; from Gawlik, K. S., Melnyk, B. M., & Teall, A. M. (2020). *Evidence-based physical examination: Best practices for health and well-being assessment.* New York, NY: Springer Publishing Company.

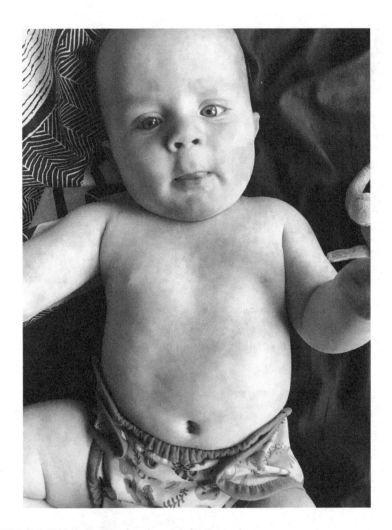

FIGURE 9.5 Fifth's disease (erythema infectiosum).

SOURCE: From Gawlik, K. S., Melnyk, B. M., & Teall, A. M. (2020). *Evidence-based physical examination: Best practices for health and well-being assessment.* New York, NY: Springer Publishing Company.

Streptococcal Throat Infection

Description: The student will experience a red, sore throat, general malaise, and possible elevated body temperature.

Causes: Streptococcal throat infection is cause most commonly by Group A *Streptococcus*. Other streptococcal groups (B, C, and G) can also cause similar symptoms. Group B *Streptococcus* is associated with meningitis and sepsis in neonates and peri-partum fever in women.

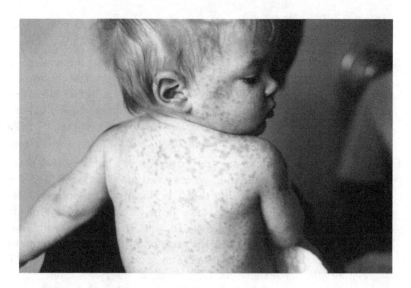

FIGURE 9.6 Roseola (exanthem subitem).

SOURCE: From Gawlik, K. S., Melnyk, B. M., & Teall, A. M. (2020). *Evidence-based physical examination: Best practices for health and well-being assessment.* New York, NY: Springer Publishing Company.

Signs and Symptoms: The incubation period after exposure to Group A *Streptococcus* is 1 to 4 days. The patient complains of fever, chills, weakness, and sore throat.

Evaluation: Check the student's vital signs for high temperature, tachycardia. Examine the throat for erythema, swollen tonsils, and an exudate.

First Aid/Treatment: It will be difficult in the school setting to determine the actual cause of the symptoms. The student should have evaluation by their primary care provider. Throat culture is the standard to determine if there is infection. There is a rapid Strep test available for providers. Definitive treatment is with antibiotics (Johns Hopkins Medicine, 2020).

Follow-Up: The student may return to the class room when they have been fever free for 24 hours on treatment.

▇ Traumatic Causes of Injury

Lacerations

Description: Lacerations can be nonurgent to emergent issues that require evaluation and stabilization.

Causes: Lacerations are caused by trauma to the body resulting in a break in the integrity of the skin.

Signs and Symptoms: Pain and bleeding at the site are the main symptoms. Students may also have nerve damage distal to the laceration.

Evaluation: Begin your assessment with scene safety and call for assistance if needed. Observe the student for alertness, site of injury, and continued bleeding. For facial or oral lacerations observe the student for blood in the mouth or nose. For lacerations on other body areas, check distal to the wound for pulses and check to see if the neurological exam is intact. Check the student's vital signs with attention to pulse. Perform a pain assessment.

First Aid/Treatment: First put on personal protective equipment such as gloves and, if excessive bleeding, wear a gown and face mask. The initial goal is to stop the bleeding. This should be done by direct pressure to the laceration. For small lacerations, once the bleeding has been controlled, clean the wound with soap and water and pat dry. Apply a dressing and if necessary elevate the body part. The need for EMS should be determined by the extent of the injury and its location. Have a staff member call 911 and notify the parents/guardians of the injury. Observe the student for continued bleeding, change in mental status, or other change in condition that may indicate significant blood loss (American College of Surgeons, Committee on Trauma, n.d.; Department of Homeland Security, 2020; Illinois Department of Public Health, 2017).

Follow-Up: The student should be referred for a tetanus booster if it has been greater than 5 years since the last tetanus vaccination.

Bites: Insect, Human, Animal

Description: Bites from most sources will be classified as puncture wounds. Puncture wounds are deeper than they are wide.

Causes: Bites can be caused by insects, mammals including humans, and reptiles.

Signs and Symptoms: Most bites cause minor discomfort. Initial symptoms include pain and possibly bleeding at the site depending on the source of the bite. Injuries can be significant with large animal bites. Some bites can cause allergic reactions when venom from the insect or reptile is injected into the skin. Other symptoms include itching or warmth around the site; in more serious cases, students may have a severe allergic reaction such as anaphylaxis (see Urgent and Potentially Life-Threatening Conditions) and may require immediate treatment with epinephrine.

Evaluation: Move the student to a safe area away from where the bite occurred. Check vital signs. Observe for changes in respiration, breathing, mental status. Most students with bites will have normal vital signs and not be in any distress.

First Aid/Treatment: Most bites and stings can be treated without going to the hospital or to a healthcare provider. Check the bite site for stingers or other foreign bodies that might be left in the wound. If possible, remove the stinger/foreign body. One way to do this is to use transparent tape to lift the stinger out. Wash the affected area with soap and water and pat dry. An ice pack may be used for comfort as well as topical creams and ointments for itching, infection, and pain. In animal or human bites as noted with other bites and stings, clean the wound with soap and water. Animal and human bites are more prone to develop infection. Snake and other reptile bites should be treated the same as other bites initially. Depending on the season and your location, specific types of snakes may be present and dangerous. If the type of snake is not known it is best to be cautious and send the student to the emergency department for evaluation (Healthline, 2016; Mayo Clinic Staff, 2020a; Schneir & Clark, 2015).

Follow-Up: Immediately report the occurrence to the parents/guardians.

Burns

Causes: Burns can be caused by heat, sun overexposure, chemicals, radiation, and electrical contact. These modalities can cause tissue damage. Burns can range from minor to fatal.

Signs and Symptoms: Symptoms of a burn injury depend on how deep the burn is. Burns are classified as first degree, second degree, or third degree. First degree burns are minor affecting the outer layer of skin. This can be caused by hot water, soup, chemicals, radiation, and electricity. The patient will have some redness to the area and some pain. Second degree burns involve the second layer of skin and patients can have swelling, redness, splotchy areas, and blisters. Pain is more severe in second degree burns and the patient can have scarring as well. Third degree burns are full skin thickness. Burned areas are black, brown, or white and the skin can look like leather. Since third degree burns are full thickness, the nerves are also destroyed and the patient has no pain and may have numbness of the area (Mayo Clinic Staff, 2016, 2018a).

Evaluation: Move the student to a safe and secure area. Assess the student for the area of burns. Look for blisters as signs of second degree burns. Students will be in pain.

First Aid/Treatment: If the burns involve the hands, face, groin, or cover a large area call 911 for immediate transfer to an emergency department. Most second degree and all third degree burns regardless of size should be evaluated in the emergency department. With other causes such as chemical or electrical burns and if the student is having trouble breathing, the student should be transported to the emergency department. For minor burns you can run the area under cool water, and apply a cool wet compress to help with pain. If the burn involves the hand or fingers remove jewelry from the affected area. If permissible, administer weight-based dose of acetaminophen or ibuprofen.

Follow-Up: Depending on the severity and location of the burn, the student may be out of school for some time. Students should be cleared to return to school although there should be no specific requirement for a note from the provider.

Sprains/Strains

Description: A sprain is an injury (tearing or stretching) of the tissue that binds two bones together. A strain is an injury to muscles or where muscle attaches to bone.

Causes: Most sprains and strains are caused during some physical activity. Exercise, school sports such as basketball, skiing, tennis, and falls are all potential causes of sprains and strains.

Signs and Symptoms: Symptoms of sprains and strains include pain, swelling, ecchymosis and if the injury involves the ankles or knees can result in pain on walking.

Evaluation: Assess vital signs. Check the injured extremity for discoloration, swelling, deformity, and pulses. Note if the student was ambulatory after the injury.

First Aid/Treatment: Initial treatment is rest, ice, and elevation of the injured body part. Compression with an elastic bandage can also be helpful. If the sprain or strain is mild it can be treated conservatively at home with ambulation as tolerated. If the student is unable to bear weight, has pain on the bone, or numbness, exclude for evaluation by a provider (Mayo Clinic Staff, 2018b).

Follow-Up: Students may require permission to use crutches or, in schools with multiple floors, to use an elevator. A note should be provided by the provider if this is required.

Eye Injury

Description: A physical or chemical wound to the eye or eye socket.

Causes: Eye injuries can be caused by many mechanisms. Commonly, blunt trauma from a punch, blows from sports equipment can cause eye injury. Additional causes include chemical splashes and flying objects from various sources can cause abrasions or puncture wounds.

Signs and Symptoms: Signs and symptoms may depend on the mechanism of injury. Students with eye injury may have ongoing pain in the eye, blurred vision, abrasions to the cornea, foreign body, lacerations to the eyelids, protuberance of one eye more than the other, or the eyes do not move in synchrony after the injury. Pupil size alteration is also a possible sign of significant injury.

Evaluation: Carefully check the face and the eyes for any visible foreign body, visible blood or fluid protruding out from the globe. Be cautious and do not touch the globe.

First Aid/Treatment: In students with a possible corneal abrasion rinse the eye with saline or clean water, have the student blink, and check for lashes in the eye. Don't permit the student to rub the eye or touch it with any objects. Don't put any commercially available drops in the eye (Boyd & Gudgel, 2019). For other injuries to the eye instruct the student to not rub, touch, or put pressure on the eye. Do not apply drops or ointments. If a student has had a blunt injury to the eye a cool compress can help with swelling and pain. Place a protective cover over the eye and send the student to the emergency department or have the parents/guardians take the student to an eye doctor. If there is a chemical splash or burn, begin flushing the eye with copious amounts of clean water. Contact 911 for transport to an emergency department. Try to obtain information about the chemical or compound involved and provide that information to the EMS providers (American Academy of Ophthalmology, 2019).

Follow-Up: No specific follow up is needed. Students should not be required to provide notes from the provider unless there is specific activities that are restricted such as sports for a period of time.

Head Trauma

Description: Head trauma results from direct force to the head. This may occur in many activities in the school setting including organized sports, gym class, and recess. This is frequently referred to as a closed head injury. Depending on the severity of the trauma students may have traumatic brain injury. Concussion is the result of direct head trauma and should be considered if the student has symptoms after head injury.

Causes: Direct force to the head results in head trauma. Most head trauma does not result in breaks to the skin on the scalp. This injury is more common in males and peaks up to 4 years old and again in 15 to 24 year olds.

Signs and Symptoms: Signs and symptoms may be as minimal as tenderness to the scalp and minor swelling to the injured area. Other symptoms may include confusion or trouble concentrating, headache, irritability, nausea or vomiting, difficulty remembering, feeling tired, and sleep disturbance. These symptoms may occur at the time of injury or days later.

Evaluation: First, place the student in a safe and secure area which may be the location where the injury occurred. Get a good description of the mechanism of injury from the student and any witnesses. Check the head for location of the injury, look for scalp lacerations. Check the pupils and look for response to light and equal pupils.

First Aid/Treatment: If the student is awake and alert, consider administering ice packs to the injured area of the head. If the student had any loss of consciousness, is unconscious, or is confused or lethargic at the time of your evaluation, call 911 and activate the emergency response system. Have staff contact the parent/guardian and make them aware of the incident and the condition of the student and if 911 has been contacted. If the student is unconscious, do not move the student but provide support at the student's location. Report all head trauma, even if it appears minor, to the parent.

Follow-Up: Students with head trauma should have an evaluation by the primary care provider. The primary care provider should clear the student to return to gym or sports activities (CDC, 2019; NASN, 2016a).

Dental Trauma

Description: The management of dental trauma depends on the extent of the injury and the student's age.

Causes: The majority of dental injuries are due to direct impact from a fall, sports injury, or fighting. You should consider additional injuries to other parts of the body depending on the mechanism of injury.

Signs and Symptoms: Students with dental trauma may have many different symptoms based on the mechanism of injury and the type of injury sustained. Pain and bleeding are common. Difficulty chewing, infection, and pain in the jaw may be present and can be addressed with local wound care.

Evaluation: It is important to determine the mechanism of injury to the tooth in order to determine possible types of injury. Assess if there is pain or tenderness to a tooth. Look for an obvious chipped, broken, or missing tooth. If there is a missing tooth, consider that it may have been swallowed or inhaled if it cannot be found where the student was injured. Check for bleeding and lacerations of the lips or inside the mouth. If a child continues to bleed following the loss of a tooth, report this to parents as there could be an underlying cause.

First Aid/Treatment: If there is bleeding have the student apply pressure for about 10 minutes. If the bleeding does not stop call the parent and recommend they take the child for medical attention. For primary teeth, the most common injury is dislocation. If the primary tooth is loose it may be left in place and most will heal. Very loose primary teeth may be removed to prevent choking or swallowing the tooth if it becomes dislodged. Refer to the child's dentist for removal. If a primary tooth is knocked out it should not be replaced. Replacing it may cause damage to the permanent teeth. Any broken or fractured tooth should be referred to the dentist. In the event a permanent tooth is knocked out, this is a dental emergency. The knocked out tooth should be placed back in the socket within 15 minutes, provided that the child is capable of not swallowing the tooth. It may be replaced within 1 hour if stored in cold milk or in a dental preserve container. Eighty-five percent of permanent teeth placed back in the socket will survive (McTigue, Thompson, & Azadani, 2019).

Follow-Up: No specific follow-up is required. Students may return to class without delay. Restriction from participation in sports may require a note from the dentist.

Common Complaints

Headache

Description: Headaches are a common complaint. More than 90% of adolescents report headaches. Headache is considered pain above the eyes. When students with headache miss school or social activities, parents frequently have them evaluated.

Causes: Headaches in students are not often caused by serious disorders. Headaches are classified as primary such as migraine or cluster headaches and tension type. These are probably underdiagnosed. Secondary headaches can be caused by viral illness and fever, post-trauma (see Head Trauma), medication, and more serious conditions.

Signs and Symptoms: Some symptoms of headache include pain, anxiety, depression, and behavioral problems. Other symptoms can include dizziness, blurred vision, nausea, photophobia.

Evaluation: All students should have vital signs taken with particular attention to blood pressure. Assess the severity of the pain and other symptoms that the student presents with.

First Aid/Treatment: Most students will benefit from analgesics. If permissible or with parental consent, administer appropriate weight-based dose of acetaminophen or ibuprofen. Monitor the student for 15 to 30 minutes. If the headache persists or worsens, then consider contacting the parent/guardian and sending the student home (Bonthius & Hershey, 2020).

Follow-Up: Once the student has returned to school, monitor how frequently the student reports to the nursing office with complaints of headaches. Notify the parent/guardian if the frequency increases.

Nosebleed/Epistaxis

Description: Epistaxis is bleeding from the nose. It can be from minor to life-threatening.

Causes: The most common cause of nose bleed or epistaxis is local trauma such as nose picking. Other types of trauma such as falls, sports injuries, and fights can lead to nose bleeds. Also in people who blow their nose hard they can also have bleeding. Other causes such as hypertension would not be common in the school setting.

Signs and Symptoms: Active bleeding from one or both nares can be present. Students may be nervous about the bleeding as well. If there has been significant bleeding the student can swallow blood. Blood in the stomach and gastrointestinal tract can cause nausea, vomiting, and black tarry stools.

Evaluation: A history should be taken with attention to what the was student doing when the bleeding started. You should ask about other bleeding episodes, easy bruising, and any known bleeding disorders. You would also want to get a medication history, looking for antiplatelet and anticoagulation medications such as aspirin, Eliquis, and others. If students are on these medications for medical reasons, this information should be available to the school nurse before the school year starts. It is difficult to examine the nares when there is active bleeding. In order to evaluate the nares, you must first stop the bleeding. You can look into the nose once the bleeding has stopped. Most bleeding is from the anterior portion vessels known as Kiesselbach's plexus. It is very superficial to the mucous membranes of the nose.

First Aid/Treatment: Check vital signs. You should evaluate for tachycardia and hypotension, which might indicate significant blood loss. Attempts to stop the bleeding in the school setting should be attempted if the bleeding has continued. With the student in the upright position have them pinch their nose closed for at least 10 minutes. Most bleeding will have stopped at that point. If bleeding continues, continue compression, notify parents, and contact 911 to transport the student to the emergency department.

Follow-Up: No specific follow-up is needed. For those students on anticoagulant or antiplatelet medication, an updated medication list should be in the student's health record.

Chalazion/Sty

Description: A sty is inflammation of the eyelid due to blockage of oil glands near the eyelashes. It is usually painless but can be very irritating to the student.

Causes: Acute or chronic inflammation.

Signs and Symptoms: Painless lump on the eyelid. Occasionally there will be mild erythema of the lid and redness of the eye.

Evaluation: Use personal protective equipment and check the eyes with the lids open and closed.

First Aid/Treatment: Treatment is typically warm soaks on and off. This may take several days to resolve. Antibiotics are not indicated (MedlinePlus, 2019). If the child complains of pain, notify the parent.

Follow-Up: There is no indication to restrict the student's activities or school attendance. Once resolved, no follow-up is required. If the student's physician recommends the student not attend school while the sty is present, request a note clearing the student to return to class without restrictions.

Diarrhea

Description: Diarrhea is the sudden onset of an increase in the water content of stool and increase in frequency of bowel movements. May be up to 20 times a day.

Causes: Diarrhea is most likely a viral illness such as norovirus or rota virus and happens during the winter months. Diarrhea can also be caused by bacteria and parasites. Some antibiotics can lead to diarrhea typically caused by *Clostridium difficile* (also known as *Clostridioides difficile*). Other medication can cause diarrhea as well, such as laxatives and NSAIDs. Inflammatory bowel disease can also present with diarrhea. Less common causes of diarrhea include bleeding, thyroid disease, and exposure to toxins.

Signs and Symptoms: Most students will present with increased frequency of loose stool with or without abdominal pain. Prolonged diarrhea will cause weight loss and poor appetite.

Evaluation: Try to characterize the diarrhea: watery, bloody, dark, and tarry. Take a history of food and medication intake the previous 24 hours if available. Check a recent travel history as this is associated with an 80% chance that the diarrhea is caused by bacteria.

First Aid/Treatment: Allow the student to be in a position of comfort. If there is no associated vomiting the student may drink small sips of water. Perform vital signs and document in the record. Note if the blood pressure is low and the pulse elevated out of range for the child's age; this may indicate dehydration (Mayo Clinic Staff, 2020b). If there is more than one episode of diarrhea, or the child is nauseous as well, exclude from school.

Follow-Up: Monitor other students with similar symptoms during the same period of time. Request note for return to school as per school policy.

Vomiting/Nausea/Stomach Ache

Description: Nausea, vomiting, and stomach ache are symptoms that can be caused by many conditions. Nausea is a feeling of unease or upset in the stomach area. It may be associated with a feeling of needing to vomit. Students may also have pain sensation in the stomach area.

Causes: There are many potential causes of nausea and vomiting. In the school setting, stress and anxiety may be a culprit. Intense pain from trauma due to sports or a fall including concussions can cause nausea and vomiting. Infectious processes such as viral infection can cause these symptoms. Other causes can include food poisoning, indigestion, odors, and smells.

Signs and Symptoms: The symptoms are nausea and vomiting. At times students may have stomach pain associated with the nausea and vomiting.

Evaluation: Take a history to try to determine the cause. Many times the cause will be elusive and treatment can be instituted. If a specific cause can be determined, then treating the cause should help alleviate the symptoms. Serious causes will prompt notifying the parents/guardians or contacting 911. Check vital signs for possible infectious cause and possible dehydration if the student has been vomiting profusely.

First Aid/Treatment: Initial attempts to ease the symptoms include having the student take sips of cold water very slowly. Drinks with sugar can also calm the stomach. Allow the student to rest in a quiet area. Once the nausea and vomiting (if present) have resolved with minimal treatment, the student can return to normal school activities. Consider having the student avoid participation in sports for the day. If the student has fever and vomiting, the student should be sent home and have a medical evaluation (Cleveland Clinic, 2019).

Follow-Up: No specific follow-up is indicated. If the treating provider thinks there is a potential for an infectious cause a note to return to school should be requested.

Splinters

Description: Splinters are sharp small objects that penetrate the skin. They can be painful.

Causes: Most students get splinters when running hands and fingers over wooden benches or wooden play structures. Splinters can also be metal or other objects from classes such as science or vocational classes.

Signs and Symptoms: Splinters can cause a lot of pain for the size of the imbedded object.

Evaluation: Observe the injured area and attempt to identify the splinter. Assess the student for last tetanus administration.

First Aid/Treatment: Wash and dry the affected area with warm water and soap. A magnifying glass may be needed to see the splinter. If you have tweezers available, then wipe them down with rubbing alcohol or an alcohol pad. Once you have located the splinter use the tweezers to pull it out slowly, provided you do not have to further break the skin. Once the splinter is removed wash and dry the area again and cover the area with a band-aid. If the splinter is too deep on the bottom of the foot or too large refer to the primary physician. If tetanus is out of date recommend to the parent/guardian to have the vaccination updated (American Academy of Dermatology, n.d.).

Follow-Up: If the splinter is removed by the school nurse the student may return to class.

Menstrual Cramps

Description: Menstrual cramps are painful throbbing pain in the lower abdomen that occur before or during menstruation. It can be mild to severe and disabling.

Causes: Some conditions that cause menstrual cramping include uterine fibroids (noncancerous muscle tumor) and endometriosis.

Signs and Symptoms: Throbbing pain in the lower abdomen. The pain may radiate to the back and legs as well. Other symptoms include nausea, headache, and dizziness.

Evaluation: No specific evaluation is required by the school nurse. Students with severe menstrual cramps may miss school during the menstrual cycle due to pain.

First Aid/Treatment: If menstrual cramps begin while a student is in class, the goal is to relieve the pain and discomfort with oral analgesics. The school nurse may, if permitted by the parent, administer acetaminophen or ibuprofen for the pain. If no improvement in 30 to 45 minutes consider an appropriate disposition (Mayo Clinic Staff, n.d.-b).

Follow-Up: No specific follow up is required.

Fever

Description: Fever is a temporary increase in the body's temperature.

Causes: Fever can be caused by a number of conditions. Infections, both viral or bacterial, inflammatory conditions such as rheumatoid arthritis (check to see if the student has juvenile rheumatoid arthritis associated with fever), recent immunizations, and some medications. Many times the cause of the fever will remain unknown.

Signs and Symptoms: When the body temperature rises above normal (98.6°F, 37°C) you have a fever. In addition to elevated body temperature the student may have associated symptoms such as sweating, chills, bodyache, weakness, and headache. Younger children up to about 5 years old can develop seizures as a result of the fever (see Seizure section).

Evaluation: If the child feels warm to touch and is having other symptoms such as those noted, consider that the child has a fever. If you are equipped with a thermometer then take and record the temperature. Check to make sure the student is able to make eye contact and follow verbal instructions. If the student is listless, has poor eye contact with or without vomiting, this may be of concern. Notify the parents and consider contacting emergency medical services.

First Aid/Treatment: If the parent/guardian has provided prior consent to administer medication such as acetaminophen or ibuprofen, administer the correct weight-based dose. Keep the student comfortable. Provide cool fluids as tolerated. If the student is still in school after receiving acetaminophen or ibuprofen, retake the temperature 45 to 60 minutes after the initial temperature.

Follow-Up: Students should be able to return to school when fever free for 24 hours. There is no specific reason to require a doctor's note unless it is school policy.

Plant Dermatosis (Poison Ivy/Sumac)

Description: Rashes from plant contact can be itchy.

Causes: Causes of plant dermatosis include immunologic, toxin related, mechanical, chemical, and allergic. One might see students with poison ivy or poison oak depending on the season and geographic location. Poison ivy is found all across the United States; poison oak is found in southern and western states; and poison sumac is found mostly on the eastern North American continent. The scientific name for poison ivy is *Toxicodendron radicans*. These common dermatoses can cause an allergic contact dermatitis or an irritant contact dermatitis (Mayo Clinic Staff, n.d.-e).

Signs and Symptoms: Students may present with rash that resembles small weeping blisters (blister fluid is not contagious), bumps, and patches (Figure 9.7).

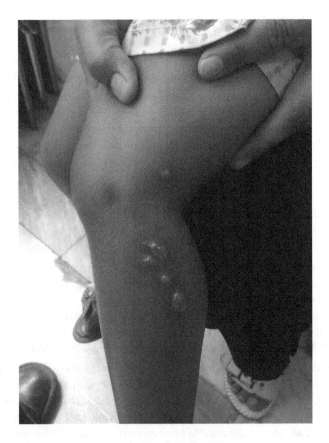

FIGURE 9.7 Weeping blisters from contact with poison ivy.

SOURCE: Courtesy of Alborz Fallah; from Gawlik, K. S., Melnyk, B. M., & Teall, A. M. (2020). *Evidence-based physical examination: Best practices for health and well-being assessment.* New York, NY: Springer Publishing Company.

Blisters are usually in a linear arrangement due to the mechanism of contact through brushing up against a plant. Severe itching may be present along with swelling of the area. Typically the rash will spread through scratching and then touching other areas of skin.

Evaluation: Perform a visual examination of the areas of the skin that is affected. Avoid touching the involved area without the use of gloves to protect the school nurse. Encourage the child not to touch the involved area.

First Aid/Treatment: Immediately rinse skin with water, rubbing alcohol, or poison plant washes if available. Degreasing soap such as dishwashing soap can be used and may be available in the school. Apply wet compresses to the affected areas. Oral antihistamines may be needed for itching. Calamine lotion and other over-the-counter remedies may be beneficial. If severe, a physician may need to prescribe oral or topical steroids to help resolve the rash (CDC, 2018).

Follow-Up: No follow-up is required.

References

American Academy of Dermatology. (n.d.). *How to remove a splinter*. Retrieved from https://www.aad.org/injured-skin/remove-splinters

American Academy of Ophthalmology. (2019). *Recognizing and treating eye injuries*. Retrieved from https://www.aao.org/eye-health/tips-prevention/injuries

American College of Surgeons, Committee on Trauma. (n.d.). *Stop the bleed*. Retrieved from https://www.bleedingcontrol.org/

American Family Physician. (2019). Lice and scabies: Treatment update. Retrieved from https://www.aafp.org/afp/2019/0515/p635.html

Bonthius, D. J., & Hershey, A. D. (2020). Headache in children: Approach to evaluation and general management strategies. *UpToDate*. Retrieved from https://www.uptodate.com/contents/headache-in-children-approach-to-evaluation-and-general-management-strategies?search=headache%20in%20children&source=search_result&selectedTitle=1~150&usage_type=default&display_rank=1

Boyd, K., & Gudgel, D. (2019). *First aid for eye scratches*. Retrieved from https://www.aao.org/eye-health/tips-prevention/first-aid-eye-scratches

Brutsaert, E. F. (n.d.-a). *Diabetes mellitus*. Retrieved from https://www.merckmanuals.com/home/hormonal-and-metabolic-disorders/diabetes-mellitus-dm-and-disorders-of-blood-sugar-metabolism/diabetes-mellitus-dm

Brutsaert, E. F. (n.d.-b). *Hypoglycemia*. Retrieved from https://www.merckmanuals.com/home/quick-facts-hormonal-and-metabolic-disorders/diabetes-mellitus-dm-and-disorders-of-blood-sugar-metabolism/hypoglycemia?query=hypoglycemia#v32365104

Centers for Disease Control and Prevention. (2015). *Head lice information for schools*. Retrieved from https://www.cdc.gov/parasites/lice/head/schools.html

Centers for Disease Control and Prevention. (2018). *Poisonous plants*. Retrieved from https://www.cdc.gov/niosh/topics/plants/symptoms.html

Centers for Disease Control and Prevention. (2019). *Traumatic brain injury & concussion*. Retrieved from https://www.cdc.gov/traumaticbraininjury/symptoms.html

Chamberlain, N. (2013). *Skin rashes: Diseases 1-6.* Retrieved from https://www.atsu.edu/faculty/chamberlain/exanthems.htm

Clayton, G. C. (2019). Seizure and status epilepticus. *Society of Academic Emergency Medicine.* Retrieved from https://www.saem.org/cdem/education/online-education /m4-curriculum/group-m4-neurology/seizure-status-epilepticus. https://www.hopkins medicine.org/health/conditions-and-diseases/status-epilepticus

Cleveland Clinic. (2019). *Nausea and vomiting.* Retrieved from https://my.clevelandclinic .org/health/symptoms/8106-nausea--vomiting

Contra Costa Health Services. (2014, August). *Communicable disease guide for schools and child care settings. School/childcare guidance: Impetigo.* Retrieved from https://cchealth .org/impetigo/pdf/school-childcare.pdf.

Department of Homeland Security. (2020). *Stop the bleed.* Retrieved from https://www .dhs.gov/stopthebleed

Healthline. (2016). *Bug bites and stings.* Retrieved from https://www.healthline.com/health/bug-bites#treatment

healthychildren.org. (2016). *Hand, foot & mouth disease: Parent FAQs.* Retrieved from https://www.healthychildren.org/English/health-issues/conditions/infections/Pages/Hand-Foot-and-Mouth-Disease.aspx

Illinois Department of Public Health. (2017). *Guidelines for the nurse in the school setting* (3rd ed.). Maywood, IL: Illinois Emergency Medical Services for Children. Retrieved from https://ssom.luc.edu/media/stritchschoolofmedicine/emergencymedicine/emsforchildren/documents/resources/practiceguidelinestools/Guidelines%20for%20the%20Nurse%20in%20the%20School%20Setting%203rd%20Edition%20April%202017%20Final.pdf

InformedHealth.org. (2006). *Impetigo: Overview.* Cologne, Germany: Institute for Quality and Efficiency in Health Care. Retrieved from https://www.ncbi.nlm.nih.gov/books/NBK279537/

Johns Hopkins Medicine. (2019). *Health: Conditions and diseases: Upper respiratory infection (URI or common cold).* Retrieved from https://www.hopkinsmedicine.org/health/conditions-and-diseases/upper-respiratory-infection-uri-or-common-cold

Johns Hopkins Medicine. (2020). Staphylococcal scalded skin syndrome. Retrieved from https://www.hopkinsmedicine.org/health/conditions-and-diseases/staphylococcal-scalded-skin-syndrome

Lice and Scabies: Treatment Update. American Family Physician. May 15, 2019. https://www.aafp.org/afp/2019/0515/p635.html. Accessed July 3, 2020.

Mayo Clinic Staff. (2016). *Patient care & health information: Burns.* Retrieved from https://www.mayoclinic.org/diseases-conditions/burns/symptoms-causes/syc-20370539

Mayo Clinic Staff. (2018a). *Patient care & health information: Burns: First aid.* Retrieved from https://www.mayoclinic.org/first-aid/first-aid-burns/basics/art-20056649

Mayo Clinic Staff. (2018b). *Patient care & health information: Sprains.* Retrieved from https://www.mayoclinic.org/diseases-conditions/sprains/symptoms-causes/syc-20377938

Mayo Clinic Staff. (2019a). *Patient care & health information: Impetigo.* Retrieved from https://www.mayoclinic.org/diseases-conditions/impetigo/diagnosis-treatment/drc-20352358

Mayo Clinic Staff. (2019b). *Patient care & health information: Pink eye (conjunctivitis).* Retrieved from https://www.mayoclinic.org/diseases-conditions/pink-eye/symptoms-causes/syc-20376355

Mayo Clinic Staff. (2020). *Snakebites: First aid.* Retrieved from https://www.mayoclinic .org/first-aid/first-aid-snake-bites/basics/art-20056681

Mayo Clinic Staff. (2020b). *Diarrhea*. Retrieved from https://www.mayoclinic.org/diseases-conditions/diarrhea/symptoms-causes/syc-20352241

Mayo Clinic Staff. (n.d.-a). *Choking: First aid*. Retrieved from https://www.mayoclinic.org/first-aid/first-aid-choking/basics/art-20056637

Mayo Clinic Staff. (n.d.-b). *Patient care & health information: Menstrual cramps*. Retrieved from https://www.mayoclinic.org/diseases-conditions/menstrual-cramps/symptoms-causes/syc-20374938

Mayo Clinic Staff. (n.d.-c). *Type 1 diabetes in children*. Retrieved from https://www.mayoclinic.org/diseases-conditions/type-1-diabetes-in-children/symptoms-causes/syc-20355306

Mayo Clinic Staff. (n.d.-d). *Type 2 diabetes in children*. Retrieved from https://www.mayoclinic.org/diseases-conditions/type-2-diabetes-in-children/symptoms-causes/syc-20355318

Mayo Clinic Staff. (n.d.-e). *Contact dermatitis*. Retrieved from https://www.mayoclinic.org/diseases-conditions/contact-dermatitis/symptoms-causes/syc-20352742

McTigue, D. J., Thompson, A., & Azadani, E. (2019). Patient education: Mouth and dental injuries in children (Beyond the Basics). *UpToDate*. Retrieved from https://www.uptodate.com/contents/mouth-and-dental-injuries-in-children-beyond-the-basics

MedlinePlus. (2019). Eye emergencies. Retrieved from https://medlineplus.gov/ency/article/000054.htm

National Association of School Nurses. (2015). *Naloxone use in the school setting: The role of the school nurse* (Position Statement). Silver Spring, MD: Author. Retrieved from https://www.nasn.org/advocacy/professional-practice-documents/position-statements/ps-naloxone

National Association of School Nurses. (2016a). *Position statements: Concussion—Role of the school nurse*. Retrieved from https://www.nasn.org/nasn/advocacy/professional-practice-documents/position-statements/ps-concussions

National Association of School Nurses. (2016b). *Position statements: Diabetes management in the school setting*. Retrieved from https://www.nasn.org/nasn/advocacy/professional-practice-documents/position-statements/ps-diabetes

National Association of School Nurses. (2019). *Position statement: Head lice management in the school setting*. Retrieved from https://www.nasn.org/nasn/advocacy/professional-practice-documents/position-statements/ps-head-lice

Schneir, A., & Clark, R. F. (2016). Bites and stings. In J. E. Tintinalli, J. S. Stapczynski, O. J. Ma, D. M. Yealy, G. D. Meckler, & D. M. Cline (Eds.), *Tintinalli's emergency medicine: A comprehensive study guide* (8th ed.). New York, NY: McGraw-Hill.

Substance Abuse and Mental Health Services Administration. (2018). Key substance use and mental health indicators in the United States: Results from the 2018 National Survey on Drug Use and Health. Retrieved from https://www.samhsa.gov/data/sites/default/files/cbhsq-reports/NSDUHNationalFindingsReport2018/NSDUHNationalFindingsReport2018.pdf

World Health Organization. (2018). *Management of substance abuse*. Retrieved from https://www.who.int/substance_abuse/information-sheet/en/

10

CHRONIC CONDITIONS IN THE SCHOOL-AGED CHILD

LEWIS W. MARSHALL, JR.

LEARNING OBJECTIVES

- Identify chronic conditions that may be encountered in the school setting.
- Apply appropriate management issues in the chronically ill school-aged child.
- Recognize when there is a significant change in a student's condition and immediate care is indicated.

▓ Introduction

It is estimated that one in four school-aged children in the United States have chronic medical conditions. Centers for Disease Control and Prevention (CDC), 2015b; National Association of School Nurses (NASN), 2017. Chronic health conditions in children require managing daily issues and anticipating potential emergencies. Chronic illnesses in the school setting require collaboration with the student, parents, healthcare provider, and the school nurse to ensure that the student is in the best place medically to be successful in school.

The school must be prepared to address children's needs in order to help them stay healthy and perform well in school. Chronic conditions present many challenges including just getting to school and staying in school (Vaughn, Salas-Wright, & Maynard, 2014). The school nurse plays a pivotal role providing treatments and medications, and alleviating anxiety for the parents, teachers and students. The overriding goal is that the child remains in school alongside siblings and peers.

This section provides readers with information on specific chronic conditions likely to be encountered in the school setting. It discusses common management, frequently used medications, and cautions regarding activity restriction if any. We also discuss potential changes in the chronic condition that may require intervention by the school nurse, what those interventions might include, and appropriate follow-up. The author offers only basic, information for the school nurse to reference. The student's private physician and parents determine the necessary course of treatment for each child.

▧ Scope of Chapter

This chapter is organized into four subchapters. Chronic conditions have been classified based on the source: neurological, pulmonary, hematologic, and various other conditions. These conditions are not exclusive but represent those most commonly seen in the school-aged child.

The school nurse must remain cognizant of the fact that each child with a chronic condition must have a specific plan of care, individualized health care, with clearly identified nursing diagnosis, student goals, intervention, and evaluation timeline.

Children today are placed in the least restrictive environment and will learn and thrive with a sound support system balanced by the school nurse.

▧ Neurological Conditions

Epilepsy

Description: Epilepsy is a neurological condition of the brain characterized by increased neuronal activity. Over two thirds of all epileptic seizures begin in childhood; it is one of the most common disorders in childhood. The word *epilepsy* is derived from Greek words meaning "to seize upon." In the past it was referred to it as the "falling sickness." *Seizure* may be a preferable term because it embraces all paroxysmal electrical discharges of the brain. Epilepsy can develop in anyone and affects males and female of all races and ethnic backgrounds.

Symptoms: Symptoms vary based on the type of epilepsy and the type and location of neuronal activity. Some people can have absence episodes where they stare off for a few seconds. Others may have uncontrolled twitching of the arms and legs which is called grand mal or tonic–clonic seizures. Still others may have loss of consciousness, sensations of fear or anxiety. Most people will have the same type of seizure each time. Seizures are classified by how they begin in the brain. It can be a focal or small area of the brain where the seizure begins or the entire brain can be involved in what is known as a generalized seizure. Focal seizures can be with or without loss of consciousness. There are many types of generalized seizures. Absence seizures which often occur in children is where the child may stare into space, have subtle body movements, and have a loss of awareness. Other types include tonic or muscle tightening, atonic or drop seizures, clonic or jerking movements of the face or arms, myoclonic or jerking of the arms and legs, and tonic–clonic also known as grand mal associated with loss of consciousness.

Causes: There are many potential causes of epilepsy. Some causes in school-aged children include febrile seizures, head trauma, infections, and disorders such as autism and neurofibromatosis.

Treatment: Most patients with epilepsy can be seizure-free with medication. The student should have a current medication list available in the student records. Patients may require multiple medications to control seizures. Many of the anti-seizure medications may have side effects that are obvious in the school setting including fatigue, dizziness, rashes, memory problems, and depression. The school nurse should have knowledge of the medication that the student is taking and the common side effects should a student seek help. With parental permission and under a physician order, medication may be given at school.

Disposition: Students with epilepsy who are controlled on medications may enjoy full participation in all school activities. Some may have restrictions on activities. In this instance, the student should supply a note from their provider outlining the restricted activity. Students may need emotional support due to misconceptions other students may have about people with epilepsy. The school nurse may also need to provide education to the teachers who have more exposure to the student and are more likely to be present if a seizure occurs (Miller & Goodkin, 1991).

Cerebral Palsy

Description: Cerebral palsy (CP) is a condition that appears early in life. Those with CP have movement disorders and problems with muscle tone and posture. These students can have abnormal reflexes, unsteady walking, or problems with any combination of muscular tone and coordination.

Causes: CP symptoms result from problems with brain development in utero. Most of the time the cause is unknown. Some possible factors include gene mutations, maternal infections such as the recent Zika virus outbreak, infant infections including meningitis and encephalitis, bleeding into the brain of the fetus, or trauma and lack of oxygen during labor or delivery. Other risk factors include breech presentation, multiple births, and premature births (Mayo Clinic, 2019c).

Treatment: Students with CP may need resources during the school day. Resources may include a mental health specialist or counselor, physical and occupational therapy, speech and language therapy, and recreational therapy. These services may help the student to be successful academically. Students with CP may also be on medication to help alleviate some of the symptoms such as muscle spasm. These medications may cause drowsiness in some students and this should be taken into consideration when students appear tired.

Disposition: There should be an up to date medication list. This should include not only those medications taken at home but also any medication that the student may need to take during the day. The school nurse should be familiar with any medication that the student needs assistance with administering during the school day. There should be a review of current medications at the beginning of the school year and any time a medication is added, discontinued, or reduced (Mayo Clinic, 2019b).

Muscular Dystrophy

Description: Muscular dystrophy (MD) is characterized by progressive muscle weakness and its associated effects.

Causes: MD is caused by defects in genes that control the production of muscle proteins. This defect leads to death of muscle cells (Huml, 2015). There are many varieties of MD. Symptoms begin in childhood and appear mostly in males. There is no cure for MD. The types include Duchenne MD, Becker MD, myotonic, facioscpulohumeral (FSHD) MD, limb-girdle, and congenital. In Duchenne MD, students may have falls, trouble getting up from their desks, trouble running, muscle pain, and learning disabilities. If the school nurse sees students with these symptoms frequenting the nursing office, it should raise some suspicion and recommendation to the parent/guardian to have the child evaluated. Becker MD presents with similar symptoms as Duchenne but they begin in the teen years. Another variety that begins in the teen years is FSHD MD. This presents with face and shoulder muscle weakness. The student's shoulder blades may stick out when they raise their hands. Limb-girdle type can also begin in the teen years. Students with this type may have frequent trips and falls as a clue to the condition. Congenital MD is apparent at birth or by age 2 and the school district should be aware when the child enters the school system. Myotonic MD is seen in adults and the patient has trouble relaxing muscles after contractions.

Treatment: There is no treatment but some therapy can improve the quality of life. Students may benefit from having some of these services in school. Low impact exercise and some weight lifting may be beneficial. The school nurse should obtain a note from the medical provider with specific types of exercise that can be utilized and which ones need to be avoided. Range of motion and stretching can also be helpful. Mobility assist devices may also be beneficial; a cane, walker, and motorized wheel chair may help keep the student as active as possible during the school day (Mayo Clinic, 2020a).

Disposition: The school nurse should have a complete medical record on students with MD. If physical or occupational therapy is provided in the school, the nurse should be notified if a student has any complaints of pain or discomfort. Contact the parents/guardians for acute changes in condition.

Pulmonary Conditions

Asthma/Reactive Airway

Description: Asthma is a chronic lung condition with reversible inflammation and narrowing of the airways. Asthma is one of the most common lung diseases in children.

Causes: Asthma attacks include symptoms of shortness of breath with or without wheezing, chest tightness, and cough. Many conditions have been linked to the development of asthma including genetic, environmental, and occupational exposures. Some people can have symptoms as a result of exercise (exercise-induced asthma), cold air, indoor and outdoor allergens such as tobacco smoke, dust mites, and cockroach allergen. Pets and mold can aggravate symptoms.

Treatment: The goal in patients with asthma is to control the condition and prevent acute attacks. This can be accomplished by having an asthma action plan. There are several good asthma actions plans available from health organizations such as the American Lung Association and from your local health department (Centers for Disease Control, 2020; National Heart, Blood and Lung Institute, n.d.). All students with asthma should be encouraged to have their own action plan. Student may be on controller medication (long-acting beta agonists) for asthma to reduce inflammation and prevent acute attacks. Acute asthma attacks with shortness of breath and wheezing can be treated with short acting bronchodilators such as Albuterol. The CDC has a National Asthma Control Program to promote asthma-friendly schools (CDC, 2015a).

Disposition: Many students will be able to carry their own medication including controller and rescue medication. School districts may require a note from the parent or medical provider to allow them to carry their own medication in school. Students who are aware of their triggers can try to avoid the triggers but this is not always possible. For students with exercise or cold-induced asthma they should take their rescue inhaler before beginning to exercise or before going out in the cold. A nebulizer should be available in the school for use as directed by a physician for students in need.

Cystic Fibrosis

Description: Cystic fibrosis (CF) is a genetic disease that can affect many systems. We commonly hear about pulmonary and gastrointestinal disease. CF is diagnosed clinically in patients who are symptomatic. It should be in the differential diagnosis list of newborns and children with frequent respiratory infections and inability to gain weight. Once CF is suspected, a sweat chloride test can help support the diagnosis. In the medieval times folk tales described infants with salty skin who would die early (Filbrun, Lahiri, & Ren, 2016). Milder disease with more subtle onset may occur in older children. These children can present with frequent lung infections, chronic productive cough, and new onset diabetes. Children with difficult-to-control asthma with mucous production should also lead to a high index of suspicion.

Causes: CF is caused by genetic mutations. There are so many mutations identified that it is difficult to predict genotype and phenotype.

Treatment: Treatment is aimed at mediating organ dysfunction. In pulmonary CF, medications such as Ivacaftor, which can increase chloride transport, and Lumacaftor, which stabilizes protein on cell surfaces, are prescribed. Chest physiotherapy is also utilized to mobilize thick secretions. This is usually done at home but may be needed at school. Chest physiotherapy in the form of clapping the back can be performed by the school nurse. Nutrition is a key element in any CF treatment plan. Annual blood tests may also be needed to assess vitamin levels (Castellani, 2018).

Disposition: School nurses should be aware of students with a diagnosis of CF. There should be clear understanding of medications and other treatments being provided to the student. Students with CF may be on multiple medications including IV medications and may present with an IV line. The nurse should be made aware of any indwelling IV lines prior to the student coming to school. CF or its treatment may make the student tired and fatigued at times leading to decreased school performance. If the student needs to take medication during the school day, the medical provider should provide a note in support of allowing the student to carry their own medication. One common oral medication is pancreatic enzymes; this is in tablet or capsule form and is not dangerous to other students. Nurses should be made aware of all children who carry and self-administer medication in the school. Students will need time to eat meals and may require snacks between meals. This should be encouraged and allowed.

Hematologic Conditions

Sickle Cell Anemia and Thalassemia

Description: Sickle cell anemia is a blood condition where red blood cells are damaged and as a result deform and stick to the endothelium leading to vaso-occlusion. When deformed, cells can be sequestered in vascular organs. The spleen is involved because red blood cells (RBCs) flow through the spleen for removal of RBC membranes and other abnormalities. When the sickled cells build up, damage and vascular obstruction occur. The spleen is typically the first organ to stop working. Other organs that can be affected include the liver, the heart, and the penis. Sickle cell disease RBCs have a reduced lifespan and with the breakdown of the cells can lead to hemolytic anemia. With this hemolysis we can also see an increase in bilirubin which can cause the student's eyes to have yellow sclera. Students may present with joint and bone pain when in painful crisis and may miss school frequently. There are several different genotypes that have variable degrees of symptoms. There is hemoglobin SC disease, sickle thalassemia, hemoglobin SD (Punjab), and hemoglobin SO (Arab; Mayo Clinic, 2020b). The discussion of these genotypes is beyond the scope of this chapter.

Causes: These hemoglobinopathies are caused by a genetic mutation that results in cell deformity or dysfunction.

Treatment: The best treatment is of course prevention of acute complications and chronic organ damage. Promoting healthy eating habits as well as maintaining hydration are important. Other treatments include medication such as hydroxyurea and blood transfusion. Stem cell transplant and gene therapy are also becoming more available (Mayo Clinic: Sickle Cell Anemia).

Disposition: Students in crisis may present to the nursing office with painful joints and bones with fatigue and weakness. These students may require oral hydration. If the student appears ill with fever, contact the parent/guardian to have the student evaluated urgently. For students with minor painful crises, acetaminophen or ibuprofen may be sufficient to alleviate the pain and allow the student to return to class. Older students may keep and take their medication as needed with the medical provider's approval.

Iron-Deficiency Anemia

Description: There many other types of anemia that result in low blood count, weakness, fatigue, and other symptoms. Iron deficiency is one type of anemia in which there are low blood counts (hemoglobin and hematocrit) due to low dietary iron or increased loss such as bleeding from the intestinal tract and in female students with heavy menses (Worwood, May, & Bain, 2017). Other types include pernicious anemia, aplastic anemia and hemolytic anemias. These types of anemia can be found in different disease processes and chronic conditions.

Causes: Anemia can be inherited or acquired and both can lead to variable symptoms depending on the specific type of anemia.

Treatment: No specific in school treatment would be required. Students should be encouraged to have a healthy diet at school and at home.

Disposition: If a student becomes excessively tired or weak, dizzy, with rapid pulse contact the parent/guardian. While waiting have the student sit or lie down in the nursing office. Encourage oral fluid intake while the student is in the nursing office/area (Mayo Clinic, 2019a; National Institute of Health: National Heart, Lung and Blood Institute, 2011).

Bleeding Disorders (Hemophilia, von Willebrand)

Description: The ability of blood to clot is a life-saving mechanism. The body must be able to keep blood circulating and to stop bleeding at the site of injury. This process is known as hemostatis (Laffan & Manning, 2017). Bleeding disorders result from a disruption in the normal clotting mechanism.

Causes: Bleeding disorders develop when there are deficiencies or problems with the function of clotting proteins and platelets and specific deficiencies of clotting factors II, V, VII, X, and XII. Most bleeding disorders are inherited and students with bleeding disorders will be well known to the school system and the school nursing staff. Other causes include medication, vitamin K deficiency, and low blood counts. Common known bleeding disorders include hemophilia A and B and von Willebrand disease. Hemophilia is typically a disease of males since the genetic mutation is on the X chromosome. There are two types. hemophilia A which is a factor VIII deficiency and B which is a factor IX deficiency. The two types have the same symptoms (Drew Clare & Hemphill, 2016). Von Willebrand's disease is the most common bleeding disorder. Most patients have mild disease. In the student age group, bruising skin and bleeding gums can be seen.

Treatment: The main treatment for the bleeding disorders is replacement of clotting factors. For students with mild disease there are medications that can be used as well. Transfusion therapy is also an option for some. Students may present to the nurse with other complaints not related to the bleeding disorder. In these cases, if treating fever or pain, do not administer aspirin or nonsteroidal anti-inflammatory medicines. Contact the parent/guardian for further treatment options.

Disposition: All students with bleeding disorders should be very knowledgeable about their condition including self-treatment and emergency management of bleeding episodes. Many will have the factor replacement done at home. Students should be taught to seek care for all injuries including minor ones that may seem insignificant to others. Nurses should be aware of the student's management plan for bleeding episodes (Drew Clare & Hemphill, 2016).

Clotting Disorders

Description: Clotting disorders are also genetic and students with these conditions are at higher risk of forming blood clots inappropriately.

Causes: There are several types of genetic conditions that lead to abnormal clotting. Factor V Leiden is the most common and results in clotting due to continuous functioning of Factor V (Mayo Clinic, 2018). Most students with this condition will not get clots. Prothrombin mutation is also common in children. There are rare deficiencies of proteins known as C and S which result in increased clotting. Antithrombin prevents the development of clots in the body and a deficiency can lead to clots in children and teens (Children's Hospital Los Angeles, n.d.).

Treatment: Students with clotting disorders may not be on any specific medication or treatment absent active clotting. Blood thinning medication may be ordered for students with one or more episodes of abnormal clotting.

Disposition: These students will be asymptomatic unless active clotting is present. If a student with a known clotting disorder develops pain and swelling in one leg, they may be developing a clot and if they present to the nurse, the parents or guardians should be contacted.Consider having the student evaluated by their provider.

■ Other Chronic Conditions

Diabetes

Description: Diabetes is an endocrine disorder involving insulin that results in alterations in blood glucose levels. Many students with diabetes will be identified early in life. In the school setting the risk to the student is elevated or decreased glucose levels. Both of these extremes can cause symptoms in many patients. In many diabetic patients the blood glucose level will vary and symptoms will vary as well.

Causes: Diabetes affects how your body uses glucose. In type 1 diabetes the body does not produce insulin and these students will require insulin injections or through an insulin pump. It is also known as juvenile or insulin-dependent diabetes (Mayo Clinic, n.d.-a). Type 2 diabetes is more common in adults but the incidence in children is increasing due to increased obesity in school-aged groups. In type 2 diabetes the body makes insulin but the cells are not as responsive to the insulin (Mayo Clinic, n.d.-b; NASN, 2016).

Signs and Symptoms: As glucose blood levels increase students may begin to have increased thirst and hunger and increased urination. Other symptoms that may occur with hyperglycemia are blurred vision, tiredness, not participating in break/gym activities and nausea. In a student with known diabetes who is asking to go to the bathroom more frequently than normal, doesn't want to participate in gym, or complains of vision disturbance, consider notifying the parents and suggest checking sugar (Brutsaert, n.d.-a). Students with diabetes may also have low blood sugar. This may be due to medication, decreased food intake, or increased exercise. The symptoms that may occur include sweating, feeling shaky or having tremors, feeling lightheaded and hungry. If the blood sugar continues to go down other symptoms such as dizziness, confusion, slurred speech, and syncope may occur (Brutsaert, n.d.-b).

Treatment: Some student will be very adept at monitoring their blood glucose. Technology is used more and more in monitoring and treating hyperglycemia. Systems with constant monitoring capability give students more control of their disease and its management. This may help improve the students' independence as they get older. It may also give students better insight into the management.

Disposition: Nurses should be aware of students with diabetes and how it is being managed in order to be prepared in the event a student develops symptoms of hyperglycemia or hypoglycemia.

Eating Disorders

Description: Eating disorders comprise a spectrum of conditions. These include anorexia nervosa, bulimia nervosa, binge-eating disorder (BED), and avoidant/restrictive food intake disorder (ARFID). These conditions are described in the *Diagnostic and Statistical Manual of Mental Disorders, Fifth Edition* (*DSM-5*; American Psychiatric Association [APA], 2013). Anorexia nervosa is weight loss by dieting, over-exercising, and laxative/diuretic abuse that is medically significant. Bulimia nervosa is described as binge eating at least once a week followed by purging. BED is binge eating without purging or other compensatory behavior to lose weight. ARFID is abnormal feeding behavior not associated with desire to lose weight. All of these conditions may be associated with psycho-social conditions that should be addressed (Mehler & Andersen, 2017).

Causes: Eating disorders develop to deal with problems such as self-esteem, emotions, fears, conflicts in relationships, to name a few. Eating disorders serve as strategies and have little to do with eating.

Treatment: Eating disorders are complex and will require an interdisciplinary team of medical and mental health specialists, nutritionists, and dieticians.

Disposition: School staff should be educated on eating disorders in school-aged children and be observant. Students who appear to lose weight quickly or who present to the nurse's office with frequent complaints of vomiting may be at risk. Poor academic performance with other symptoms such as weight loss and isolation may also be clues to a developing condition related to eating disorders. School nurses should refer these students to medical and mental health professionals familiar with eating disorders.

Gastrointestinal Disease

Description: Gastrointestinal (GI) disease can be broadly classified as functional and structural.

Causes: Functional GI conditions are identified by symptoms due to improperly working but normal looking GI tract. These conditions include irritable bowel syndrome (IBS), constipation, and chronic diarrhea. Some things that lead to functional GI complaints include poor diet, stress, overuse of medication to treat constipation, and other medications such as iron and opioid pain medication. In structural GI conditions the GI system is abnormal and doesn't work properly. Common conditions such as hemorrhoids and IBS may be seen in the student population. Many of these conditions have similar symptoms. There could be as many as 14% of high school students and 6% of middle school students with IBS. Symptoms include abdominal discomfort, cramping, diarrhea, and bloating feeling (Cleveland Clinic, 2016).

Treatment: Treatment for many functional and structural GI conditions may include modification of diet and nutrition, and medication to control symptoms; probiotics might also be of value.

Disposition: Most students with these conditions should be able to have full participation in school activities. No specific treatment need be available at school (National Institute of Diabetes and Digestive and Kidney Disease, 2014).

HIV/AIDS

Description: HIV is well known. Children under 13 with HIV were typically infected by mother-to-child transmission. Older children who have HIV were infected through sex. In 2016, 21% of all new HIV positive cases were in the 13- to 24-year-old age group. Adolescents are at increased risk of becoming infected because of a low rate of condom use, high rates of sexually transmitted disease, and an increase in risky behavior when intoxication is in the mix. AIDS is a spectrum of conditions secondary to infection from HIV. It is characterized by weight loss and fever.

Causes: HIV is caused by a retrovirus that attacks the body's immune system.

Treatment: There are several antiretroviral treatments available and they are recommended for all people living with HIV. Medication adherence is critical to keeping viral load undetectable in those with HIV.

Disposition: The school nurse can serve as a resource for youth with HIV and those who are at risk (U.S. Department of Health and Human Services, 2020).

Oral Health

Description: Oral health is important as it affects many areas of our lives. Poor oral health can affect the ability to speak and eat. Decay and improper teeth placement can also affect self-esteem which is important in the school-aged group. Pain associated with dental disease can also affect academic performance and attendance in school.

Causes: Tooth decay or cavities are the most common chronic disease in America. They are caused by demineralization of the tooth enamel from bacteria-produced acids on the tooth.

Treatment: There is no specific in-school treatment unless the school district provides dental services.

Disposition: School nurses can be student advocates for good oral health. When students have dental pain or bleeding, they may go to see the nurse. This is an opportunity to educate the student (CDC, 2019a). Dental examinations can be required as part of the physical exam and screenings can be conducted at the school with administrative approval.

Juvenile Arthritis

Description: Juvenile arthritis (JA) is caused by joint inflammation which causes pain, swelling, stiffness, and decreased range of motion of the joint. This condition can limit the student's activities in school and after school. School work can also be affected. School staff may notice students with JA limping or appearing clumsy. When the arthritis is active students may present with fever and rash.

Causes: JA is a rheumatologic disease usually with an autoimmune basis.

Treatment: One of the key treatments is exercise to maintain flexibility and range of motion. Some students may need medication such as nonsteroidal anti-inflammatory drugs (NSAIDs) or steroids.

Disposition: The school nurse should be informed about which students may have this condition and what medication if any they are taking. If there is a flare up while in school the student may be able to take their own medication if available or the school nurse may offer and administer NSAIDs or acetaminophen if appropriate (National Institute of Arthritis and Musculoskeletal and Skin Diseases, 2015).

Childhood Cancers

Description: Childhood cancers are rare. There are many different types of childhood cancer and, with current treatment children, are living full lives.

Causes: Common childhood cancers include leukemia, lymphoma, tumors of the brain (neuroblastoma), eye (retinoblastoma) and kidney (Wilms tumor; National Cancer Institute, 2019).

Treatment: Childhood cancers are treated like many adult cancers with chemotherapy, radiation therapy, immunotherapy, and stem cell transplant.

Disposition: Students with childhood cancers in remission can be full participants in school activities with approval of the students' provider. The school nurse will need to know which students have been treated or are being treated and in school. If there is a high level of illness, parents should be informed and the student granted an excused absence. A current medication list must be made available to the school nurse. It is imperative that the nurse be aware of the side effects or increased risk to the students who are undergoing cancer treatment.

Obesity and Overweight

Description: Obesity and overweight are serious problems in the United States and have been categorized as a chronic disease. Obesity and overweight places people at long- and short-term risk for serious health issues. Obesity affects millions of children and adolescents.

Causes: The cause of obesity is complex. Behavior and genetics can play a role. Where people live also affects their ability to make healthy choices. Some behaviors include eating poorly and a sedentary lifestyle. Obesity can lead to the development of other serious disease including diabetes, hypertension, and high cholesterol. Other conditions can also develop such as asthma, sleep apnea, and GI problems. Many children and adolescents can have associated psychological problems, low self-esteem, and be victims of bullying. Some medications used to treat psychological conditions have weight gain as a side effect.

Treatment: There are treatment options available. Improving diet and increasing exercise are central to any treatment plan. There are some medications that help with a comprehensive weight loss program but many of them are not approved for use in children and adolescents.

Disposition: Obese and overweight students can receive nutritional counseling and life-style modification information. School nurses can be a moving force in encouraging obese students to understand the long-term health effects of obesity. The student should be referred to school and community resources to help them achieve a healthy lifestyle (CDC, 2019b).

Lupus

Description: Lupus is an autoimmune disease also known as systemic lupus erythematosus (SLE). Lupus can affect many organ systems including skin, joints, heart, lungs, and the brain. The illness can be mild with few symptoms and no treatment to severe and life-threatening. Lupus is seen in children 15 and older and in young adults. Lupus can cause nonspecific symptoms including fever, rash, joint involvement, weight loss, and low energy among others.

Causes: Similar to JA, lupus is an autoimmune disorder affecting normal cells and tissue. Lupus can be caused by genetics and the environment.

Treatment: When children with lupus have a flare with joint pain while in school, NSAIDs can be given to alleviate symptoms. If a fever is present an infectious process needs to be considered. There is no cure for lupus at this time.

Disposition: If the student has mild symptoms limited to the joints then treatment can be given in school and the student can complete the school day. If the symptoms are moderate to severe and the student has fever, contact the parents/guardians to have the student evaluated by the medical provider. Students may return to school and participate fully as symptoms resolve (Children's Hospital of Philadelphia, 2019).

Hypertension

Description: Hypertension or high blood pressure can be seen in school-aged children. It is characterized by blood pressure greater than 120/80 in older children. In younger children there is no specific blood pressure reading that can be called high. It is based on normal ranges as children grow. Hypertension can be insidious because in the majority of cases there are no symptoms. In some students symptoms of headaches may suggest the pressure is elevated. In students with known hypertension with serious symptoms such as vomiting, seizures, or chest pain, 911 should be contacted to transport the student to the emergency department.

Causes: Causes of primary hypertension in students is similar to causes in adults, namely obesity, diet, sedentary lifestyle, smoking, or second-hand smoke. Hypertension caused by other conditions is known as secondary hypertension. Causes of secondary hypertension may include kidney diseases, endocrine abnormalities, medication, and illicit drugs.

Treatment: Students may have good blood pressure control with lifestyle changes such as exercise, eating less salt, and losing weight. Other students will require medication to control their blood pressure.

Disposition: Every student should have their blood pressure checked annually at school by the school nurse. The school nurse should have the student's information in the school record including the medication list. If the student has moderate to severe complaints consistent with hypertension, 911 should be called. The parents/guardians need to be informed of the students status (Mayo Clinic, 2019d).

Conclusion

School nurses should consider the children diagnosed with a chronic condition part of a special class. Every school nurse strives to do a *good* job with all students but these particular students depend on the nurse to do a *great* job. Meeting their many needs is a most rewarding challenge.

References

American Psychiatric Association. (2013). *Diagnostic and statistical manual of mental disorders: DSM-5* (5th ed.). Arlington, VA: American Psychiatric Publishing.

Brutsaert, E. F. (n.d.-a). *Diabetes mellitus*. Retrieved from https://www.merckmanuals.com/home/hormonal-and-metabolic-disorders/diabetes-mellitus-dm-and-disorders-of-blood-sugar-metabolism/diabetes-mellitus-dm

Brutsaert, E. F. (n.d.-b). *Hypoglycemia*. Retrieved from https://www.merckmanuals.com/home/quick-facts-hormonal-and-metabolic-disorders/diabetes-mellitus-dm-and-disorders-of-blood-sugar-metabolism/hypoglycemia?query=hypoglycemia#v32365104

Castellani, C., Duff, A., Bell, S. C., Heijerman, H., Munck, A., Ratjen, F., ... Drevinek, P. (2018). ECFS best practice guidelines: The 2018 revision. *Journal of Cystic Fibrosis, 17*(2), 153–178. doi:10.1016/j.jcf.2018.02.006

Centers for Disease Control and Prevention. (2015a). *Controlling asthma in schools.* Retrieved from https://www.cdc.gov/asthma/awareness_month/schools.htm. (See also the fact sheet at https://www.cdc.gov/asthma/pdfs/schools_fact_sheet.pdf)

Centers for Disease Control and Prevention. (2015b). *Managing chronic health conditions.* Retrieved from https://www.cdc.gov/healthyschools/chronicconditions.htm

Centers for Disease Control and Prevention. (2019a). *Children's oral health.* Retrieved from https://www.cdc.gov/oralhealth/basics/childrens-oral-health/index.html

Centers for Disease Control and Prevention. (2019b). *Overweight & obesity: Childhood Obesity causes & consequences.* Retrieved from https://www.cdc.gov/obesity/childhood/causes.html

Centers for Disease Control and Prevention. (2020). *Asthma action plans.* Retrieved from https://www.cdc.gov/asthma/actionplan.html

Children's Hospital Los Angeles. (n.d.). *Genetic clotting disorders.* Retrieved from https://www.chla.org/genetic-clotting-disorders

Children's Hospital of Philadelphia. (2019). *Pediatric lupus.* Retrieved from https://www.chop.edu/conditions-diseases/systemic-lupus-erythematosus-lupus

Cleveland Clinic. (2016). *Gastrointestinal disorders.* Retrieved from https://my.clevelandclinic.org/health/articles/7040-gastrointestinal-disorders

Drew Clare, J. A., & Hemphill, R. R. (2016). Hemophilias and von Willebrand's disease. In J. E. Tintinalli, J. S. Stapczynski, O. J. Ma, D. M. Yealy, G. D. Meckler, & D. M. Cline (Eds.), *Tintinalli's emergency medicine: A comprehensive study guide* (8th ed.). New York, NY: McGraw-Hill. Retrieved from https://accessmedicine-mhmedical-com.ezproxy.med.nyu.edu/content.aspx?sectionid=109444198&bookid=1658&jumpsectionid=109444199&Resultclick=2#1121514957

Filbrun, A. G., Lahiri, T., & Ren, C. L. (2016). Introduction and epidemiology of cystic fibrosis. In *Handbook of cystic fibrosis* (p. 2). Cham, Switzerland: Adis International Limited.

Howard, J., & Telfer, P. (2015b). Treatment of sickle cell disease. In *Clinical practice: Sickle cell disease in clinical practice.* London, UK: Springer. Retrieved from https://link-springer-com.ezproxy.med.nyu.edu/chapter/10.1007/978-1-4471-2473-3_18

Huml, R. A. (2015). Introduction to muscular dystrophy. In R. Huml (Eds.), *Muscular dystrophy.* Cham, Switzerland: Springer.

Laffan, M. A., & Manning, R. A. (2017). Investigation of haemostasis. In B. Bain, I. Bates, & M. Laffan (Eds.), *Dacie and Lewis practical haematology* (12th ed., pp. 366–409). Amsterdam, The Netherlands: Elsevier.

Mayo Clinic. (2018). *Patient care & health information: Factor V leiden.* Retrieved from https://www.mayoclinic.org/diseases-conditions/factor-v-leiden/symptoms-causes/syc-20372423

Mayo Clinic. (2019a). *Patient care & health information: Anemia.* Retrieved from https://www.mayoclinic.org/diseases-conditions/anemia/symptoms-causes/syc-20351360

Mayo Clinic. (2019b). *Patient care & health information: Cerebral palsy: Diagnosis & treatment.* Retrieved from https://www.mayoclinic.org/diseases-conditions/cerebral-palsy/diagnosis-treatment/drc-20354005

Mayo Clinic. (2019c). *Patient care & health information: Cerebral palsy: Symptoms and causes.* Retrieved from https://www.mayoclinic.org/diseases-conditions/cerebral-palsy/symptoms-causes/syc-20353999

Mayo Clinic. (2019d). *Patient care & health information: High blood pressure in children.* Retrieved from https://www.mayoclinic.org/diseases-conditions/high-blood-pressure-in-children/symptoms-causes/syc-20373440

Mayo Clinic. (2020a). *Patient care & health information: Muscular dystrophy.* Retrieved from https://www.mayoclinic.org/diseases-conditions/muscular-dystrophy/diagnosis-treatment/drc-20375394

Mayo Clinic. (2020b). *Sickle cell anemia.* Retrieved from https://www.mayoclinic.org/diseases-conditions/sickle-cell-anemia/symptoms-causes/syc-20355876

Mayo Clinic. (n.d.-a). *Type 1 diabetes in children.* Retrieved from https://www.mayoclinic.org/diseases-conditions/type-1-diabetes-in-children/symptoms-causes/syc-20355306

Mayo Clinic. (n.d.-b). *Type 2 diabetes in children.* Retrieved from https://www.mayoclinic.org/diseases-conditions/type-2-diabetes-in-children/symptoms-causes/syc-20355318

Mehler, P., & Andersen, A. E. (2017). *Eating disorders: A guide to medical care and complications* (3rd ed.). Baltimore, MD: Johns Hopkins University Press.

Miller, J. W., & Goodkin, H. P. (1991). *Epilepsy.* Hoboken, NJ: John Wiley & Sons.

National Association of School Nurses. (2016). *Position statements: Diabetes management in the school setting.* Retrieved from https://www.nasn.org/nasn/advocacy/professional-practice-documents/position-statements/ps-diabetes

National Association of School Nurses. (2017). *Students with chronic health conditions: The role of the school nurse* (Position Statement). Silver Spring, MD: Author. Retrieved from https://www.nasn.org/nasn/advocacy/professional-practice-documents/position-statements/ps-chronic-health

National Cancer Institute. (2019). *Childhood cancers.* Retrieved from https://www.cancer.gov/types/childhood-cancers

National Institute of Arthritis and Musculoskeletal and Skin Diseases. (2015). *Health topics: Juvenile arthritis.* Retrieved from https://www.niams.nih.gov/health-topics/juvenile-arthritis#tab-overview

National Institute of Diabetes and Digestive and Kidney Disease. (2014, June). *Health information: Irritable bowel syndrome (IBS) in children.* Retrieved from https://www.niddk.nih.gov/health-information/digestive-diseases/irritable-bowel-syndrome-ibs-children

National Institute of Health: National Heart, Lung and Blood Institute. (2011). *Your guide to anemia.* Retrieved from https://www.nhlbi.nih.gov/files/docs/public/blood/anemia-inbrief_yg.pdf

Nicole, C., Catherine, B., & Jill, H. (2016). Emerging treatments for severe obesity in children and adolescents. *BMJ, 354,* i4116. Retrieved from https://www.bmj.com/content/354/bmj.i4116

U.S. Department of Health and Human Services. (2020). *AIDSinfo: HIV and specific populations.* Retrieved from https://aidsinfo.nih.gov/understanding-hiv-aids/fact-sheets/25/82/hiv-and-children-and-adolescents

Vaughn, M. G., Salas-Wright, C. P., & Maynard, B. R. (2014). Dropping out of school and chronic disease in the United States. *Journal of Public Health, 22*(3), 265–270. doi:10.1007/s10389-014-0615-x

Worwood, M., May, A. M., & Bain, B. J. (2017). Iron deficiency anaemia and iron overload. In B. Bain, I. Bates, & M. Laffan (Eds.), *Dacie and Lewis practical haematology* (12th ed., pp. 165–186). Amsterdam, The Netherlands: Elsevier. doi:10.1016/B978-0-7020-6696-2.00009-6

THE NEW ALPHABET FOR SCHOOL PERSONNEL

MARY ELLEN ULLMER BOLTON

LEARNING OBJECTIVES

- Recognize standard acronyms used in the field of school nursing.
- Develop a ready reference for acronyms for the school venue.
- Describe the acronyms as they pertain to school health services and education.
- Identify priority topics, such as IEP, 504, I&RS, with a greater understanding.
- Demonstrate an understanding of nursing responsibility for IHP, ECP, and EEP.

▓ Introduction

As with any other career field—law enforcement officer (LEO), Department of Justice (DOJ), Medical Doctor (MD)—nursing has its own acronyms. A nursing student learned these shortcuts in Nursing 101: QD, BID, TID, STAT, PRN to name a few. The certified school nurse (CSN) not only uses the old, tried and true acronyms in healthcare delivery, but also incorporates acronyms from education. As the CSN is an active participant at Section 504, Intervention and Referral Services (I&RS) and Child Study Team (CST) meetings, they need to know the vernacular to sit at the table and be a valuable contributor interpreting information discussed, identifying student needs, and addressing any special accommodations the student requires to be successful in academic and nonacademic settings. School nurses, certified as instructional, are in the classroom setting on a daily basis. Lesson plans and core content standards are essential in the preparation for student instruction. Provided for reference is an overview of acronyms for health services and health education, referred to by some as "alphabet soup." They are divided into three categories: General terms (Table 11.1), resources (Table 11.2), and pediatric diseases and classifications (Table 11.3). Several areas will be addressed in greater depth throughout this chapter.

TABLE 11.1 SUMMARY OF GENERAL TERMS FOR SCHOOL PERSONNEL

ACRONYM	FULL TITLE
ABA	Applied Behavior Analysis
ADA	Americans with Disabilities Act of 1990
ADAAA	Americans Disabilities Act Amendments Act (effective 2009)
AED	Automatic External Defibrillator
AP	Advanced Placement Course
ASL	American Sign Language
AT	Assistive Technology
BOE	Board of Education
CBA	Curriculum Based Assessment
CCCS/SLS	Core Content Curriculum/Student Learning Standards
CST	Child Study Team
ECP	Emergency Care Plan
EEP	Emergency Egress Plan
ELL/ESL	English Language Learner/English as a Second Language
ESY	Extended School Year
FAPE	Free Appropriate Public Education
FERPA	Family Educational Rights Privacy Act
G&T/GATE	Gifted and Talented/Gifted and Talented Education
GE/Gen.Ed.	General Education
GED	General Education Diploma
I&RS	Intervention and Referral Services
IDEA	Individuals with Disabilities Education Act
IEP	Individualized Education Program
IHP/IHCP	Individual Healthcare Plan
LDTC	Learning Disability Teacher Consultant
LEA	Local Education Association
LGBTQIA	Lesbian, Gay, Bisexual, Transgender, Questioning. Intersexual, Asexual
LRE	Least Restrictive Environment
LST	Life Skills Training
MAT	Medication Assisted Treatment
MDT	Multidisciplinary Team
NCLB	No Child Left Behind Act (2001)
NSBA	National School Board Association
OG	Orton Gillingham Reading Program

(continued)

TABLE 11.1 SUMMARY OF GENERAL TERMS FOR SCHOOL PERSONNEL (*CONTINUED*)

ACRONYM	FULL TITLE
OT	Occupational Therapy
PARCC	Partnership for Assessment of Readiness for College and Careers
PSAT	Preliminary Scholastic Aptitude Test
PT	Physical Therapy
SAC	Substance Abuse Coordinator/Student Assistance Counselor
SAT	Scholastic Aptitude Test
SGO	Student Growth Objectives
SI	Sensory Integration
SLP (SP/LG)	Speech and Language Program
SPED	Special Education
WJ; WJ-III, WJ-IV	Woodcock-Johnson Psychosocial Battery

TABLE 11.2 RESOURCES FOR SCHOOL PERSONNEL

ACRONYM	FULL TITLE	WEBSITE
AAP	American Association of Pediatricians	https://www.aap.org
ADA	American Diabetes Association	https://www.diabetes.org/
AHA	American Heart Association	https://www.heart.org/
CDC	Centers for Disease Control and Prevention	https://www.cdc.gov
CRP	College & Career Ready Practices	http://www.state.nj.us/education/cccs/2014/career/
DHHS	Department of Health & Human Services	https://www.hhs.gov
DOE	Department of Education	https://www.ed.gov
DSM-V	*Diagnostic and Statistical Manual of Mental Disorders—Fifth Edition (DSM-5)*	https://psychcentral.com/dsm-5/
EF	Epilepsy Foundation	https://www.epilepsy.com/
ERIC	Educational Resources Information Center	https://eric.ed.gov/
ESEA	Elementary and Secondary Education Act	https://www.ed.gov/esea

(continued)

TABLE 11.2 RESOURCES FOR SCHOOL PERSONNEL (*CONTINUED*)

ACRONYM	FULL TITLE	WEBSITE
FARE	Food, Allergy Research & Education	https://www.foodallergy.org
FRC	Family Resource Center	https://thefamilyresourcecenter.org
FPIESF	The Food Protein-Induced Enterocolistis Syndrome Foundation	contact@thefpiesfoundation.org
IDA	International Dyslexia Association	https://www.cognitive-assessment.com/dyslexia
IDEA	Individuals with Disabilities Education Act	https://sites.ed.gov/idea/
LDA	Learning Disability Association	https://ldaamerica.org/types-of-learning-disabilities
NASN	National Association of School Nurses	https://www.nasn.org/home
NEA	National Education Association	http://www.nea.org/home/827.htm
NIAAA	National Institute on Alcohol Abuse and Alcoholism	https://www.niaaa.nih.gov
NIMH	Institute of Mental Health	https://www.nimh.nih.gov/index.shtml
OCR	Office of Civil Rights	https://www.hhs.gov/ocr/index.html
P&A DCCP	Protection & Advocacy: Department of Child Protection & Permanency	https://acl.gov/programs/aging-and-disability-networks/state-protection-advocacy-systems
PCC	Poison Control Center	https://www.aapcc.org/
PTO	Parent Teacher Organization	https://www.ptotoday.com/
WHO	World Health Organization	https://www.who.int

TABLE 11.3 PEDIATRIC DISEASES AND CLASSIFICATIONS FOR SCHOOL PERSONNEL

ACRONYM	FULL TITLE
ADD; AD/HD or ADHD; ADD/In	Attention Deficit Disorder; Attention Deficit/Hyperactivity Disorder; Attention Deficit, Inattentive
APD	Auditory Processing Disorder
ASD	Asperger's Syndrome Disorder
CAPD	Central Auditory Processing Disorder
DD	Developmentally Delayed/Developmentally Disabled
EB	Epidermolysis Bullosa
ED	Emotionally Disturbed

(continued)

TABLE 11.3 PEDIATRIC DISEASES AND CLASSIFICATIONS FOR SCHOOL PERSONNEL (*CONTINUED*)

ACRONYM	FULL TITLE
FPIES	Food Protein-Induced Enterocolitis Syndrome
HI	Hearing Impaired
LD	Learning Disability
MH	Multiply Handicapped
MSPI	Milk and Soy Protein Intolerance
NVLD	Nonverbal Learning Disabilities
OCD	Obsessive Compulsive Disorder
ODD	Oppositional Defiance Disorder
OHI	Other Health Impaired
PPD, PPD-NOS	Pervasive Developmental Disorder; Pervasive Developmental Disorder-Not Otherwise Specified
SLD	Specific Learning Disability

■ Working as a Team Member: 504, CST, and I&RS Team

School nursing began in 1902 in New York City as an experiment. Lina Rogers Struthers was hired as the first school nurse with the mission to single-handedly keep students in school by promoting immunizations and preventing communicable diseases. Although this appeared to be a herculean task, the nurse accomplished it beyond expectations, establishing the role of the school nurse as a "preventionist."

Often, the school nurse is the only medical professional in a school building. Their background, education and experience make them the most valuable individual, on healthcare issues, to sit at team meetings for the purpose of identifying student needs, setting priorities, and recommending special accommodations for a successful academic and nonacademic school year. The 21st century school nurse is not relegated to "Band-aids and ice packs," but an equal participant and educational professional in attendance at team meetings.

Section 504

Overview

The origin of Section 504 accommodations is found in the Rehabilitation Act of 1973, the Americans with Disabilities Act (ADA) of 1990, and the ADA Amendments Act (ADAAA) of 2008, which prohibits discrimination against any individual due to a disability. This includes equal access to academic and nonacademic activities within public and private schools in receipt of federal funding. Specifically, "this section does not provide funding for special education or services provided under an IEP, but it does permit the federal government to withdraw funding from programs that do not comply with the law" (National Center for Learning Disabilities, 2019).

Eligibility for Accommodations

Eligibility for 504 accommodations has three established criteria:

1. The individual has a physical or mental impairment, which substantially limits one or more major life activities.
2. The individual has a record of such an impairment.
3. The individual is regarded as having such impairment (28CFR Sec. 36. 104).

How to Determine Eligibility for 504 Accommodations

504 accommodations may be requested by the parent, teacher(s), and/or the school nurse. A multidisciplinary approach is used to determine eligibility to include but not be limited to input from the primary care physician, observations of parents, school nurses and teachers, as well as any other screening process deemed appropriate. The 504 team is usually composed of the 504 coordinator (designated by the school administration), the certified school nurse, parent(s), teacher(s), and the building principal, when appropriate. The team shall take into consideration any physical, psychosocial, cultural, and behavioral assessments where indicated. Each candidate's evaluation shall be totally dependent upon their individual needs. If, following the evaluation process, it is determined that the child is eligible, a 504 plan shall be created by the team to meet the identified needs of the student. The components of the plan are agreed upon by all participants. For children of tender years, this may be accomplished without the child's input, but always with parental approval. However, as a child becomes more mature, it is recommended that the child be present at the meeting and agree to the accommodations proposed. This will improve compliance and foster a sense of autonomy.

The 504 Plan

Special accommodations, under this plan, may include services and opportunities that best meet the individual needs of the student. The goal is always to assist the student to achieve a free, appropriate public education within the least restrictive environment. While a child with diabetes may have free access to the health office, a child with a fracture of the right tibia may have access to the school elevator.

A few of the more common reasonable accommodations found in a 504 plan might be:

1. Preferential seating
2. Extended time on tests and/or exams
3. Computer-aided devices
4. Reduced classroom assignments and/or homework
5. Copies of textbooks kept at home to reduce weight in the backpack
6. Scribe in the classroom
7. Graphic organizers
8. Use of technology, where indicated

9. Verbal testing

10. Adjusted class times and schedule

11. Free access to the health office

12. Home instruction with medical orders, in compliance with statutes and district policy

Timelines

A 504 Plan is a fluid, legal document. It is binding on all those individuals affected by the accommodations. It may have additions or deletions as deemed necessary for the best interest of the student. Absent of any changes, the plan should be reviewed on an annual basis with diagnosis and special accommodations being revised as necessary by all parties involved. At the onset of each school year, school personnel, with a need to know, must read and sign off on the plan to indicate their knowledge of the accommodations and intent for compliance.

School Nursing Responsibilities

Upon notification of a request for a 504 team meeting, the school nurse shall perform the following tasks:

- Perform a thorough review of the student's health history, including but not limited to routine physicals, immunizations, past screenings, medical, and parental notes, health office visits, and attendance.

- Conduct routine screening to determine current hearing, vision, height, weight, blood pressure and compare to baseline screenings of previous years, if available. Complete Health Office Reporting form (Appendix 11.1 for template).

- Determine what, if any, special accommodations are identified and/or requested by the student, parent, and primary care physician. It is not essential to have a prescription written by a physician; however, there must be documentation to support the diagnosis used for the purpose of addressing the need for special accommodations.

- Attend the 504 meeting well prepared and act in the best interest of the student; make recommendations that are in concert with the medical and behavioral history documented in the health records and personal knowledge and experience with this child.

- Sign off on the 504 plan created by the coordinator which will identify school responsibilities, parental responsibilities, and student responsibilities (note that there is no mandated form).

- Create an indivudal healthcare plan (IHP; Appendix 11.2) to reflect the accommodations in the 504 plan and ensure the IHP is available to all health office professional staff, including, but not limited to, any colleagues and/ or substitute school nurses. If indicated, create an emergency egress plan (EEP; Appendix 11.3).

Child Study Team and Creating an Individual Education Plan

Overview

The child study team (CST), which may have different titles depending upon the designation given by individual state Departments of Education, is a cohesive group of educational professionals prepared to assess, evaluate, and determine if there is a need for an individual education plan (IEP) to address the child's academic performance. Although the members may differ dependent upon student needs and district composition, the usual participants are: learning disability teaching consultant (LDTC), social worker, psychologist (any of whom may act as the case manager), classroom teacher (both general education and special education), and most importantly, the parent(s). Other specialists that may be seated at the table may include: English as a second language (ESL) specialist, occupational therapist (OT), physical therapist (PT), and speech therapist. In cases that involve or may involve medical diagnoses, and particularly for medically fragile student(s), the school nurse shall be invited to attend. In addition, upon invitation, the administrator may be in attendance. Funding for these services is provided under the Individuals with Disabilities Act (IDEA)

Eligibility

Eligibility criteria for an IEP are first limited to those children ages 3 to 21 years old. Minimally, there must be sufficient documentation that the child is experiencing/demonstrating difficulty in performing routine academic tasks and/or functions for grade level and age.

With sufficient evidence that a child is having difficulty learning, the members of the CST will determine appropriate testing to provide evidence of a need for an IEP. Evaluations may be conducted in the areas of: medical, psychosocial, cognitive, behavioral, academic, speech, and the ability to function in the school setting. For a child to be eligible for an IEP, testing must identify that success in the school setting would be improved by special services addressing one or more of the following 13 categories upon which the parent must agree to the identified category:

1. Auditory Impaired
2. Autistic
3. Communication Impaired
4. Deaf/Blind
5. Emotionally Disturbed
6. Intellectually Disabled
7. Multiply Disabled
8. Orthopedically Impaired
9. Other Health Impaired
10. Preschool Child with Disability
11. Social Maladjustment

12. Specific Learning Disability

13. Visually Impaired (NJAC 6A; 14-3.5, September 5, 2006)

The school nurse performs medical intake for all new students. This medical professional is in the ideal position to identify and educate parents on the rights for children covered under the IDEA and ADAAA.

The Individual Education Plan

An IEP shall be written by the team with coordination by the case manager. The plan will be created to assist the student to achieve success in the school setting. Accommodations may range from but not limited to:

1. General education with and/or without assistance of a personal or classroom paraprofessional

2. Push-in or pull-out services of a special education teacher for academic support

3. Self-contained classroom setting with one or more special education teachers

4. Speech, occupational therapy, and/or physical therapy

5. Transportation to and from school

6. Assistive technology

7. Extended school year programming

8. Ready access to the health office and/or one-on-one nursing services

Timelines

The individualized education program (IEP) is reviewed by the entire team on an annual basis. Every 3 years, there shall be a complete review of the components of the plan with new testing, as determined appropriate by the CST (U.S. Department of Education, 2019).

School Nursing Responsibility for a Child Study Team Meeting and Individual Education Plan

Upon notification of the need/request (by any interested party) for a CST meeting, the school nurse shall perform the following tasks:

■ Perform a thorough review of the student's health history, to include but not be limited to routine physicals, immunizations, past screenings, medical and parental notes, health office visits.

■ Conduct routine screening to determine current hearing, vision, height, weight, blood pressure, and compare to baseline screenings of previous years, if available. Where indicated, send a referral to parent or legal guardian for remediation by the personal care physician.

- Determine, what, if any medical issues warrant your attendance at the CST meeting; complete a CST reporting form to include, but not be limited to: health history, screening, heath office visits, attendance, and any other significant observations, and forward to the case manager. The case manager will request the parent/legal guardian to address any vision and/or hearing referrals with a physician prior to the first CST meeting.

- When indicated, and invited, attend the CST meeting well prepared and act in the best interest of the student; make recommendations that are in concert with the medical and behavioral history documented in records, and your personal knowledge and experience with this child.

- Sign off on the CST attendance roster; and when completed the IEP.

- Create an IHP to reflect the accommodations in the IEP and make sure the IHP is available to all health office staff, including but not limited to any colleagues and/or substitute school nurses.

Intervention and Referral Services Team

Overview

Although an intervention and referral services team (I&RS) is predominately a New Jersey concept, there is every confidence that other states have a similar, if not identical, program. The purpose of I&RS is the early identification of students having academic and/or psychosocial difficulties in the school setting. These concerns may be identified by parents, faculty, staff, and/or the school nurse with referral of the student/family to a team of educational professionals for strategies to achieve academic success. This team was previously known as the Core Team or Pupil Assistance Committee. The I&RS was introduced in 2002 and in February of 2014, readopted by the New Jersey Department of Education with amendments in NJAC 6A: 16-7 (2014).

The team is composed of specific educational professionals with the background, education, and experiences to listen to academic, behavioral, and/or medical concerns demonstrated by the student to provide useful strategies for enhanced success. It is common for this team to be made up of a general education teacher, guidance counselor, special education teacher, speech therapist, ESL teacher, school nurse, administrator, CST member, when possible, and the parents. The team maintains records, assesses outcomes of each strategy implemented, and maintains an open line of communication both at meetings and in the written word. The manual (2008 currently under revision) may be accessed at: *Scope of services for building-based I&RS teams* (2008).

Eligibility

A student is eligible for referral to I&RS team when meeting the following criteria:

1. The student is in kindergarten to grade 12, usually in general education.

2. The student demonstrates behavioral, medical, and/or academic concerns observed by any professional staff member in the building and/or by the parent.

The Plan

Although each I&RS plan is specific to the needs of the individual student, the following is a list of generic strategies that might be suggested (it must be noted that this list is not comprehensive):

1. Graphic organizers

2. Close monitoring of attendance and tardiness

3. Referral for vision and/or hearing deficits when indicated

4. Request for a physical by the primary care physician when thought appropriate and agreed upon by the parent/legal guardian

5. Assessment by the OT for hand scribing difficulties

6. Evaluation by the speech therapist for the need for individual or group therapy

7. Referral to a remedial resource when academic performance is a concern

8. Modifications in tests, homework, and method of instruction when indicated

9. Use of positive reinforcement; that is, stickers, special assignments, privileges;

10. A reminder of classroom schedule left on the student's desk in a discreet location

Timelines

I&RS meetings are routinely held on a monthly basis, in some cases more often to address new students. In addition, each student covered under an I&RS is reviewed on a monthly basis by the team for progress and need for continued monitoring, additional or new strategies, or discharge from the program. When multiple strategies have failed to demonstrate improved outcomes and sufficient documentation has been compiled, the I&RS team may refer the student to the CST for review and consideration for special services under an IEP. It must be noted that the I&RS process is not a gateway to the CST and most often is very successful in assisting the student to improved performance in the school setting.

School Nursing Responsibilities

Upon notification of the need/request for an I&RS team meeting, the school nurse shall perform the following tasks:

- Perform a thorough review of the student's health history, to include but not be limited to routine physicals, immunizations, past screenings, medical and parental notes, health office visits and attendance.
- Conduct routine screening to determine current hearing, vision, height, weight, blood pressure and compare to baseline screenings of previous years, if available; submit Health Office Referral Form (sample found in Appendix 11.1 of this chapter).

■ Attend the I&RS meeting, well prepared and act in the best interest of the student; make recommendations that are in concert with the medical, and behavioral history documented in your records and personal knowledge and experience with this child.

■ Sign off on the I&RS attendance sheet; perform the tasks assigned by the case manger specifically for students with medical needs;

■ Create an IHP to reflect the accommodations in the I&RS plan and make sure the IHP is available to all health office medical professional staff, including but not limited to any colleagues and/or substitute school nurses.

Comparing and Contrasting I&RS, 504 Plan, and IEP

Table 11.4 compares and contrasts each type of team the school nurse may be asked to have an active role.

TABLE 11.4 COMPARISON OF I&RS, 504 PLAN, AND IEP

CRITERIA	I&RS	504 PLAN	IEP
Source documents	NJAC 6A: 16	Rehabilitation Act of 1973 ADA of 1990 ADAAA 2009	IDEA (Individuals with Disabilities Education Act, 20 U.S.C. § 1400 (2004))
Purpose	Provide any student with academic or psychosocial difficulties with strategies to succeed in the school	Prevent discrimination due to disability by providing equal access and reasonable accommodations	Identify, assess, and provide eligible students with special education services to meet their needs
Age	Kindergarten to Grade 12	Lifetime	Birth to graduation or age 21
Funding	School district budget	School district budget	State and federal funding
Requirements	Provide early intervention for identified academic or psychosocial concerns in the school setting	The individual has: a physical or mental impairment, which substantially limits one or more major life activities; a record of such an impairment; or is regarded as having such impairment (28CFR Sec. 36. 104)	Child has one of 13 disabilities listed in IDEA which has an impact on the ability to learn from the general education curriculum: Auditory Impaired, Autistic, Intellectually Disabled, Communication Impaired, Emotionally Disturbed, Multiply Disabled, Deaf/Blind, Orthopedically Impaired, Other Health Impaired,

(continued)

TABLE 11.4 COMPARISON OF I&RS, 504 PLAN, AND IEP (*CONTINUED*)

CRITERIA	I&RS	504 PLAN	IEP
Require- ments (*cont.*)			Preschool Child with Disability, Social Maladjustment, Specific Learning Disability Visually Impaired (NJAC 6A; 14-3.5, September 5, 2006)
Signature of Approval	Required	Required	Required

I&RS, intervention and referral services; IEP, individualized education program.

◼ Health Services: An In-Depth Look at IHP, ECP, and EEP

Individual Healthcare Plan

Overview

"It is the responsibility of the registered professional school nurse to develop an IHP and ECP for students with healthcare needs that affect or have the potential to affect safe and optimal school attendance and academic performance. The IHP is developed by the school nurse using the nursing process in collaboration with the student, family, and healthcare providers. The school nurse utilizes the IHP to provide care coordination, to facilitate the management of the student's health condition in the school setting, to inform school-educational plans, and to promote academic success." (National Association of School Nurses [NASN], 2015)

Eligibility

Any student with healthcare needs is eligible for an IHP. The following criteria might be helpful in knowing where to start:

1. Children with medications administered in school (QD and PRN)
2. Children with chronic healthcare needs with or without medication
3. Children with an IEP, 504, or on home instruction as a result of chronic or acute healthcare needs

The Individual Healthcare Plan

Common elements of the IHP would include, but certainly not be limited to:

1. Parental/legal guardian contact information (home, work and cell phone numbers)
2. Additional contacts, approved by the parent/legal guardian, who may be called in urgent cases when the parent/legal guardian is not available

3. Assessment: Review of student's health history to identify the need for an IHP (diabetes, asthma, food allergy, anxiety, seizure disorder, etc.)

4. Nursing diagnosis: Individual health needs of the student as a result of the presenting diagnosis stated by the primary care provider

5. Goals: Measurable, clear, short- and long-term reasonable, outcomes

6. Interventions: Those actions to prevent and/or treat current and anticipated healthcare needs (medication and treatments prescribed by the primary care provider, education, etc.)

7. Expected outcomes: Primary and secondary prevention of symptomatology

8. Evaluations: After following the IHP as itemized in the preceding, one must determine if the actions taken met the expected outcomes—if yes, continue with the IHP; if no, revise the plan to reflect a more positive outcome in the future. Consider utilizing all resources available to the health office in the evaluation and revision process

Timelines

After identifying the need, the school nurse creates and implements the IHP. The IHP is a working document which can be revised, as needed, throughout the school year. On an annual basis, the school nurse shall review the IHP for completeness and accuracy in meeting the individual student's needs. In some cases, the student's needs or medications may be changed or be discontinued; for example, a student may no longer be allergic to a particular food, according to the allergist's written notation. This annual review will usually be completed at the onset of the school year, due to the fact that new medication orders are required at that time. It is routine and customary to sign/initial and date the IHP at the time of the review to indicate the completion of this nursing task.

School Nursing Responsibilities

The school nurse's responsibilities may include but are not limited to:

■ Review the student records to determine the need for an IHP.

■ Collect data on the physician's diagnosis and prescribed treatments available to the school nurse.

■ Create the IHP in concert with the student and parent(s); indicate if an ECP or EEP is in place.

■ Sign and date the IHP at the completion of the document and update or review on an annual basis or more often, when indicated.

■ Store the IHP in a safe, locked location, which is readily accessible to all licensed professional school nurses; a binder of IHPs, in alphabetical order, by grade level, stored in the locked file cabinet would be readily accessible and more often referred to than in each individual file folder. A sample IHP may be found in the Appendix 11.2 to this chapter.

Emergency Care Plan

Overview

"The ECP, written by the school nurse, is for support staff with an individual plan for emergency care for the student. These plans are kept confidential yet accessible to appropriate staff." NASN (2015)

Eligibility

Any student at risk for a medical emergency in any location outside of the health office, should not only have and IHP but also an ECP. This document would provide the faculty and staff with a template for care of the student in the classroom until the licensed professional school nurse arrives.

After reviewing the confidential list and IHPs, the school nurse determines which students require an ECP. The following categories should be considered: (a) medications delegated; (b) equipment/procedures delegated; (c) fragile medical conditions.

Three life-saving medications most often delegated to trained faculty and staff are: epinephrine auto-injector, glucagon, and Narcan (naloxone). The list of legally delegated medications may be greater or less comprehensive depending upon the state legislation (e.g., some states authorize the delegation of Diastat while other states do not). Equipment and procedures that might be delegated include CPR and use of the automated external defibrillator (AED). In addition, students with fragile medical conditions, mobility concerns, seizure disorders, and severe sensitivity to loud noises should be considered for an ECP.

The Emergency Care Plan

There is no one formalized format or template for this plan; in general, the essential components may be but are not limited to:

1. Student's name, address, and parent/legal guardian contact information
2. Diagnosis (shared with faculty and staff with parental consent on a need-to-know basis)
3. Individual medical needs to support the student with a potential emergency in the school setting
4. Education/staff development of designees
5. Signature(s) of employee(s) to document completion of educational component and knowledge of care

Timelines

An ECP may be written at any time during the school year, needs to be reviewed on an annual basis, and staff development conducted annually as delegates and staffing assignments may change.

Nursing Responsibilities

The nursing responsibilities may include but are not limited to:

- Identify need for an ECP for each student as identified in the preceding;
- Research federal and state statutes and school board policies regarding those tasks that may be legally delegated by the school nurse to nonmedical personnel.
- Create the ECP including but not limited to actions to be taken by non-nursing staff until the school nurse arrives.
- Include the parental consent form for medication administration to be delegated to nonnursing personnel.
- Research available resources to assist in training: American Heart Association, Epilepsy Foundation, American Diabetes Association, Food Allergy Research and Education are a few examples.
- Conduct training in accordance with needs of students and guidelines established.
- Complete each ECP with signatures indicating training completed, consent for responsibilities.
- Make sure a copy of the ECP is kept in the student's permanent file, as well as a copy given to the delegate(s); document that an ECP has been created on their permanent health record.

Emergency Egress Plan

Overview

An individual emergency egress plan (EEP), for the purpose of this chapter, is a document created for the safe and secure evacuation from the building for an individual who may have difficulty leaving the school during emergency conditions. This is not to imply that the school nurse does not have responsibilities for emergency egress, shelter in place, or lockdown for the entire school population. This is paramount, especially at a time of catastrophic events. In some cases, this information may be included in the IHP or the ECP and a separate document may not be necessary.

Eligibility

Any individual who has a mobility issue—that is, wheel chair user, student with crutches, faculty with limited mobility, child highly sensitive to loud noises such as the fire drill alarm, students that may not follow instructions or are an "escape" risk, to name a few—should be considered appropriate for an EEP.

The Plan

Although there is no required format or template for this plan (an example is found in Appendix 11.3), in general, the essential elements should be, but are not limited to:

1. Student's name, address, and parent/legal guardian contact information;

2. Diagnosis (to remain confidential, yet accessible to staff with a need-to-know and parental consent);

3. Individual medical needs to support the student during a potential emergency in the school setting;

4. Staff development of designees regarding evacuation procedure and use of equipment to maintain the individual's safety;

5. Signature(s) of employee(s) to document completion of training and knowledge of care required.

Timelines

An EEP may be written at any time during the school year but needs to be reviewed on an annual basis with staff development conducted annually, as delegates and staffing assignments may change.

School Nursing Responsibilities

The responsibilities of the school nurse may include but are not limited to:

- Identify those in need of assistance during an emergency egress; include anyone that requires the use of the elevator, has limited mobility, and/or difficulty during a crisis (whether real or a drill).

- Assess the equipment available and the need to purchase assistive devices to transport the child down stairs.

- Study the building egress plan in relation to the multiple locations the child will have classes.

- Identify the delegate(s) to be responsible for the assisted transport.

- Consult administration, the local police department, EMS, and local fire department in the creation of the plan; these outside agencies must be aware of the EEP for special needs individuals and the location of the students' classrooms.

- Create the plan in concert with recommendations of all individuals involved.

- Conduct training of delegates and obtain signatures of delegates following training confirming their commitment to their role and responsibilities for the EEP for this student.

- Monitor effectiveness of training during monthly fire drills and revise the plan as needed.

- File a copy of the EEP in the student's permanent record and provide a copy to the delegate(s).

References

Eligibility for Section 504 Accommodations: 28CFR Sec.36.104.

Determination of Eligibility for Special Education and Related Services; N.J.S.A. 6A: 14-3.5 p. 67–75 (2006, September 5).

Intervention and Referral Services: NJAC. 6A:16-7 (2014).

National Association of School Nurses. (2015). *Individual healthcare plans. The role of the school nurse.* Retrieved from https://www.nasn.org/advocacy/professional-practice -documents/position-statements/ps-ihps

Scope of services for building-based I&RS teams. (2008). Retrieved from https://www .state.nj.us/education/students/irs/scope.pdf

Section 504 IDEA funding is contingent upon compliance with Section 504. (National Center for Learning Disabilities). (2019, August 3). Retrieved from https://www.ncld .org

U.S. Department of Education. A guide to the individualized education program. Retrieved from https://www2.ed.gov/parents/needs/speced/iepguide/index.html

Online Resources

A Parent's Guide to Special Education. (2019, August 3). Retrieved from https://www2 .ed.gov/parents/needs/speced/iepguide/index.html

A Sample Diabetes Medical Management Plan. (2019, October 23). Retrieved from http:// main.diabetes.org/dorg/PDFs/Advocacy/Discrimination/dmmp-form.pdf

Intervention and Referral Services Code. (2019, October 25). Retrieved from http://www .state.nj.us/education/code/current/title6a/chap16.pdf

National Association of School Nurses, Position Paper on Individual Healthcare Plans. (2019, August 3) (with written consent). Retrieved from https://www.nasn.org/ advocacy/professional-practice-documents/position-statements/ps-ihps

Sample Emergency Care Plan for Anaphylaxis. (June 2020). Retrieved from https://www .foodallergy.org/living-food-allergies/food-allergy-essentials/food-allergy -anaphylaxis-emergency-care-plan

Sample Emergency Care Plan for Asthma. (2019, September 5). Retrieved from https:// portal.ct.gov/-/media/Departments-and-Agencies/DPH/dph/hems/asthma/pdf/ PEDAAPEngSpanpdf.pdf?la=en

Sample School Nurse Health Form for Intervention & Referral Services. (2019, September 17). Retrieved from https://www.nj.gov/education/students/irs/

Sample Seizure Response Plan. (2019, October 23). Retrieved from https://www.epilepsy .com/learn/schools-and-seizure-preparedness

Section 504 IDEA funding is contingent upon compliance with Section 504. (National Center for Learning Disabilities). (2019, August 3). Retrieved from https://www.ncld .org

The Nursing Process. (2019, October 24). Retrieved from https://www.nursingprocess.org/ Nursing-Process-Steps.html

APPENDIX 11.1

INTERVENTIONAL AND REFERRAL SERVICES

Sample School Nurse/School Health Form (This template may also be used for IEP and 504 Reporting)

Confidential

To: _____

From: _____

Reference _____

Date: _____

Please complete and return this form to the I&RS team by: _____

Health History—Is the student currently taking any medication(s)? If yes, please identify.

_____

Are you aware of any prior use of medication(s) by the student? If yes, identify each medication and condition treated.

_____

Are you aware of any medical or other condition(s) that could interfere with the student's ability to perform in school? If yes, please describe the condition(s) and its implications.

_____

_____

Health Assessment

Date of birth: _____

Height: _____   Weight: _____

Vision: _____   Hearing: _____

Skin: _____   Posture: _____

Comments: _____

Socialization observable behaviors: _____

Behavioral changes: _____

Comments: _____

Physical appearance (e.g., personal hygiene, fatigue, odor of smoke, attire)

_____

_____

_____

Visits to Nurse

Frequency/Number: _____

Reasons: _____

Physical Education Excuses

Frequency/Number: _____

Reasons: _____

Comments: _____

Student's Strengths/Skills:

_____

_____

_____

Positive Characteristics:

_____

_____

_____

Environmental Supports:

_____

_____

_____

Other: _____

Other Pertinent Information: _____

_____

SOURCE: New Jersey Department of Education—I&RS Manual (2008-under revision).
May be used for School Nurse Reporting to the 504 Team, I&RS Team and CST.

APPENDIX 11.2

INDIVIDUALIZED HEALTHCARE PLAN

Student Name: _____

Address: _____

Home Phone: _____   Mother's Cell: _____   Father's Cell: _____

Other Emergency Contacts: _____

Healthcare Provider: _____   Provider's Phone: _____

IHP Written By: _____   Date: _____

Teacher: _____   Grade: _____   Classroom: _____

Diagnosis:

Assessment Data*	Nursing Diagnosis*	Planning*	Nursing Interventions*	Evaluation Criteria*

Reviewed/Revised Date & Initials	Reviewed/Revised Date & Initials

Emergency Egress Plan Indicated: _____ NO _____ YES and attached
*Using the Nursing Process(https://www.nursingprocess.org/Nursing-Process-Steps.html)

APPENDIX 11.3

INDIVIDUAL EMERGENCY EVACUATION PLAN

Student Name: _____ DOB: _____ Date: _____

Grade: _____ Classroom Room #: _____

In case of an emergency, the above-named student   *shall evacuate the building in the following manner:*
1. Student shall remain with one-on-one aide at all times; weekly class schedule is attached;
2. Student shall exit the building via the classroom with fellow students in a wheelchair (w/c) utilizing the existing ramp; if the student is not in the w/c at the time of the emergency, the student will be immediately transferred to the w/c to facilitate movement on blacktop away from the building;
3. Aide shall make an effort for student to be the last person on line to avoid injury and provide time for a safe transfer to the w/c;
4. Student and aide shall move away from the building to the far side of the blacktop and then turn to face the building;
5. Student shall remain silent and focused until otherwise instructed by teacher to return to the building or alternate site;
6. When indicated, the student and aide shall lead the line to return to the building via the ramped entrance to the classroom;
7. One student shall enter the building via the north corridor doors near the 4C classroom and unlock the 40 classroom exterior doors.

The above outlined EEP has been reviewed and approved by:

_____

Signatures: Principal Teacher School Nurse 1:1 Personnel

_____

Signatures: Additional School Personnel Responsible for this Student

_____

THE POTENTIALLY
MARGINALIZED CHILD

12

MENTAL HEALTH DISORDERS IN SCHOOL-AGED CHILDREN

BRENDA MARSHALL

LEARNING OBJECTIVES

- Demonstrate familiarity with the current statistics related to mental disorders in school-aged children.
- Identify the most frequently seen diagnoses of mental illness in children.
- Assess suicidality and non-suicidal self-injury.
- Engage techniques to encourage honest expression of fears/anxiety.

▨ Introduction

Mental illness in children is more common than cancer, diabetes, and HIV/AIDS together, making it the most common disease category of childhood. Approximately 22% of American children have, or have had, a psychiatric disorder (Merikangas et al., 2010). The symptoms of these disorders present in 50% of the affected children by age 14 with another 25% presenting by age 24 (World Health Organization [WHO], 2014). The distress that is caused by psychiatric disorders in children impacts learning, behavior, and socializing by the child and the greater learning community. These disorders, which range from attention deficit hyperactivity disorder (ADHD) to psychotic episodes, often go undiagnosed in children, making their daily existence one of fear and extreme anxiety. Stigma toward mental illness has kept children and their families from accessing treatments that could change the course of their disease as well as their futures. Undiagnosed and untreated mental illness increases a child's risk for substance use, academic failure, unlawful behaviors that could result in incarceration, and suicide. The keys to opening a better future for them, their families and the community rests in providing a safe place for these children to express their concerns and early identification and referral for treatment. This chapter introduces the common psychiatric disorders seen in children and provides references and resources for assessment and referral.

▧ Stigma and Mental Illness: Critical Definitions and the Words We Use

Mental health disorders usually present prior to age 18. This would imply that most children will come in contact with a peer with mental illness. The following words are critical for understanding the stigma that comes with mental illness. The school nurse often will be the person to educate other adults and children about mental health and mental illness, serving as a role model in creating a safe and accepting environment. The American Psychiatric Association (APA) provides useful tips that can be utilized effectively by the school nurse to decrease the stigma felt by people with mental illness (APA, 2018).

▧ Critical Words and Word Placement

Avoid offensive slang terms or insulting language: Listed herein are common terms to be used when talking about mental health disorders. Stopping the use of derogatory terms like psycho, junkie, nuts, cookoo, nutcase in the school environment helps to restore dignity to the person with a mental illness.

Person first identification of a mental health condition: *A person with depression* in lieu of *a depressed person.* Placing the focus on the person not the diagnosis reminds the speaker of the person's humanity and identifies the illness as a piece of the person's life, not a defining characteristic.

Disorder specific vocabulary: Rather than the generalized moniker of mental illness, use the specific diagnosis: *She was diagnosed with an anxiety disorder* instead of *he was mentally ill.*

▧ Current Statistics Related to Mental Disorders in School-Aged Children

Recent statistics gathered by the Centers for Disease Control and Prevention (CDC), paints a critical picture of mental health and mental disorders in children under 18 years of age (Figure 12.1). Globally, the prevalence of mental illness in children has increased within the last few years (Polanczyk, Slum, Sugaya, Caye, & Rohde, 2015). The most commonly diagnosed disorders for American children are anxiety, depression, behavioral problems, and attention deficit hyperactivity disorder (ADHD; Merikangas et al., 2010). Co-occurring disorders (existence of two or more diagnoses) are common. One illustration of this is that three out of four children between the ages of 3 and 17 diagnosed with depression also have an anxiety disorder, and of those children, half have a diagnosable behavioral problem (Ghandour et al., 2018). These disorders, including developmental and behavioral disorders in addition to mental disorders change with age, with the diagnosis of depression and anxiety increasing as the child gets older while developmental and behavioral disorders decrease after age 12 (Ghandour et al., 2018). Symptoms of mental illness usually appear by 14 years of age in 50% of the population, with another 25% by the age of 24.

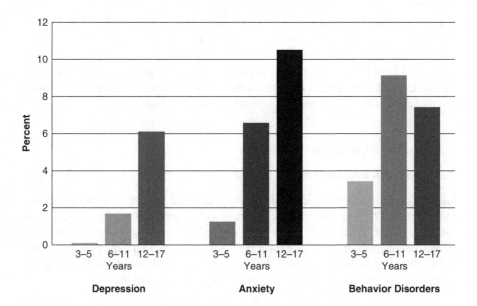

FIGURE 12.1 Mental illness by age in the United States.

SOURCE: Centers for Disease Control and Prevention. (2019). *Data and statistics on children's mental health*. Retrieved from https://www.cdc.gov/childrensmentalhealth/data.html

■ The Role of Genetics and Epigenetics: Determinants of Mental Illness in Children

Genetics: Genetics, or the study of hereditary traits passed on in the DNA, is believed by some theorists to play a role in the development of some mental disorders. This is due, in part, to the fact that some psychiatric diagnoses can be found more frequently in family groups (Marshall, 2018). Currently there is not, according to the National Institute of Mental Health (NIMH), a single gene that will explain why one out of five Americans has mental illness (NIMH, n.d.). The consensus is that the interplay between gene susceptibility and environmental factors increases the likelihood of an emergent mental illness in certain individuals (Haworth, Carter, Eley, & Plomin, 2017). Haworth et al. (2017) posit that it is as important to assess a person's well-being as well as their susceptibility to mental illness. Approximately 40% of "internalizing symptoms" by an adolescent can be related to that person's sense of well-being (Haworth et al., 2017). Their theory is that understanding what supports positive mental health in youth can help reduce the symptoms of mental illness that erupt during adolescence.

Epigenetics refers to how environmental stressors can alter genetic functions without altering the DNA sequence itself, producing what are called markers, or tags, that impact the functioning of the gene. This phenotype change actually alters the way the organism appears and behaves. Epigenetics are at the foundation of gene regulation (Nestler, Pena, Kundakovic, Mitchell, & Akbarian, 2016). Adverse childhood experiences (ACEs) are identified as environmental stressors, potentially impacting the epigenetic landscape and thereby changing the mental health future of the child (Lang et al., 2019). Nestler et al. (2016) identify how the impact of environmental stressors, specifically early in life, can increase a person's vulnerability to psychiatric disorders which then translates into a lifetime of mental illness.

Mental Illnesses in Children

Definition and Prevalence

Mental illnesses are the most common diseases diagnosed in childhood with one in five adolescents (22.2%) experiencing a severe mental disorder (Merikangas et al., 2010). In children between the ages of 2 and 8 years, one in six (17.4%) have a mental, developmental, or behavioral disorder (Bitsko et al., 2018). The CDC (n.d.) describes childhood mental illness as "serious changes in the way children typically learn, behave or handle their emotions, which cause distress and problems getting through the day."

Statistics

Over 4.5 million (7.4%) children between ages 3 and 17 years are diagnosed with a behavior problem, approximately the same number (4.4 million) have an anxiety disorder and 1.9 million (3.2%) have depression (CDC, 2019a). Developmental disorders, behavioral disorders, and mental disorders are more prevalent in boys between the ages of 2 to 8 and in children living in poverty (Cree et al., 2018). Prevalence rates of diagnosis, similar to anxiety and depression, are increasing. In 2003 the percentage of children between 6 and 17 years of age diagnosed with anxiety was 5.4%, which increased to 7.1 % in 2018.

Disparities

Four determinants related to race and ethnicity have been identified as foundational in creating disparities for the diagnosis and receipt of services for children with mental illnesses. They consist of socio-economic, ACEs/childhood adversity (CA), the role of family structure, and the differential role of factors from neighborhoods like violence, drug use, and low quality housing (Alegria, Green, McLaughlin, & Loder, 2015).

Common Mental Illnesses in Childhood

A number of mental illnesses affecting children are described in the following. This is not an exhaustive list, but reflects the commonly diagnosed mental illnesses that will be seen by the school nurse.

Anxiety Disorders

Of children between the ages of 3 and 17, 7.1% experience an anxiety disorder (Ghandour et al., 2018). It is best to consider anxiety as the umbrella under which also exists generalized anxiety disorder (GAD), phobias, separation anxiety disorder, obsessive compulsive disorder, and panic disorder. What distinguishes normal anxiety or worry from a diagnosable disorder is that the child with an anxiety disorder has an impairment in normal daily functioning including social and familial relationships and academic performance. As noted in Table 12.1, some common problems are present in children with anxiety disorders including:

- The child might not understand or be able to explain why there is the feeling of anxiety, this in and of itself can become a cause of worry, both to the child and the guardians.
- There is no logical reason for the worry, and no logical method to help reduce the feeling of anxiety that has taken hold.
- The child becomes preoccupied with the fear, unable to shake the sense of dread to the extent that it begins to interfere with activities of daily living. The fear does not get better over time and can worsen.

Etiology of Anxiety Disorders

Risk factors for anxiety disorders are both genetic and environmental. they include early ACEs or other negative life events for children and a family history of anxiety or mental illness.

Assessment and Evaluation

It is important to take a good history. Medical conditions that should be considered when conducting an assessment are use of caffeine, nicotine, thyroid conditions, and over-the-counter (OTC) and prescription drug use.

Treatment and Therapies

Refer to a psychologist, psychiatrist or psychiatric nurse practitioner (NP) for diagnosis and treatment with medication and/or psychotherapy. Stress management techniques can be discussed with the child ranging from breathing exercises to aerobic activities, but should not be in lieu of formal treatment with standard care.

Attention Deficit Hyperactivity Disorder

ADHD is a neurodevelopmental disorder which is usually diagnosed in childhood and continues into adulthood. Almost 1 in 10 (9.4%) children in the United States between the ages of 2 to 17 (6.1 million) are diagnosed with ADHD (Danielson, Bitsko, Ghandour, Holbrook, & Blumberg, 2016). Boys are diagnosed more frequently with ADHD (12.9%) than girls (5.6%; Danielson et al., 2016). It is not unusual for a child diagnosed with ADHD to have other comorbid mental health diagnoses (Table 12.2).

TABLE 12.1 SIGNS AND SYMPTOMS OF SPECIFIC ANXIETY DISORDERS IN CHILDREN

DISORDER	SIGNS AND SYMPTOMS
General anxiety disorder (GAD)	This general category of anxiety exhibits symptoms of restlessness, difficulty concentrating, irritability, unable to control worry, problems with sleeping, fatigue, and being constantly on edge.
Panic disorder	Persons experiencing panic attacks, or moments when there is sudden intense fear. The attacks might be triggered by objects or situations or might be unexplainable. There is often fear of recurrence so the person might avoid specific situations or places. Symptoms: Sweating, trembling, heart palpitations, sense of impending doom, loss of control, shortness of breath, and may complain of chest discomfort.
Phobia-related disorders	General phobias are fears of specific situations or objects. The fear is not proportional to the situation. The fear of contact with the object/situation causes excessive (and often) irrational intrusive worry. Anxiety level exacerbates on contact with the object/situation. Specific phobias (simple phobias) fear of: ■ Heights ■ Animals or insects ■ Needles/injections ■ Blood ■ Flying
Separation anxiety disorder	Fear of having to be apart from someone important, with whom a strong attachment has been formed fearing that something bad might happen to the person. Symptoms include stomachaches and other physical symptoms and nightmares.
Selective mutism	This disorder is rare. The symptoms are the inability of a person to speak in certain, specific social environments and situations even though they are able to speak. Usually seen with children under 5 years of age. Behaviors: Extreme shyness, withdrawal, clinging behaviors, temper tantrums, and other compulsive traits.
Social anxiety disorder and agoraphobia	Anxiety related to social situations or expectation of performance in front of others. The behaviors might be withdrawal from social situations or avoidance of engaging with people, which might cause negative reactions from others and heightened sense of embarrassment. Agoraphobia presents as fearing two or more specific situations including open spaces, public transportation, public spaces, being in a crowd, being alone (either inside or outside), and being in enclosed spaces.

SOURCE: Adapted from National Institute of Mental Health. (2018). *Mental health information: Anxiety disorders*. Retrieved from https://www.nimh.nih.gov/health/topics/anxiety-disorders/index.shtml

Etiology of ADHD

It is believed that genetics play a role in the development of ADHD with increased risk for immediate biological family members, but no specific gene has been identified (Yearwood, Pearson, & Newland, 2012). Epigenetics like maternal exposure to

TABLE 12.2 PERCENTAGE OF U.S. CHILDREN WITH ADHD AND ANOTHER DISORDER

Any mental, emotional, or behavioral disorder: 64%
Behavior or conduct problems: 52%
Anxiety: 33%
Depression: 17%
Autism spectrum disorder: 14%
Tourette syndrome: 1%

SOURCE: Centers for Disease Control and Prevention. (2019). Attention deficit/hyperactivity disorder (ADHD): Data & statistics about ADHD. Retrieved from https://www.cdc.gov/ncbddd/adhd/data.html

lead during pregnancy, maternal smoking leading to low birth weight, maternal use of alcohol during pregnancy, and exposure to lead in early childhood have been identified as risk factors. Other causes like traumatic brain injury, environmental adversity, and poverty have been thought to be contributors (Yearwood et al., 2012).

Signs and Symptoms of ADHD

There are three cardinal groups of symptoms in ADHD—inattention, hyperactivity, and impulsivity. These behaviors can be severe and negatively impact school, home, and social environments. *Inattention:* Makes careless mistakes, doesn't follow directions, high risk taking/impulsivity, daydreams, loses things, neglects to follow through on things, easily distracted, talkative, does not enjoy prolonged requirement of mental effort. *Hyperactivity:* Squirms and fidgets, excessive running/climbing, difficulty remaining seated for extended time periods, constant movement. *Impulsivity:* Lack of premeditation or consideration to outcomes or consequences of a behavior.

Types of ADHD

Predominantly inattentive, predominantly hyperactive-impulsive, or a combination of both: The impact of the inattentive presentation impedes the child's ability to organize, follow directions, self-monitor, pay attention in class, and stay focused. The impact of the hyperactive impulsive behaviors can present as class disruptions when the child is running around, climbing on things, not following directions, not respecting boundaries, and speaking out of turn. The combined presentation presents behaviors from both the previous descriptions.

Assessment and Evaluation

There are a number of assessment tools that are utilized to identify ADHD in youth. These tools usually assess the child in multiple environments by those who are with the child (i.e., parents/teachers/self-report for older children). Rating scales include the Connors Rating Scales (ages 3–17), the Brown Attention Deficit Disorder Scale for Children and Adolescents (BADDS) for multiple age groups, the Vanderbilt ADHD Rating Scale (ages 6–12), and the Swanson, Nolan, and Pelham IV (SNAP) scale (ages 11–15).

Treatment and Therapies

Referral to a psychologist, psychiatrist, or psychiatric NP for diagnosis and treatment with medication and/or behavior therapy. Behavior therapy models that include parents and teachers can help the child have consistent support. Children with ADHD should be encouraged to have adequate sleep, a healthy diet, hydration, and physical activity.

Autism Spectrum Disorder

The prevalence of autism spectrum disorder (ASD) in the United States in 2018 was determined to be 1 in 59, an increase of 15% from 2016 (Baio et al., 2018). New Jersey has the highest rate of 1:34, representing a 20% increase over 2 years, possible due to better access to student records. ASD appears in all ethnic, racial, and socioeconomic groups (Baio et al., 2018). There is a four to one likelihood that boys have ASD than girls, with most children being diagnosed by age 4 (Baio et al., 2018). ASD presents on a continuum or spectrum with a wide heterogeneity of clinical symptoms. Some children may present with giftedness in academics or another field while others may be severely challenged in multiple areas.

Etiology of ASD

ASD is a neurobehavioral disorder, based in biology, that presents with developmental disabilities. As with most of the disorders that have been discussed, there are both genetic and epigenetic components.

Signs and Symptoms of ASD

Delayed or difficulties in communication, social interaction, and emotional regulation are seen in children with ASD. Some of the children demonstrate repetitive behaviors while others communicate in ways that appear different from others of their own age group. The impairment in socializing, where the child is not bothered (or actually prefers) to play alone and has a hard time to establish eye contact when communicating with others. There might be difficulties in talking about feelings or understanding when others speak about feelings. Changes in routines often are difficult for children with ASD to adapt to.

Spectrum of ASD

ASD can impact thinking, problem-solving, and learning abilities ranging from severely impacting activities of daily living (dressing, bathing, toilet training) while others excel academically and require ongoing social skills therapy to improve communication skills.

Assessment and Evaluation

The school nurse will probably not be the first to have assess to the child with ASD, as it is usually diagnosed between the ages of 2 to 4. Children with ASD, who are mainstreamed at school, may experience some anxiety and turn to the school nurse for a safe place. The nurse might notice that the child has a flat, non-modulated speech pattern and appear to be emotionless. This child might also not properly interpret the non-verbal nuances in everyday social interaction.

Treatment and Therapies

Referral to an agency where psychologists, psychiatrists, social workers, and psychiatric NPs can assess and treat as an interdisciplinary team. The child might already be receiving specialized assistance in the school environment in the areas of speech and language, social skills, and occupational therapy.

Behavior/Conduct Problems

Behaviors that are aggressive and defiant can be more than just disruptive to the classroom. When children have these behaviors over time, demonstrating unwanted behaviors and not being concerned about consequences, it is called externalizing disorders. Over 7% of children between 3 and 17 years of age display an externalizing disorder, but it is most commonly seen between the ages of 6 and 11. Two types of externalizing disorders—oppositional defiant disorder (ODD) and conduct disorder (CD)—are presented in Table 12.3. These diagnoses present problems in all areas of the child's life—home, school, and the social environment.

Etiology of Disruptive Behavior Disorders

Development of disruptive behavior disorders is multifactorial and includes developmental, social/learned, and biological factors. Genetics and epigenetics play a role and it is not uncommon for there to be a family history of substance use problems, personality disorders, mood disorders, or schizophrenia.

Assessment and Evaluation

Often, it is the school nurse who will be the first person to identify behavioral and mental health needs of children. The unique role the school nurse can play in mental health screening, promoting mental health wellness programs and decreasing stigma demonstrated to students with mental health needs can improve outcomes through early identification and intervention. Recognizing behavioral problems and making referrals to appropriate mental health specialists underscores the important impact school nurses can have on a student's mental health and academic success.

TABLE 12.3 DISRUPTIVE BEHAVIOR DISORDERS AND THEIR ASSOCIATED BEHAVIORS

Disruptive disorder	Associated behaviors may include (but are not limited to):
Oppositional defiant disorder (ODD)	Opposing or defying figures of authority, frequent angry outbursts, resentful and spiteful to others, easily irritated or annoyed, deflects blame onto others, temper tantrums, behaviors focused on revenge
Conduct disorder	Persistent disobeying of serious rules including but not limited to truancy and running away. Aggressive behaviors that harm others (people and animals), and conscious, chronic, purposeful lying, stealing, and/or causing damage to the person and property of others. Conduct disorder may be diagnosed after a person with ODD becomes violent or aggressive.

Treatment and Therapies

Treatment should be sought as soon as the behaviors become consistently apparent and needs to be tailored to the needs of both the child and the family. The child should be evaluated to eliminate other possible triggers for the behaviors (learning difficulties or comorbid psychiatric diagnosis). The treatment should be consistent between school and home environments and include parents and other family members.

Eating Disorders

Eating disorders are serious psychiatric disorders with acute and chronic episodes that impact the youth's psychological, social and physical well-being (APA, 2013). Youth with eating disorders are typically preoccupied with food and their body weight. The course of these diseases are severe, chronic, and can be life-threatening (de Vos, Radstaak, Bohlmeijer, & Westerhof, 2018).

Mood Disorders

Mood disorders include diagnosis of major depressive disorder (MDD), dysthymia, severe mood dysregulation, hypomania, mania, and bipolar disorder. This affective dysregulation is estimated to affect an estimated 14.3% adolescents between the ages 13 and 18 years and is higher among female adolescents (18.3%) than male adolescents (10.5%; Merikangas et al., 2010). The episodes, either elevated or depressed, vary in both duration and intensity, and impact behaviors and cognitions. Early onset of mood disorders can predict long-term disease lasting into adulthood (Yearwood et al., 2012; Figure 12.2). It is not uncommon to find comorbid mental illnesses diagnosis present.

Etiology of Mood Dysregulation Disorders

Multifactorial etiology include genetic, epigenetic, environmental (external, internal, and relational), cognitive, and personality. It is the combination of these factors coupled with duration and intensity during a child's critical developmental stage that becomes a determinant of the disease (U.S. Preventive Services Task Force [PSTF], 2016). In the United States, 3.2% of children between ages 3 and 17 (1.9 million) have depression. Characteristics and common comorbidities of mood disorders can be found in Table 12.4.

Suicidality

Assessing Suicidal Thoughts and Behaviors

Suicide, or taking one's own life, is a public health problem that devastates individuals and families. Suicide attempts are when the act to kill oneself is not completed and the person does not die. Risk for suicide is higher among persons who have experienced child abuse, bullying, or sexual violence. It is the 10th leading cause of

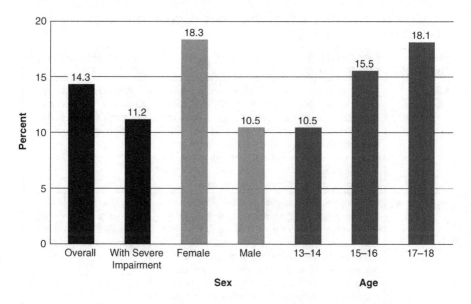

FIGURE 12.2 Lifetime prevalence of any mood disorder among US adolescents.

SOURCE: Data from Harvard Medical School: National Comorbidity Survey. (2017, August 21). Data table 1: Lifetime prevalence *DSM-IV*/WMH-CIDI disorders by sex and cohort. Retrieved from https://www.hcp.med.harvard.edu/ncs/ftpdir/NCS-R_Lifetime_Prevalence_Estimates.pdf

TABLE 12.4 MOOD DISORDERS:CHARACTERISTIC SYMPTOMS AND COMMON COMORBIDITIES

MOOD DISORDER	CHARACTERISTIC SYMPTOMS AND SCREENINGS	SYMPTOMS SEEN IN SCHOOL
Major depressive disorder (MDD)	Sadness, feeling down most of the day, every-day. Change in weight, eating, and sleeping lasting more than 2 weeks. Chronic and recurring. Can be mild, moderate or severe. Fatigue, sense of worthlessness, indecisive, anhedonia causing distress impacting daily function. Suicidal ideations or attempts. Screening should start at age 12 and continue to age 18 (U.S. Preventive Services Task Force, 2016).	Stomachaches, poor concentration, impaired academic functioning, impaired socialization, tantrums, crying, social isolation. Suicide threats. Comorbidities: Anxiety, substance use, conduct disorder, eating disorder, attention deficit hyperactivity disorder.
Dysthymia	Similar to MDD, low energy, changes in eating and sleeping, low self-worth, hopelessness, poor concentration; lasting for at least 2 years.	Same as MDD.

(continued)

TABLE 12.4 MOOD DISORDERS:CHARACTERISTIC SYMPTOMS AND COMMON COMORBIDITIES (*CONTINUED*)

MOOD DISORDER	CHARACTERISTIC SYMPTOMS AND SCREENINGS	SYMPTOMS SEEN IN SCHOOL
Severe mood dys-regulation	Usually seen before age 12. Abnormally angry or sad mood coupled with three of the following symptoms: insomnia, racing thoughts, agitation, intrusiveness, pressured speech, restlessness, distractibility or flight of ideas. Lasting for at least a year (12 months) with symptoms continuous and observed in home, school, or in social environments (must have two domains).	Fights, crying, inability to concentrate in class, academic failure, social isolation, exhaustion.
Hypomania	Expansive or irritable mood, different from usual mood and lasting a minimum of 4 days coupled with three of the following symptoms: Grandiosity, talkativeness, increased goal activities, increased seeking of pleasurable experiences, flight of ideas, decreased need for sleep, inflated self-esteem. Not attributable to substances, medicine, or a medical condition. No psychotic features. Changes in mood and behaviors seen by others.	Injury due to risk taking, poor judgment, inflated self-opinion leading to arguments and fights.
Mania	Persistently elevated and abnormal mood that lasts at least 1 week with three of the following symptoms: decreased need for sleep, grandiosity, very talkative, flight of ideas, engaging in pleasurable activities, distractible, increased goal activities which are not attributable to substances, medicine, or a medical condition. May have psychotic features. Severe impairment of normal functioning that may require hospitalization.	Injury due to risk taking, may present with psychotic symptoms including auditory or other sensory hallucinations. Weakness due to physical exhaustion, weight loss, and dehydration.
Bipolar disorder	*MDD + mania—Bipolar 1* *MDD + hypomania—Bipolar 2* Alternating episodes of depression, mania, or hypomania and euthymia.	Dependent upon what kind of episode the child is experiencing.

SOURCE: Adapted from Yearwood, E. L., Pearson, G. S., & Newland, J. A. (2012). *Child and adolescent behavioral health* (pp. 168–169). West Sussex, UK: Wiley-Blackwell.

death in the United States, affecting all races, ethnicities, and ages and the second leading cause of death in youth ages 10 to 24. Non-Hispanic American Indian/Alaskan Natives and non-Hispanic Whites have the highest rates of suicide. Veterans and other military workers and sexual minority youth are also at higher risk for suicide. Suicidal thoughts are often episodic, coming up in the child's thought quickly and having a relatively short duration (Kleiman & Nock, 2018). Suicide ideations are not uncommon in children and should be listened to without placing guilt on the child (Yearwood et al., 2012).

Warning Signs

Children who are considering suicide may exhibit signs at school including: changes in academic performance with a drop in grades; withdrawing from interacting with teachers, staff, and students; loss of interest in activities; absenteeism; dropping out of extracurricular activities. When they speak with the school nurse they might be preoccupied with death, asking questions about different ways to die or asking questions about what happens when a child dies. The child may have hopelessness, begin to give away personal items, write or draw pictures about death, and exhibit significant changes in mood.

Risk factors that increase the likelihood of a suicide attempt include previous suicide attempts, major depressive disorder, a loss of a loved one or divorce in the family, chronic bullying behaviors, family members who have committed or attempted suicide, ACEs, witnessing or experiencing violence, sexual abuse, access to firearms or pills, impulsivity, feeling like a burden, feeling hopeless, or experiencing acute rejection.

Do not be afraid to ask, "Are you feeling depressed or sad lately?" and "Are you thinking about hurting or killing yourself?" Contrary to some beliefs, directly asking the child may provide a sense of relief and an adult to speak with. The NIMH provides a tool kit for school nurses and juvenile detention centers that includes suicide screening information sheets, a suicide survey, educational videos, and resource lists in multiple languages (CDC, 2020).

Substance Use Disorders

The substance of greatest abuse for youth, according to the 2018 National Survey on Drug Use and Health (NSDUH) was alcohol, with about 7.1 million adolescents and young adults (12–20 years of age) illegally consuming alcohol. Drinking patterns in 2017 from eighth grade to 12th grade reflect higher consumption by older children, which may be related to access (Figure 12.3). Alcohol use has been declining since 2009 (U.S. Department of Health and Human Services, Substance Abuse and Mental Health Services Administration, Center for Behavioral Health Statistics and Quality, 2018).

Vaping, or use of e-cigarettes, by middle and high school students increased between 2017 and 2018, with Cullen et al. (2018) reporting that over 3.6 million youth now use e-cigarettes. The rapid increase in vaping by middle and high school students has become a national concern (Figure 12.4).

Treatment of youth with substance use disorders is different from adults, as the child's brain is still growing (Kaminer & Godley, 2010). There are different outcome patterns depending on the youth, which have been divided into three categories; one third have excellent treatment response with cessation of substances; one third alternate between recovery and relapse; and the last third do not have good treatment response with the substance use disorder progressively increasing (Kaminer, Winters, & Kelly, 2015).

Schizophrenia

Schizophrenia is a chronic and debilitating mental illness that has thought disorder as a key characteristic. There is a typical lack of insight and disruption in perceptions that impact a person's ability to be emotionally responsive, impeding social interac-

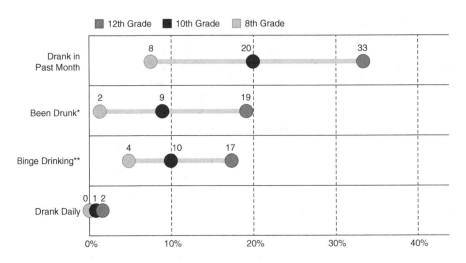

FIGURE 12.3 Reported drinking patterns among eighth, 10th and 12th grade students, 2017 (numbers in percentages).

*Been drunk in the previous 30 days.
**Five or more drinks in a row in the previous 14 days.
SOURCE: Data from responsibility.org. Retrieved from https://files.eric.ed.gov/fulltext/ED589764.pdf

tions and the ability to function in activities of daily living. It is rare in childhood, with symptoms generally first appearing in adolescence.

Etiology of Schizophrenia

Schizophrenia has a multifactorial etiology inducing brain changes including biochemical, genetic, epigenetic, and environmental factors.

Signs and Symptoms of Schizophrenia

Positive symptoms of schizophrenia are hallucinations; bizarre thoughts; confusion of reality, dreams, and television/social media; confusion; moodiness; personality changes; delusions; and paranoia. Negative symptoms include withdrawal from social situations and relationships, increasing isolation, decreased personal grooming, increased fearfulness and anxiety. These symptoms impact relationships and academic capacity. Onset might be slow, beginning with negative symptoms that are easy to mistake for adolescent moodiness. These changes are also frightening for the youth, who may not be willing to share the fear and anxiety with anyone.

Assessment and Evaluation

Changes in a student's normal behaviors from being social and outgoing to shy and withdrawn may be the first signs. Speech that does not make sense, responding to

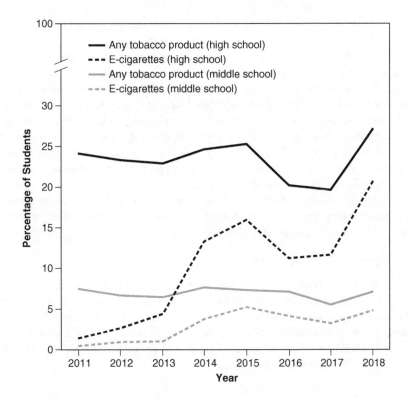

FIGURE 12.4 Percentage of middle and high school students who currently use e-cigarettes and any tobacco product.

SOURCE: Cullen, K. A., Ambrose, B. K., Gentzke, A. S., Apelberg, B. J., Jamal, A., & King, B. A. (2018). Notes from the field: Use of electronic cigarettes and any tobacco product among middle and high school students—United States, 2011–2018. *Morbidity and Mortality Weekly Report, 67*, 1276–1277. doi:10.15585/mmwr.mm6745a5

voices or people who are not present, and eccentric behaviors or speech should alert the school nurse to the possibility of emerging signs of schizophrenia.

Treatment and Therapies

Refer to a psychiatrist or agency that can work with the student, family, and school. Treatment can include psycho-pharmacy, individual therapy, family therapy and specialized plan of academic programs (American Academy of Child and Adolescent Psychiatry [AACAP], 2019).

Non-Suicidal Self-Injury

Non-suicidal self-injury (NSSI) is the intentional and non-socially sanctioned harm to one's own body, without intending to commit suicide. NSSI occurs at the rate of

15% to 20% in adolescents and young adults with an average age of onset of 13 or 14 (Klonsky, Victor, & Saffer, 2014). NSSI is highest in those with a psychiatric diagnosis and is usually associated with emotional dysregulation, depression, and anxiety. It is more common in women, and there is a difference in the chosen type of NSSI between females (cutting) ad males (burning and hitting). It is also more common with White youth sexually identifying as gay, bisexual, and questioning (Sornberger, Smith, Toste, & Heath, 2013). Acts of self-harm may present as cutting, scalding of skin, hair pulling, burning one's skin, or other methods of inflicting pain on self. The belief is that this helps to alleviate their emotional pain or sense of emptiness. These youth do not want to kill themselves, they are engaging in a deliberate act to destroy their own body tissues (Yearwood et al., 2012). Some common reasons that youth engage in NSSI are as an act of self-punishment, in order to exert influence over others, as a negative coping strategy to stop dissociation, and to feel the rush of excitement at the time of injury (Yearwood et al., 2012).

Assessment and Evaluation

NSSI is often comorbid with other psychiatric diagnosis like mood disorders and anxiety. Children should be evaluated for unexplained injuries and hiding their arms and legs to conceal wounds. Asking about suicidal thoughts, examining the types of wounds, finding out when the NSSI behaviors began, and assessing the intensity of the urges will allow the school nurse to be able to provide a detailed report to the physician or other mental health practitioner.

Protective Factors

While mental illness and suicide are serious challenges facing today's youth, there are some determinants of mental health that can act to protect mental health. These protective factors can assist in improving the lives of all children. Whereas risk factors like ACEs and environmental violence increase the likelihood of emotional problems protective factors like reliable and consistent support from caregivers, emotional self-regulation, and developing problem-solving skills can promote well-being. The office of the school nurse is a place for a child to experience nonjudgmental, empathy and compassion. The unique role of the school nurse to provide support and encouragement as well as education and resources to students, staff, and families can serve to remove barriers to help and promote emotional well-being.

▨ References

Alegria, M., Green, J., McLaughlin, K., & Loder, S. (2015). *Disparities in child and adolescent mental health and mental health services in the U.S.* New York, NY: William T. Grant Foundation.

American Academy of Child and Adolescent Psychiatry. (2019). Recommendations for pediatricians, family practitioners, psychiatrists, and non-physician mental health practitioners. Retrieved from https://www.aacap.org/AACAP/Member_Resources/Practice_Information/When_to_Seek_Referral_or_Consultation_with_a_CAP.aspx

American Psychiatric Association. (2013). *Diagnostic and statistical manual of mental disorders: DSM-5* (5th ed.). Arlington, VA: American Psychiatric Publishing.

American Psychiatric Association. (2018). *Warning signs of mental illness.* Retrieved from https://www.psychiatry.org/patients-families/warning-signs-of-mental-illness

Baio, J., Wiggins, L., Christensen, D. L., Maenner, M., Daniels, J., Warren, Z., … Dowling, N. F. (2018). Prevalence of autism spectrum disorder among children aged 8 years— Autism and developmental disabilities monitoring network, 11 sites, United States, 2014. *MMWR Surveillance Summaries, 67*(No. SS-6), 1–23. doi: 10.15585/mmwr.ss6706a1

Bitsko, R. H., Holbrook, J. R., Ghandour, R. M., Blumberg, S. J., Visser, S. N., Perou, R., & Walkup, J. (2018). Epidemiology and impact of healthcare provider diagnosed anxiety and depression among US children. *Journal of Developmental and Behavioral Pediatrics, 39*(5), 395–403. doi:10.1097/DBP.0000000000000571

Centers for Disease Control and Prevention. (2019a). *Children's mental health data & statistics.* Retrieved from https://www.cdc.gov/childrensmentalhealth/data.html

Centers for Disease Control and Prevention. (2019b). *Attention deficit/hyperactivity disorder (ADHD): Data & statistics about ADHD.* Retrieved from https://www.cdc.gov/ncbddd/adhd/data.html

Centers for Disease Control and Prevention. (2020). *Preventing suicide.* Retrieved from https://www.cdc.gov/violenceprevention/suicide/fastfact.html

Centers for Disease Control and Prevention. (n.d.). *Children's mental health.* Retrieved from https://www.cdc.gov/childrensmentalhealth/basics.html

Cree, R. A., Bitsko, R. H., Robinson, L. R., Holbrook, J. R., Danielson, M. L., Smith, D. S., … Peacock, G. (2018). Health care, family, and community factors associated with mental, behavioral, and developmental disorders and poverty among children aged 2–8 years—United States, 2016. *Morbidity and Mortality Weekly Report, 67*(50), 1377–1383. doi:10.15585/mmwr.mm6750a1

Cullen, K. A., Ambrose, B. K., Gentzke, A. S., Apelberg, B. J., Jamal, A., & King, B. A. (2018). Notes from the field: Use of electronic cigarettes and any tobacco product among middle and high school students—United States, 2011–2018. *Morbidity and Mortality Weekly Report, 67*, 1276–1277. doi :10.15585/mmwr.mm6745a5

Danielson, M. L., Bitsko, R. H., Ghandour, R. M., Holbrook, J. R., & Blumberg, S. J. (2016). Prevalence of parent-reported ADHD diagnosis and associated treatment among U.S. children and adolescents. *Journal of Clinical Child & Adolescent Psychology, 47* (2), 199–212, doi:10.1080/15374416.2017.1417860

de Vos, J. A., Radstaak, M., Bohlmeijer, E. T., & Westerhof, G. J. (2018). Having an eating disorder and still being able to flourish? Examination of pathological symptoms and well-being as two continua of mental health in a clinical sample. *Frontiers in Psychology, 9*, 2145. doi:10.3389/fpsyg.2018.02145

Ghandour, R. M., Sherman, L. J., Vladutiu, C. J., Ali, M. M., Lynch, S. E., Bitsko, R. H., & Blumberg, S. J. (2018). Prevalence and treatment of depression, anxiety, and conduct problems in U.S. children. *Journal of Pediatrics, 206*, 256–267.e3. doi:10.1016/j.jpeds.2018.09.021

Harvard Medical School: National Comorbidity Survey. (2017, August 21). *Data table 1: Lifetime prevalence DSM-IV/WMH-CIDI disorders by sex and cohort.* Retrieved from https://www.hcp.med.harvard.edu/ncs/ftpdir/NCS-R_Lifetime_Prevalence_Estimates.pdf

Haworth, C., Carter, K., Eley, T., & Plomin, R. (2017). Understanding the genetic and environmental specificity and overlap between well-being and internalizing symptoms in adolescence. *Developmental Science, 20*, e12376. doi:10.1111/desc.12376

Kaminer, Y., & Godley, M. (2010). Adolescent substance use disorders: From assessment reactivity to post treatment aftercare: Are we there yet? *Child & Adolescent Psychiatric Clinics North America, 19*, 577–590. doi:10.1016/j.chc.2010.03.009

Kaminer, Y., Winters, K. C., & Kelly, J. (2015). Screening, assessment, and treatment options for youth with substance use disorder. In Y. Kaminer (Ed.), *Youth substance abuse and co-occurring disorders*. Washington, DC: American Psychiatric Publishing.

Kleiman, E., & Nock, M. (2018). Real-time assessment of suicidal thoughts and behaviors. *Opinion in Psychology, 22*, 33–37. doi:10.1016/j.copsyc.2017.07.026

Klonsky, E. D., Victor, S. E., & Saffer, B. Y. (2014). Nonsuicidal self-injury: What we know, and what we need to know. *Canadian Journal of Psychiatry, 59*(11), 565–568. doi:10.1177/070674371405901101

Lang, J., McKie, J., Smith, H., McLaughlin, A., Gillberg, C., Shiels, P., & Minnis, H. (2019). Adverse childhood experiences, epigenetics and telomere length variation in childhood and beyond: A systematic review of the literature. *European Child & Adolescent Psychiatry*, 1–10. doi:10.1007/s00787-019-01329-1

Marshall, B. (2018). *Fast facts for managing patients with a psychiatric disorder*. New York, NY: Springer Publishing Company.

Merikangas, K. R., He, J. P., Burstein, M., Swanson, S. A., Avenevoli, S., Cui, L., … Swendsen, J. (2010). Lifetime prevalence of mental disorders in U.S. adolescents: Results from the National Comorbidity Survey Replication-Adolescent Supplement (NCS-A). *Journal of the American Academy of Child and Adolescent Psychiatry, 49*(10), 980–989. doi:10.1016/j.jaac.2010.05.017

National Institute of Mental Health. (2018). *Mental health information: Anxiety disorders*. Retrieved from https://www.nimh.nih.gov/health/topics/anxiety-disorders/index.shtml

National Institute of Mental Health. (n.d.). *Genetics and mental disorders: Report of the National Institute of Mental Health's Genetics Workgroup*. Retrieved from https://www.nimh.nih.gov/about/advisory-boards-and-groups/namhc/reports/genetics-and-mental-disorders-report-of-the-national-institute-of-mental-healths-genetics-workgroup.shtml

Nestler, E., Pena, C., Kundakovic, M., Mitchell, A., & Akbarian, S. (2016). Epigenetic basis of mental Illness. *Neuroscience in Translation, 22*(5), 447–463. doi:10.1177/1073858415608147

Polanczyk, G. V., Salum, G. A., Sugaya, L. S., Caye, A., & Rohde, L. A. (2015). Annual research review: A meta-analysis of the worldwide prevalence of mental disorders in children and adolescents. *Journal of Child Psychology and Psychiatry, 56*, 345–365. doi:10.1111/jcpp.12381

Sornberger, M. J., Smith, N. G., Toste, J. R., & Heath, N. L. (2013). Nonsuicidal self-injury, coping strategies, and sexual orientation. *Journal of Clinical Psychology, 69*(6), 571–583. doi:10.1002/jclp.21947

U.S. Department of Health and Human Services, Substance Abuse and Mental Health Services Administration, Center for Behavioral Health Statistics and Quality. (2018). *National survey on drug use and health 2016 (NSDUH-2016-DS0001)*. Retrieved from https://www.samhsa.gov/data/sites/default/files/NSDUH-DetTabs-2016/NSDUH-DetTabs-2016.pdf

U.S. Preventive Services Task Force. (2016). *Final recommendation statement: Depression in children and adolescents: Screening*. Retrieved from https://www.uspreventiveservicestaskforce.org/Page/Document/RecommendationStatementFinal/depression-in-children-and-adolescents-screening1

World Health Organization. (2014). *Health for the world's adolescents—A second chance in the second decade*. Geneva, Switzerland: Author.

Yearwood, E. L., Pearson, G. S., & Newland, J. A. (2012). *Child and adolescent behavioral health*. West Sussex, UK: Wiley-Blackwell.

▧ Online Resources

The American Academy of Child and Adolescent Psychiatry. Oppositional defiant disorder: Facts for families: https://www.aacap.org/aacap/families_and_youth/facts _for_families/fff-guide/Children-With-Oppositional-Defiant-Disorder-072.aspx

The American Academy of Child and Adolescent Psychiatry. Schizophrenia in children. Facts for families: https://www.aacap.org/AACAP/Families_and_Youth/Facts_for _Families/FFF-Guide/Schizophrenia-In-Children-049.aspx

Centers for Disease Control and Prevention. ADHD fact sheet: https://www.cdc.gov/ ncbddd/adhd/documents/adhdfactsheetenglish.pdf

The National Institute of Mental Health. Ask suicide-screening questions (ASQ) toolkit: https://www.nimh.nih.gov/research/research-conducted-at-nimh/asq-toolkit -materials/index.shtml

National Institutes of Health. Autism spectrum disorder fact sheet: https://www.ninds.nih .gov/Disorders/Patient-Caregiver-Education/Fact-Sheets/Autism-Spectrum-Disorder -Fact-Sheet

Substance Abuse and Mental Health Services Administration. Risk and protective factors 2019: https://www.samhsa.gov/sites/default/files/20190718-samhsa-risk-protective-factors .pdf

Suicide Assessment Five-Step Evaluation and Triage for Mental Health Professionals SAFE-T: https://www.integration.samhsa.gov/images/res/SAFE_T.pdf

CULTURAL DIVERSITY

WILLIAM DAVID KERNAN

LEARNING OBJECTIVES

1. Define culture, diversity, and cultural competence.
2. Explain how cultural identity influences the health and learning of school-aged children.
3. Discuss how the social determinants of health influence the presence of health disparities.
4. Recognize how the school nurse can enhance student success by addressing the cultural influences on health.

▇ Introduction

There is no doubt that our schools comprise a greater diversity of student than at any other point in U.S. history. These students bring with them distinct cultural identities influenced by traditions and practices from around the globe. The changing demographics and increased diversity of school-aged children in the United States creates unique opportunities for learning, particularly as children are exposed to others from backgrounds and experiences different from their own.

All students have a cultural identity defined by myriad factors, including their nationality, race, ethnicity, life experiences, familial norms, spiritual beliefs, socioeconomic status, abilities (and limitations), gender/gender identity, sexuality, and a host of other factors, many of which influence the ways in which health is conceptualized by the student and the family.

Learning and health are inextricably linked and reciprocally related—students learn best in an environment where their health is optimized and they are healthiest when they know how best to protect and maintain their health. This relationship between learning and health is often significantly influenced by cultural traditions, beliefs, and practices, and it is important for the school nurse to understand the ways in which culture influences student health and learning.

Schools are where these different children meet, and ideally learn from, and about, each other. In this chapter the reader will learn information which will help celebrate the richness culturally diversity can bring for all students.

▨ Key Concepts Related to Culture and Health

Culture is an important consideration for those working in the school setting, as it often defines the ways in which people interact with other people and their environments. In schools, culture is ubiquitous. Each person in the school—the children, teachers, support staff, and administrators—all bring with them a unique cultural perspective and identity. Further, the school environment itself is a "culture," with defined standards of conduct and expectations of behavior.

When discussing how the school nurse can develop a greater understanding of the ways that culture might play a role in the health experiences of a student, it is important to begin with an understanding of basic terminology. This is necessary because, for some terms, there are several operational definitions and, for others, no universally accepted definition.

Culture

Multiple definitions of culture exist, each often reflecting a particular discipline or point of view. Culture, in the context of health and illness, broadly refers to a body of knowledge, beliefs, values, and guidelines for behavior shared by members of a particular group of people (Satcher, 2001). Cultural identity often influences how individuals conceptualize their health and their experiences with illness, as well as dictate what they do to protect, enhance, and/or restore their health. In fact, the definitions of *health* and *illness* sometimes vary between cultures (Spector, 2016). For example, some cultures view illness as the influence of an outside force (such as a microorganism or a malevolent spirit) while other cultures view illness as an imbalance between, for example, the physical body and the natural world.

Culturally defined traditions and customs often influence a person's approach to an illness or what they do to maintain their health. Folklore and history are elements of one's cultural identity that may influence their health. For many, culture is manifest in their use of traditional healers, folk medicine, prayer, talismans, herbal remedies, healing rituals, or complementary and alternative medicine (CAM) (Spector, 2016).

For the school nurse, culture can be viewed as a system of "rules" that informs how the child and the family manage their health. As different cultures often have different "rules," it can be challenging for the school nurse to deliver quality healthcare while simultaneously acknowledging and respecting each child's unique cultural identity.

Culture is learned and it develops over time. In the early years, the major influences on a child's culture include the connections that they have with other people and the environment(s) in which they are raised (Office of Disease Prevention and Health Promotion, 2019a). During this time, the child begins to learn the "rules" associated with the culture in which they are raised. They learn when and with whom to communicate, how to behave in social situations, and the consequences related to breaking a "rule."

It is also during this time when culture exerts a great influence on patterns of health-related behaviors, including food selection and other dietary behaviors, the importance of physical activity, and the ways in which the child copes with stress or hardship (National Research Council, 2004). As these behaviors set the foundation for life-long well-being, understanding the influence of culture on health is of paramount importance to those who work with and care for young people.

A child's cultural identity is influenced by many factors, including, but not limited to, their group affiliations, life experiences, and socioeconomic circumstances. The Office of Minority Health (NPIN, 2015, p. 1) acknowledges the importance of group membership, defining culture as "integrated patterns of human behavior that include the language, thoughts, communications, actions, customs, beliefs, values, and institutions of racial, ethnic, religious, or social groups." Therefore, group membership, such as one's racial or ethnic identity, is a central component of one's cultural identity.

Group membership may also be defined in a geographical context (urban/rural or East coast/Midwest, e.g.) or by a common language spoken (Centers for Disease Control and Prevention [CDC], 2019). While each of these group affiliations may, in part, define a child's cultural identity, the school setting often provides new opportunities for group membership. Therefore, a child's cultural identity is further shaped when that child decides to become an athlete, a musician, or a peer leader, for example.

Culture is a filter through which the individual receives and processes health-related information. Culture influences the ways in which people communicate about health, including the language and vocabulary used. Standards about who may communicate with whom, acceptable terminology that may be used, or when communication about a health-related issue may occur are often defined by one's culture. Communication of health-related information is further influenced by an individual's health literacy, which can directly influence whether or not health information is successfully communicated (CDC, 2019).

Health and learning are interrelated. Young people learn best when they are healthy, and health is optimized when students learn to how care for their health (CDC, 2018). Culture plays a significant role in the health experiences of schoolchildren. Therefore, it is critical that the school nurse work to increase cultural understanding and enhance cross-cultural communication skills in order to develop strategies to work with students and families from diverse cultures in support of the learning mission of the school setting.

Cultural Competence

Understanding a student's cultural identity is a necessary step when providing effective healthcare in schools. Therefore, it is important for the school nurse to build upon their understanding of other cultures and develop additional skills to work with students and parents from diverse backgrounds. Possessing the skills to work effectively with individuals from other cultures is a main feature of cultural competence. In order to develop the skills necessary for culturally competent school nursing practice, the school nurse must expand cultural awareness, acquire cultural knowledge, and develop cultural sensitivity (Brownlee & Lee, 2019).

Cultural awareness involves the exploration of one's own cultural identity, including the identification and acknowledgment of any biases toward cultures other than one's own. Acknowledgment of stereotypes, prejudice, and discrimination, and the resultant effect that these have on the health of individuals from other cultures, is an important step in developing cultural awareness (see definitions in Table 13.1).

Cultural knowledge refers to the body of information that the school nurse possesses about a certain cultural group, including its:

- History
- Rules for communication
- Concepts of health and illness
- Dietary practices
- Holidays and cultural celebrations
- Views on mental health, birth, and death
- Systems of healing, including folk medicine or use of traditional healers

Given this long (albeit incomplete) list of culturally informed characteristics, it should be evident that it is not possible for the school nurse to know everything about the cultural identity of each child with whom they work. Cultural knowledge is a process of information acquisition over the period of one's career as a school nurse—it is constantly being learned.

TABLE 13.1 KEY DEFINITIONS RELATED TO CULTURAL AWARENESS

TERM	DEFINITION
Assumption	Something that is accepted as true, even in the absence of evidence to substantiate the claim.
Social bias	Favoring one group over another. Stereotypes, prejudice, and discrimination are all forms of social bias.
Stereotype	The belief that all members of a particular cultural group share the same characteristics.
Prejudice	Possessing an attitude or opinion about a particular cultural group without sufficient preexisting knowledge about that group.
Discrimination	To treat people differently because of their membership in a particular cultural group.
Isms	A belief that differences based on some defining characteristic of a person produce superiority over other people based on that same defining characteristic. These can include: race (racism), sex (sexism), sexuality (heterosexism), age (ageism), etc....

Cultural sensitivity is the recognition that differences and similarities based on culture exist and necessitates an openness to learning about different cultural groups (Brownlee & Lee, 2019). A culturally sensitive school nurse considers cultural factors as an important facet in the delivery of healthcare and does not assign value (i.e., good or bad, or right or wrong) to the differences between cultures.

Culturally competent care is an approach to caring for the health of diverse groups of individuals that values and responds to their health-related beliefs, behaviors, and needs in cultural context. Developing these skills is a life-long process and involves a commitment to learning about the diverse cultural influences on health and understanding the differences among and within cultural groups.

When developing cultural competency, the goal for the school nurse is the delivery of culturally competent care, defined as "care that respects diversity in the patient population and cultural factors that can affect health and healthcare, such as language, communication styles, beliefs, attitudes, and behaviors" (Agency for Healthcare Research and Quality, 2014, p. 1).

Diversity

Culture is a complex concept and no one definition fully expresses the myriad factors that might define an individual's cultural identity. This is true because there are so many factors that comprise an individual's cultural identity, and these factors often differ from individual to individual.

Diversity, in the context of human health, refers to the ranges of differences seen among groups of people. Our schools reflect these differences, resulting in the most diverse population of school children likely ever seen in the United States. This diversity presents unique opportunities and challenges for the school nurse. Therefore, broadening one's understanding of the important role that diversity plays in schools is an essential component of the school nurse's responsibilities.

What factors contribute to the diversity seen in our schools? As mentioned previously, race, ethnicity, and religion represent group affiliations that often influence a child's cultural identity. However, there are many other factors that contribute to the diversity of our schools, including a child's age, gender and gender expression, sexuality, language, health status, physical and intellectual abilities/limitations, and family experiences, among others.

The diversity of our schools can also be viewed in a geographic context. Where children were raised and where they currently live can have a profound influence on their cultural identity. This is often tied to another important component of diversity, socioeconomic status (SES). A child's SES can greatly influence their cultural identity and, in turn, their experiences with health and illness. Moreover, geography and SES are often closely related to health disparities experienced by children (CDC, 2018).

▣ Demography and Demographic Shifts Among School-Aged Children

The diversity of our schools is measured by the science of demography, or the statistical study of populations of people based on some defining characteristic(s) of those people. Several demographic variables are frequently used to classify or count groups of people and often these variables are elements of one's cultural identity. In the United States, demographic data about race, ethnicity, religion, and SES can aid the school nurse in better understanding the diverse cultural identities of school-aged children in the United States and in their community.

Race and Ethnicity

Race and ethnicity are two common classifications of groups of people that carry cultural significance. However, when attempting to describe an individual's cultural identity, it is important to note that race and ethnicity are not synonymous concepts. Multiple definitions of each concept exist, and there is not always agreement on the best definition.

When census data about race is collected in the United States, race refers to "a person's self-identification with one or more social groups. An individual can report as White, Black or African American, Asian, American Indian and Alaska Native, Native Hawaiian and Other Pacific Islander, or some other race" (United States Census Bureau, 2017, p. 1).

As with race, there is no universal definition of ethnicity. In the context of the study of health and illness, a useful definition of ethnicity is the sharing of a strong sense of identity with people who share common characteristics, which could include:

- ▪ Race
- ▪ Religion
- ▪ Nationality or geographic origin
- ▪ Language
- ▪ Culture (dietary practices, values, art, symbols, etc…)

Ethnicity often serves to tie groups of people together around common cultural themes, including celebrations, rites of passage, holidays, political views, and community associations (Spector, 2016). While ethnicity is a multifactorial concept, when census data are collected in the United States, ethnicity measures whether a person is, or is not, of Hispanic descent (U.S. Census Bureau, 2017).

The United States is becoming more racially and ethnically diverse. By the year 2050, the majority of Americans will be non-White. The changing demographic profile of the school-aged population in the United States reflects this overall trend. These changes include:

- ▪ An increase in enrollment in U.S. public schools (including both traditional public schools and public charter schools) from 47.2 million students in fall 2000 to 50.4 million students in fall 2015 (Parker, Morin, & Horowitz, 2019), and

- An increasing racial and ethnic diversity of parents, resulting in a more diverse population of school-aged children (Devine, 2017).
- As illustrated in Figure 13.1,
  - A substantial decrease in the number of White students between 2000 and 2015, and a much smaller decline in Black students during that same time period;
  - A substantial increase in the number of Hispanic students, from 16% to 26%; and
  - Increases, although much smaller in magnitude, among Asian/Pacific Islanders (National Center for Education Statistics, 2019).

Figure 13.1 further displays enrollment predictions for fall 2027 indicting a continued decline in enrollment among White students and a sustained increase in the number of Hispanic students (National Center for Education Statistics, 2019). This predictive model indicates that U.S. schools will continue to enroll an increasingly diverse and multicultural group of students.

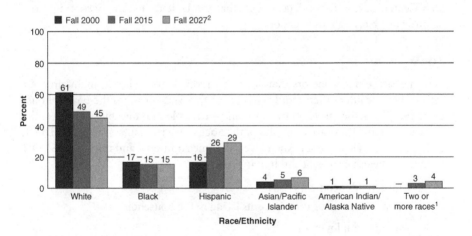

FIGURE 13.1 Percentage distribution of public school students enrolled in pre-kindergarten through 12th grade, by race/ethnicity: Fall 2000, fall 2015, and fall 2027.

—, NOT AVAILABLE.

[1] In 2000, data on students of two or more races were not collected.

[2] Projected.

NOTE: Race categories exclude persons of Hispanic ethnicity. Although rounded numbers are displayed, the figures are based on unrounded estimates. Detail may not sum to totals because of rounding. SOURCE: U.S. Department of Education, National Center for Education Statistics, Common Core of Data (CCD), "State Nonfiscal Survey of Public Elementary and Secondary Education," 2000–01 and 2015–16 (https://nces.ed.gov/programs/raceindicators/indicator_rbb.asp); and National Elementary and Secondary Enrollment Projection Model, 1972 through 2027.

Religion

With frequent national debates about school prayer, creationism, and evolution in the curriculum, and the Pledge of Allegiance, religion has long been a contentious issue within U.S. public schools. Nevertheless, the school nurse must take into consideration the important role that religion plays in the lives and well-being of students. In fact, a recent survey of American teenagers indicated that religious activities are part of the typical school day for many students. Often these activities involve wearing jewelry or clothing with religious significance or engaging in prayer before eating or prior to a sporting event (PEW Research Center, 2019).

As with race and ethnicity, shifts are occurring in terms of the numbers of Americans of different faith affiliations. In 2014, 70.6% of Americans identified as a member of one of the Christian faiths. However, in 2007 this percentage was 78.4%, representing a 7.8% decline in the number of Christians in the U.S. during that time. During that same period, the number of Americans reporting no religious affiliation (atheist, agnostic, or nothing) rose from 16.1% to 22.8% (a 6.7% increase). Furthermore, the number of American's practicing a non-Christian faith rose 1.2% (from 4.7% to 5.9%), with increases seen among the Jewish, Muslim, and Hindu faiths (PEW Research Center, 2015). These data suggest that the United States is becoming more religiously diverse, as are our schools.

Poverty

SES is one of the major factors that affects an individual's ability to maintain their health and the health of their family (CDC, 2014). SES determines the type of housing one can afford, the modes of transportation available, and the ability to access the healthcare system. These are examples of the Social Determinants of Health (SDOH; see Figure 13.2). While not an exhaustive list, some additional and important SDOH related to the health of school children include:

- Household income
- Presence of one or more parents living in the household
- Parental employment
- Level of parental education
- Parental health literacy
- Neighborhood safety, crime, violence
- Food security, access to healthy food
- Parental incarceration
- Social cohesion
- Pollution, access to clean air and drinking water

Due to the significant influence of the SDOH on individual health, *Healthy People 2020*, the nation's health agenda, identifies several specific objectives in this area, and tracks data to measure progress toward meeting each objective. As shown in

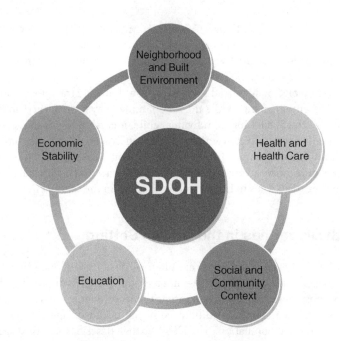

FIGURE 13.2 The Social Determinants of Health (SDOH).

SOURCE: Office of Disease Prevention and Health Promotion. (2019c, October 25). *Healthy People 2020:* Social determinants of health. Retrieved from https://www.healthypeople.gov/2020/topics -objectives/topic/social-determinants-of-health

TABLE 13.2 SELECT SDOH OBJECTIVES FROM *HEALTHY PEOPLE 2020*

	2010	2011	2012	2013	2014	2015	2016	2017
Percentage of children aged 0–17 years living with at least one parent employed year round, full time	71	71	73	73	74	75	77	78
Percentage of children aged 0–17 years living in poverty	22.0	21.9	21.8	21.5	21.1	19.7	18.0	17.5

SDOH, social determinants of health.
SOURCE: Office of Disease Prevention and Health Promotion. (2019b, October 25). *Healthy People 2020:* Social determinants of health data report. Retrieved from https://www.healthypeople.gov/ 2020/data-search/Search-the-Data#topic-area=3499

Table 13.2, *Healthy People 2020* data indicates a decrease in the proportion of children in the United States living in poverty since 2010 (Office of Disease Prevention and Health Promotion, 2019b). A continued decline in childhood poverty rates was reported between 2017 and 2018, with 16.2% of children under the age of 18 living in poverty in 2018 (Semega, Kollar, Creamer, & Mohanty, 2019). Reducing the proportion of children who live in poverty is of critical importance in the school setting, as poverty has been associated with poor learning and health outcomes (Robinson et al., 2017).

The SDOH involve major social systems, such as housing, transportation, law enforcement, and employment. While the school nurse may have limited ability to influence many of the SDOH for an individual child, it is essential for the school nurse to understand that the conditions in which children live, learn, and play have a direct and significant impact on their health and well-being. Furthermore, it is important for the school nurse to be aware that these social influences on health can be a driving force behind the disparities in health among children in the school environment.

▉ Health Disparities in the School Setting

The terms "diversity" and "disparity" are often confused. As defined previously, diversity refers to a range of differences within a group. The term disparity is the quantification of those differences, where a disparity means a *large* difference. Therefore, a health disparity is a significant difference in the health of one population when compared to another population. The CDC further describes health disparities as "preventable differences in the burden of disease, injury, violence, or opportunities to achieve optimal health that are experienced by socially disadvantaged populations" (2018, p. 1).

Two major forms of health disparity exist. A disparity in *health status* occurs when one group of disadvantaged individuals experiences a disproportionate burden of disease or injury. A disparity in *healthcare* exists when individuals from disadvantaged populations do not have equal access to the healthcare necessary to meet their needs. Both types of health disparities are important to identify and address when working with the school-aged population.

Health disparities exist because of many complex and interrelated factors, most of which have roots in historic and contemporary sociocultural inequalities. Social class, often defined by socioeconomic factors such as income, wealth, employment, and level of education, is a powerful driver of health disparities. As a resultant, disparities in health are directly linked to the unequal distribution of resources and experiences with poverty, segregation, and racism (LaVeist, 2005).

Because health disparities are most often associated with race, ethnicity, and SES, children of color and children from low-income families experience health disparities at greater rates than do other groups of children. Addressing the health disparities that exist among U.S. school children is of critical importance as health issues early in life can result in poorer health outcomes later in life (Robinson et al., 2017).

When addressing health disparities in the school setting, the goal is to create an equitable environment for students that acknowledges their unique cultural identity. Therefore, it is important to move beyond the idea of providing equal access to health services for students, as this may not adequately address the health disparities that are present. In many instances, the equal distribution of resources, services, and/or opportunities is not enough for each student to achieve optimal health. However, some students need a bigger boost than others. Therefore, an equitable distribution of resources, services, and/or opportunities based on the unique characteristics and needs of each student does provide access to all. Achieving an equitable environment in the school setting can help address health disparities.

Culture in Transition

Some aspects of a child's culture are inherited from previous generations while others are learned through life experiences. As a result, a child's cultural identity often changes over time to reflect new experiences, environments, or social situations (Kim, 2017). This is particularly true for children who move from one geographic location to another during their school years. The process of adapting to a new culture is particularly important for the school nurse to understand, as there are many reasons why children may relocate during the school years.

The school nurse may work with children who are in transition for a variety of reasons, including:

- Children whose home environment has changed, including adoptees and children in the foster system;
- Children who have moved geographically from one location to another, including foreign exchange students, immigrants, refugees, and asylees;
- Children who move because of their parent's employment, such as the children of migrant workers, military parents, missionaries, and foreign diplomats. Third-culture kids, referring to children who were raised in a culture other than that of their parent, is a subpopulation of this group.

A child who transitions from one living environment to another may face a number of challenges, including the loss of social connections, isolation, stress, and culture shock. It is common for a child to experience shifts in cultural identity when they begin to live within a new culture, particularly if that new culture has one dominant cultural group identity.

While some children retain their cultural identities when in transition, others do not. The process by which individuals from one cultural group adopt the standards and practices of another group is called acculturation. This process can be difficult for many, as they must interact with a dominant culture where the language, clothing, food, and healthcare systems may be very different from their home culture (Kim, 2017). The school nurse has an important role in supporting students as they transition into a new school setting and, possibly, a new culture.

Six Cultural Phenomena That Affect Health

The school nurse's role in the delivery of culturally competent services can seem overwhelming, as it involves:

- Understanding one's own culture as well as the cultural identities of others;
- Recognizing the diversity that exists within a multicultural school environment;
- Identifying and addressing health disparities; and
- Supporting students who may be experiencing transition in their cultural identities.

Given this long list of responsibilities, it is not possible for a school nurse to learn everything there is to know about every child's unique cultural identity. Furthermore, it is also important to note that not everyone who identifies with a particular culture follows all of the practices or traditions generally attributed to that culture.

One model to assist the school nurse to assess and care for students from diverse cultures is the Transcultural Assessment Model (Giger & Davidhizar, 1988). This model emphasizes that each individual has a distinctive cultural identity that is influenced by the following six phenomena that vary among cultures.

Biological Variation

Biological differences that exist among cultural groups are important to understand. Biochemical differences in susceptibility to certain diseases and nutritional differences are examples of this biological variation (Spector, 2016). It should be noted, however, that biological differences account for a very small proportion of the health disparities experienced by individuals from different cultural groups. More often, these differences can be explained by the sociocultural environment in which that person lives.

Communication

Communication can be one of the more challenging aspects of working with children and families from other cultures. As guidelines for communication are often defined by one's culture, there is great potential for miscommunication in a cross-cultural interaction. Aspects of communication to be considered by the school nurse include language differences, nonverbal forms of communication, and silence.

In some cultures, silence is used as a precursor to the delivery of bad news, while in others it is viewed as a necessary part of the exchange of information, allowing the listener time to process the new information and develop questions. Eye contact is another form of communication that often has cultural significance. In some cultures, eye contact is used to reassure someone while in other cultural settings eye contact is considered aggressive or rude. In fact, communication and culture are so interrelated that the U.S. government has established a set of standards that provide a road map for navigating communication issues during cross-cultural interactions in the healthcare setting. These are presented in the next section.

Environmental Control

An individual's locus of control may be influenced by their cultural identity. Someone with an internal locus of control believes that they possess the ability to control their environment, while someone with an external locus of control believes that they do not have a great deal of control over their environment. Therefore, environmental control refers to the ability of a person from a given cultural group to actively control nature and to direct factors in their environment (Giger & Davidhizer, 2002).

The school nurse may encounter a child whose family is using a cultural practice, such as a form of traditional healing or herbal remedy, to treat a particular illness. This may be the family's way of exerting environmental control. Likewise, environmental control is evident when a family advocates on behalf of their child with a severe allergy, physical limitation, or learning-related challenge. At times, the methods by which a family attempts to exert environmental control conflict with established school policies or procedures. It is therefore the school nurse's role to better understand the cultural context when providing care to the student.

Social Organization

Social organization refers to the patterns of behavior expressed in the family unit (Giger & Davidhizer, 2002). This may include the ways in which the family views life events, such as birth, death, child rearing, health, and illness. Rites of passage, celebrations, prayer, and participation in community events are additional elements of one's culture that relate to social organization.

In some cultures, the family unit is viewed as a central component of well-being and, therefore, attendance at celebrations, holidays, and family gatherings is regarded as more important than attendance at school. The roles that different individuals have in the family are also culturally defined. A school nurse may interact with a student who has a significant caretaking role for a younger sibling or grandparent. Knowing this will help the school nurse better understand the stressors that the student may be facing, or help explain school absences or a decline in academic achievement.

Space

Different cultures have different rules about the area surrounding a person's body as well as expectations about acceptable distance between individuals during interactions (Giger & Davidhizer, 2002). Violation of these rules and expectations can result in cross-cultural misunderstanding or conflict. The school nurse must be cognizant of personal space in order to avoid a situation where an individual feels as though their territory has been violated.

The school nurse may find that students from some cultures maintain distance during a health assessment or express discomfort when the assessment requires a more intimate interaction. Other children may exhibit behavior that indicates that they have very few space restrictions. This can manifest in the need for close proximity and physical contact, such as a reassuring hand on the shoulder or a hug.

Time

Individuals from different cultures may experience time differently. Some cultures are past-oriented, while others focus on the present or future. Culture also influences the amount of time an individual devotes to a certain activity, or how frequently they participate (Giger & Davidhizer, 2002). Because the U.S. educational system, as well as the healthcare system, are based around appointments and deadlines with expectations about attendance and timeliness, the influence of culture on time orientation can play a significant role in the interactions between the school nurse and a child and their parents.

For example, the school nurse may observe that parents from certain cultures make plans for their child's healthcare in advance, ensuring that their child receives routine medical, dental, and vision exams. This illustrates a cultural practice that is future-oriented. Individuals from a future-oriented culture are more likely to attend screening events and prevention programs. Conversely, the school nurse may interact with parents from a present-oriented culture. Individuals with this cultural perspective on time may value family obligations or social interactions more than they value being on time for an appointment at the school.

An understanding of the six cultural phenomena outlined in the Transcultural Assessment Model can assist the school nurse to better understand the sorts of things that often differ among cultures. This will allow the school nurse to perform a culturally informed health assessment and provide a plan of care for a student that takes into account their cultural identity.

▩ Cultural Competence for the School Nurse

A recent assessment of cultural competence among school nurses revealed that the majority of school nurses surveyed were familiar with the cultural composition of their student population and a large proportion (81.3%) reported that they could identify the health disparities present among the students they serve. Additionally, well over three quarters of the school nurses surveyed could describe the SDOH, indicating that most school nurses understand the underlying reasons why health disparities exist (Matza, Maughan, & Barrows, 2015).

This same study revealed several barriers faced by school nurses, including language/communication, lack of resources, and work-related constraints, such as lack of support within the school and time constraints (Matza et al., 2015). With these barriers in mind, there are several things that a school nurse can do to increase cultural competency.

Expand Cultural Awareness

A first step in expanding cultural awareness is for the school nurse to conduct a cultural self-inventory with the goal of better understanding how one's own cultural identity influences cross-cultural interactions with students and their families. The school nurse should reflect on their own feelings about the various cultural, ethnic, and religious groups present in the school setting. During this process, it is important to identify assumptions and biases. The use of a standardized self-evaluation tool can assist the school nurse in this process (Carr & Knutson, 2015).

It is also important for the school nurse to recognize that in a cross-cultural context, there are often competing philosophies about the source of an illness or the best way to treat the illness. Increasing one's awareness about these competing philosophies can assist the school nurse in developing an appropriate plan of care while simultaneously respecting that student's cultural beliefs and traditions.

Increase Cultural Knowledge

The school nurse should view the acquisition of cultural knowledge as a lifelong learning process. There are several ways to increase cultural knowledge, including:

- Seeking out continuing education opportunities that focus on cultural issues. Access to online professional development for nurses has increased in recent years. Attendance at cultural competency trainings is associated with improved self-confidence and cultural assessment skills (Matza et al., 2015),
- Asking questions. Many people enjoy sharing their cultural backgrounds and traditions. Asking questions can reveal important information during a clinical assessment. Asking students and their families about their beliefs about the source, severity, and potential treatments related to an illness can assist the school nurse in better understanding how to deliver culturally competent care. Asking questions is also important because not all individuals from the same culture share the same beliefs or engage in the same practices.

Enhance Cross-Cultural Communication Skills

Culture and language differences frequently result in miscommunication or misinterpretation in the clinical setting. Therefore, the school nurse must develop cross-cultural communication skills to minimize the potential for misunderstanding. To guide clinicians when engaged in cross-cultural communication, in 2000 the Office of Minority Health developed a set of 15 standards to guide clinicians as they work to improve cultural competency. The Culturally and Linguistically Appropriate Services (CLAS) standards (see Table 13.3) were developed to increase patient satisfaction, engagement, and their overall experience (OMH, 2018).

In addition to the CLAS standards, several other resources exist that will assist the school nurse when engaged in cross-cultural communication. These include:

- The *Guide to Providing Effective Communication and Language Assistant Services*, published by the Office of Minority Health;
- The *Cultural Competency and Health Literacy Primer*, a free resource published by the University Maryland's School of Public Health;
- The *Language Access Portal*, provided by the National Institute on Minority Health and Health Disparities; and
- If it is determined that an interpreter must be employed to facilitate communication, the *American Translators Association (ATA)* can help locate translators and interpreters.

TABLE 13.3 NATIONAL CULTURALLY AND LINGUISTICALLY APPROPRIATE SERVICES (CLAS) STANDARDS

THE NATIONAL CLAS STANDARDS ARE INTENDED TO ADVANCE HEALTH EQUITY, IMPROVE QUALITY, AND HELP ELIMINATE HEALTHCARE DISPARITIES BY ESTABLISHING A BLUEPRINT FOR HEALTH AND HEALTHCARE ORGANIZATIONS TO:	
PRINCIPAL STANDARD	
1	Provide effective, equitable, understandable, and respectful quality care and services that are responsive to diverse cultural health beliefs and practices, preferred languages, health literacy, and other communication needs.
GOVERNANCE, LEADERSHIP AND WORKFORCE	
2	Advance and sustain organizational governance and leadership that promotes CLAS and health equity through policy, practices, and allocated resources.
3	Recruit, promote, and support a culturally and linguistically diverse governance, leadership, and workforce that are responsive to the population in the service area.
4	Educate and train governance, leadership, and workforce in culturally and linguistically appropriate policies and practices on an ongoing basis.
COMMUNICATION AND LANGUAGE ASSISTANCE	
5	Offer language assistance to individuals who have limited English proficiency and/or other communication needs, at no cost to them, to facilitate timely access to all healthcare and services.
6	Inform all individuals of the availability of language assistance services clearly and in their preferred language, verbally and in writing.
7	Ensure the competence of individuals providing language assistance, recognizing that the use of untrained individuals and/or minors as interpreters should be avoided.
8	Provide easy-to-understand print and multimedia materials and signage in the languages commonly used by the populations in the service area.
ENGAGEMENT, CONTINUOUS IMPROVEMENT, AND ACCOUNTABILITY	
9	Establish culturally and linguistically appropriate goals, policies, and management accountability, and infuse them throughout the organization's planning and operations.
10	Conduct ongoing assessments of the organization's CLAS-related activities and integrate CLAS-related measures into measurement and continuous quality improvement activities.
11	Collect and maintain accurate and reliable demographic data to monitor and evaluate the impact of CLAS on health equity and outcomes and to inform service delivery.
12	Conduct regular assessments of community health assets and needs and use the results to plan and implement services that respond to the cultural and linguistic diversity of populations in the service area.
13	Partner with the community to design, implement, and evaluate policies, practices, and services to ensure cultural and linguistic appropriateness.

(continued)

TABLE 13.3 NATIONAL CULTURALLY AND LINGUISTICALLY APPROPRIATE SERVICES (CLAS) STANDARDS (*CONTINUED*)

THE NATIONAL CLAS STANDARDS ARE INTENDED TO ADVANCE HEALTH EQUITY, IMPROVE QUALITY, AND HELP ELIMINATE HEALTHCARE DISPARITIES BY ESTABLISHING A BLUEPRINT FOR HEALTH AND HEALTHCARE ORGANIZATIONS TO:	
14	Create conflict and grievance resolution processes that are culturally and linguistically appropriate to identify, prevent, and resolve conflicts or complaints.
15	Communicate the organization's progress in implementing and sustaining CLAS to all stakeholders, constituents, and the general public.

SOURCE: Office of Minority Health United States Department of Health and Human Services. (2018). *The National CLAS Standards*. Retrieved from https://minorityhealth.hhs.gov/omh/browse.aspx?lvl =2&lvlid=53

Diagnose Health Disparities

The school nurse plays an important role in the school setting when it comes to understanding the impact of sociocultural issues on health, and the resultant impact of poor health on student learning. Because the school nurse has the ability to view the child within their environmental context, the school nurse is able to both diagnose a health concern, as well as identify any health disparities that may be present for that student.

Cheng, Emmanuel, Levy, and Jenkins (2015) suggest two specific activities for clinicians related to the identification of health disparities:

1. Diagnose the disparities that are present for the individual child during the clinical encounter. This may involve asking the child about their living conditions, family structure, food access, social support, or access to healthcare outside of the school setting.

2. Diagnose the disparities that are present in the larger community by using available data about the local conditions where students live as well as the health status of children and their families. These data, available online, can assist the school nurse to understand changing demographics or disease trends in communities.

When a community assessment has identified the presence of health disparities within a given population, the school nurse can use this information to identify other children who may be at risk. Early intervention with children from disadvantaged cultural groups can provide critical connections to services that will better allow those students to reach their full potential (Robinson et al., 2017).

Serve as a School-Wide Advocate

The school nurse is well positioned to promote an atmosphere of respect, understanding, and acceptance throughout the school. This can be achieved by providing opportunities for both students and staff to share their cultural experiences (Loschiavo, 2019). When working on multidisciplinary teams within the school setting, the school nurse can ensure that culture, diversity, the social determinants of health, and health disparities remain a central part of the conversation. Further, the school nurse can support multicultural training opportunities for staff.

Conclusion

Everyone who works within the school environment is ultimately responsible for supporting the learning of the children under their care and supervision. As culture influences a student's health in a variety of ways, and as a student's health status often determines how well they are able to learn, the role of the school nurse in providing culturally competent healthcare is paramount in supporting the learning mission of the school. To achieve this, the school nurse can act as an advocate for students from all cultures and serve as a cultural liaison between the school, students, and their parents. In doing so, school nurses must offer a safe and welcoming environment for students from diverse cultures and be open to learning about each student's unique cultural identity.

References

Agency for Healthcare Research and Quality. (2014, July 9). *Improving cultural competence to reduce health disparities for priority populations*. Retrieved from https://effectivehealthcare.ahrq.gov/products/cultural-competence/research-protocol

Brownlee, T., & Lee, K. (2019). *Building culturally competent organizations*. Retrieved from https://ctb.ku.edu/en/table-of-contents/culture/cultural-competence/culturally-competent-organizations/main

Carr, B., & Knutson, S. (2015). Culturally competent school nurse practice. *NASN School Nurse, 30*(6), 336–342. doi:10.1177/1942602X15605169

Centers for Disease Control and Prevention. (2014, March 10). *NCHHSTP social determinants of health*. Retrieved from https://www.cdc.gov/nchhstp/socialdeterminants/faq.html

Centers for Disease Control and Prevention. (2018, August 17). *Health disparities*. Retrieved from https://www.cdc.gov/healthyyouth/disparities/index.htm

Centers for Disease Control and Prevention. (2019, October 17). *Culture and health literacy*. Retrieved from https://www.cdc.gov/healthliteracy/culture.html

Cheng, T. L., Emmanuel, M. A., Levy, D. J., & Jenkins, R. R. (2015). Child health disparities: What can a clinician do? *Pediatrics, 136*(5), 961–968. doi:10.1542/peds.2014-4126

Devine, J. (2017, August 9). *Birth, deaths, and migration transform communities*. Retrieved from https://www.census.gov/library/stories/2017/08/changing-nation-demographic-trends.html

Giger, J. N., & Davidhizar, R. (2002). The Giger and Davidhizar transcultural assessment model. *Journal of Transcultural Nursing, 13*(3), 185–188. doi:10.1177/10459602013003004

Giger, J. N., & Davidhizar, R. E. (Eds.). (1998). *Canadian transcultural nursing: Assessment and intervention*. St. Louis, MO: Mosby.

Kim, Y. Y. (2017). Cross-cultural adaptation. *Oxford Research Encyclopedia of Communication*. doi:10.1093/acrefore/9780190228613.013.21

LaVeist, T. A. (2005). *Minority populations and health: An introduction to health disparities in the United States* (*Vol. 4*). Hoboken, NJ: John Wiley & Sons.

Loschiavo, J. (2019). *Fast facts for the school nurse: School nursing in a nutshell*. New York, NY: Springer Publishing Company.

Matza, M., Maughan, E., & Barrows, B. M. (2015). School nurse cultural competence needs assessment: Results and response. *NASN School Nurse, 30*(6), 344–349. doi:10.1177/19 42602X15608188

National Center for Education Statistics. (2019, February). *Status and trends in the education of racial and ethnic groups—Indicator 6: Elementary and secondary enrollment*. Retrieved from https://nces.ed.gov/programs/raceindicators/indicator_rbb.asp

National Prevention Information Network, Centers for Disease Control and Prevention. (2015). *Cultural Competence*. Retrieved from https://npin.cdc.gov/pages/cultural -competence

National Research Council. (2004). *Children's health, the nation's wealth: Assessing and improving child health*. Washington, DC: National Academies Press.

Office of Disease Prevention and Health Promotion. (2019a, October 25). *Early childhood development and education*. Retrieved from https://www.healthypeople.gov/2020/topics -objectives/topic/social-determinants-health/interventions-resources/early-childhood-0

Office of Disease Prevention and Health Promotion. (2019b, October 25). *Healthy People 2020: Social determinants of health data report*. Retrieved from https://www .healthypeople.gov/2020/data-search/Search-the-Data#topic-area=3499

Office of Disease Prevention and Health Promotion. (2019c, October 25). *Healthy People 2020: Social determinants of health*. Retrieved from https://www.healthypeople .gov/2020/topics-objectives/topic/social-determinants-of-health

Office of Minority Health United States Department of Health and Human Services. (2018). *The National CLAS Standards*. Retrieved from https://minorityhealth.hhs.gov/ omh/browse.aspx?lvl=2&lvlid=53

Parker, K., Morin, R., & Horowitz, J. (2019, March 21). *Looking into the future, public sees an America in decline on many fronts*. Retrieved from the PEW Research Center website: https://www.pewsocialtrends.org/2019/03/21/public-sees-an-america-in-decline-on -many-fronts/

PEW Research Center. (2015, May 12). *America's changing religious landscape*. Retrieved from https://www.pewforum.org/2015/05/12/americas-changing-religious-landscape/

PEW Research Center. (2019, October 3). *For a lot of American teens, religion is a regular part of the public school day*. Retrieved from https://www.pewforum.org/2019/10/03/ for-a-lot-of-american-teens-religion-is-a-regular-part-of-the-public-school-day/

Robinson, L. R., Bitsko, R. H., Thompson, R. A., Dworkin, P. H., McCabe, M. A., Peacock, G., & Thorpe, P. G. (2017). CDC grand rounds: Addressing health disparities in early childhood. *MMWR Morbidity and Mortality Weekly Report, 66*(29), 769. doi:10.15585/ mmwr.mm6629a1

Satcher, D. (2001). *Mental health: Culture, race, and ethnicity—A supplement to mental health: A report of the surgeon general*. Retrieved from https://www.ncbi.nlm.nih.gov/ books/NBK44249/

Semega, J., Kollar, M., Creamer, J., & Mohanty, A. (2019, September). *Income and poverty in the United States: 2018* (Report No. P60-266). Washington, DC: United States Census Bureau.

Spector, R.E. (2016). *Cultural diversity in health and illness*. Upper Saddle River, NJ: Pearson.

U.S. Census Bureau. (2017, January). *Race and ethnicity*. Retrieved from https://www. census.gov/mso/www/training/pdf/race-ethnicity-onepager.pdf

Online Resources

Centers for Disease Control and Prevention. *Culture and health literacy*. Retrieved from https://www.cdc.gov/healthliteracy/culture.html

Healthy People 2020. Social determinants of health. Retrieved from https://www.healthypeople.gov/2020/topics-objectives/topic/social-determinants-of-health

National Association of School Nurses. *Cultural competency*. Retrieved from https://www.nasn.org/nasn-resources/practice-topics/cultural-competency

School Nurse Transcultural. *Nursing society*. Retrieved from https://tcns.org/

U.S. Department of Health and Human Services. *Office of minority health*. Retrieved from https://www.minorityhealth.hhs.gov

U.S. Department of Health and Human Services. *Think cultural health*. Retrieved from https://thinkculturalhealth.hhs.gov/

Further Reading

Fadiman, A. (2012). *The spirit catches you and you fall down: A Hmong child, her American doctors, and the collision of two cultures*. New York, NY: Macmillan.

14

SUBSTANCE ABUSE IN SCHOOL-AGED CHILDREN

WILLIAM DAVID KERNAN

LEARNING OBJECTIVES

- Define and differentiate substance misuse and substance abuse.
- Explain the reasons why youth use drugs.
- List current trends in drug use in the United States.
- Discuss vulnerable student populations in the context of drug use.
- Describe the role of the school nurse in the prevention of drug use among school children.

Introduction

Childhood and adolescence are developmental points in life where the young person is confronted with many new experiences, opportunities, and temptations. As this is naturally a time for discovery and experimentation, it should be no surprise that many youth are reporting their first experiences with drug use at increasingly younger ages.

A quick study of the history of drug use and misuse in the United States illustrates that drug trends emerge and subside over time, with new drugs coming to the fore. Present day concerns center on what many call the opioid "epidemic." Other drugs of current concern include anabolic steroids and synthetic cannabinoids, among others. However, it is important to note that the major drugs used by young people have remained relatively stable over time—alcohol, tobacco, and marijuana.

As this is a developmental period in which experimentation and drug use often occur, the school nurse will undoubtedly confront students who require assessment and treatment. The school nurse can also play a pivotal role in supporting evidence-based prevention programming in the school setting.

If anything is to be learned from history, it is that risk-taking behavior is a common feature of the developmental experience of many young people. In this chapter, the reader will learn information that will help schools better prepare for and respond to the issues that arise due to youth substance use.

History of Illegal Substance Use in the United States

Humans have used, misused, and abused drugs for many centuries; however, drug abuse research is only a few hundred years old. In 1806, a German pharmacist working with crude opium isolated morphine, representing the first addictive ingredient (aside from distilled alcohol) ever isolated from a natural product. Born from these early days of drug and addiction research was a new science that was to discover many new, but now commonly known, facts, including:

- Morphine is an effective treatment for physiological pain.
- Addiction to a drug often results in an individual prioritizing their drug use over deteriorating life circumstances.
- Giving an individual more of a drug quickly reverses the effect of withdrawal from that same drug (Musto, 1996).

Over 200 years later, a science that traces its roots back to research about a naturally occurring substance isolated from a flower native to Turkey (the poppy *Papaver somniferum*), is now struggling to solve a decades-long crisis involving that same drug. For researchers, healthcare providers, and substance abuse prevention professionals, today's opioid crisis is of great concern, particularly for those who work with youth. However, while opioids are a major drug of concern at present, drug abuse is certainly not a new social problem. In the United States, drugs trends ebb and flow. Table 14.1 presents a brief history of U.S. drug trends, major policy decisions, and federal enforcement efforts.

TABLE 14.1 A BRIEF HISTORY OF MILESTONES RELATED TO SUBSTANCE ABUSE IN THE UNITED STATES

1910	Bellevue Hospital (NYC) admitted its first case of heroin dependence.
1914	The Harrison Act caused development of positive changes in drug treatment. Narcotics were only available with a prescription.
1915	Bellevue Hospital (NYC) admitted 425 patients for heroin addiction.
1936	Federal Bureau of Narcotics was organized and took a stand against drug abuse.
1960s	Common drugs used for recreational purposes included marijuana, lysergic acid diethylamide (LSD), cocaine, heroin, and hallucinogens.
1965	Amphetamines (speed) became popular with young adults.
1971	Naloxone hydrochloride is developed as an antidote for opioid overdose.

(continued)

TABLE 14.1 A BRIEF HISTORY OF MILESTONES RELATED TO SUBSTANCE ABUSE IN THE UNITED STATES (*CONTINUED*)

1973	U.S. Drug Enforcement Administration founded.
1974	National Institute on Drug Abuse (NIDA) founded.
1980s	Hallucinogens and cocaine are commonly used in social settings. Schools adopted policies for students suspected of drug use.
1983	DARE (Drug Abuse Resistance Education) was developed as a school-based intervention taught by police officers (National Institute of Justice, 2011).
1985	Highly addictive crack cocaine was developed.
1988	Office of National Drug Control Policy founded.
Late 1980s	Drug testing began in a small number of public schools.
1990s	Methamphetamine (crystal meth) in use. Increase in heroin use—smoked and snorted.
1992	Substance Abuse and Mental Health Services Administration founded.
Late 1990s	Rise in deaths related to prescription opioids first recognized, despite the pharmaceutical industry's reassurance that patients would not become addicted to prescription opioids (NIDA, 2019a)
1996	California became the first state to legalize medical marijuana
2006	Centers for Disease Control and Prevention (CDC) implemented additional mechanisms to track and collect data about the growing opioid overdose crisis (CDC, 2019a) Electronic cigarettes first introduced in the United States.
2011	Food and Drug Administration announces regulation of e-cigarettes to be consistent with traditional cigarette regulation.
2012	Colorado and Washington become the first states to legalize recreational marijuana.
2017	Physician-directed medical use of marijuana is permitted in some schools for specific conditions. Laws are passed in all 50 states and the District of Columbia to increase public access to naloxone.
2019	CDC reports multistate outbreak of lung injury associated with the use of vaping products.

SOURCE: Adapted from Loschiavo, J. (2020). *Fast facts for the school nurse: School nursing in a nutshell* (3rd ed.). New York: NY, Springer Publishing Company.

▇ Substance Use Among Youth Today

Much is known about youth substance use today. National data about substance use among young people is readily available and collected periodically by several agencies within the federal government, including:

■ *The Youth Risk Behavior Surveillance System (YRBSS),* which collects data about alcohol, tobacco, and other drug use. Developed in 1990 and managed by the Centers for Disease Control and Prevention (CDC), the YRBSS, periodically collects data from representative samples of 9th through 12th grade students (CDC, 2018a).

■ The *Monitoring the Future Survey*, first conducted in 1975, collects nationwide data from adolescents about drug and alcohol use as well as their attitudes about substance use. This annual survey is managed by the National Institute on Drug Abuse (NIDA, 2019b).

■ The *School Health Policies and Practices Study (SHPPS)* assesses school health policies and practices. The survey is conducted periodically at one or more of the following levels: state, district, school, and classroom (CDC, 2019c).

Data from these and other ongoing studies provide important information to those who work to prevent substance use among youth and can be valuable sources of information for the school nurse.

■ Key Definitions

As with any topic, it is important to begin with an understanding of basic terminology. This is particularly important when discussing substance use because precise definitions of terms sometimes vary depending on context and setting. It is possible for a term used in substance use prevention programs to have a slightly different meaning for individuals who treat substance use disorders. Likewise, some terms have a different significance depending on the target population or the setting. The way a term might be used when working with youth in schools might vary slightly when working with adults in community settings. Therefore, the terms follow are defined in the context of a nurse who is working with youth and adolescents in the school setting.

The US Food and Drug Administration (FDA) defines a **drug** as "a substance (other than food) intended to affect the structure or any function of the body" (FDA, 2017, p. 1). Individuals for many different reasons—to prevent illness, treat disease, alter state of mind, and improve performance, among others—use drugs. When used appropriately, drugs can promote health and treat illness. However, when misused or abused, drugs can have deleterious effects on the well-being of the user. In this chapter, the terms "drug" and "substance" are used interchangeably.

Drugs are classified in several ways. Drugs can be grouped in terms of their recognized medical use as an over-the-counter (OTC) medication, a prescription medication, or a drug that has no accepted medical use (many of these are referred to as **illicit drugs**). In the United States, to protect the public from drugs that are potentially dangerous and/or addictive, since 1970, the Controlled Substances Act (CSA) classifies drugs using a Schedule based on each drug's medicinal value and potential to be harmful and/or addictive (U.S. Drug Enforcement Administration [DEA], 2017).

Drugs are also classified based on certain distinguishing properties of the drug. The DEA recognizes five classes of drugs, including:

■ Narcotics (commonly referred to as opioids)
■ Depressants

■ Stimulants

■ Hallucinogens

■ Anabolic steroids

Drugs within the same class often produce similar physiological effects in the user. As defined by the DEA (2017), **drug abuse** refers to:

■ The use of any drug that is inconsistent with its recognized medical use;

■ The non-sanctioned use of a controlled substance as defined by the CSA; or

■ The use of a pharmaceutical drug in any way other than that prescribed by a medical provider.

This last example is often referred to as **drug misuse**. Other examples of drug misuse include taking a medicine that was prescribed to another person and taking a medicine solely for the resultant intoxicating effect (NIDA, 2018).

■ Why Youth Use Drugs

As a developmental period known for self-discovery, boundary testing, and thrill seeking, it is no surprise that 90% of addictions start in the teen years (Partnership for Drug-Free Kids, 2018b). There are some fundamental reasons why youth use drugs, including:

■ To alter feelings: Different drugs act on the body in different ways, but many drugs used by young people result in feelings of pleasure, euphoria, increased energy, relaxation, increased self-confidence, and satisfaction (NIDA, 2014).

■ To reduce anxiety or stress: It is common for students to report increased levels of stress related to the expectations of their family, peers, teachers, and coaches. Some drugs produce a calming effect on the body, allowing individuals who experience social anxiety or fear of public speaking, for example, to engage more fully in those activities (NIDA, 2014).

■ To avoid, alter, or escape reality: Teens sometimes turn to drugs as a way to cope when healthier outlets do not seem readily apparent. Boredom is frequently reported by teens as a reason for their drug use (Hart & Ksir, 2018).

■ To improve performance: The school setting can introduce additional pressures on youth, particularly in an increasingly competitive society. Some drugs improve physical performance while others can enhance a student's ability to focus on schoolwork (NIDA, 2014).

■ Curiosity: Some youth report experimentation with drugs as a way to seek out new experiences or engage in new behaviors that they perceive as exciting or daring. Teenagers who see their parents or other adults enjoying drinking alcohol and smoking cigarettes may be curious to experience those same effects (Partnership for Drug-Free Kids, 2018a).

■ To mitigate social pressures: The influence of peers, especially during youth and adolescence, is a powerful force behind many health-related behaviors, including substance use (Hart & Ksir, 2018).

Additional reasons often reported by young people for their drug use include rebellion, the desire for instant gratification, self-medication to alleviate physical pain, and messages received from the media and popular culture (Partnership for Drug-Free Kids, 2018a). It is important for the school nurse to understand the constellation of reasons why a student may initiate, and then continue, using a drug. These "root causes" of drug use are often complex and difficult to address in the school setting alone. Assisting a young person with a substance use disorder requires a team effort within the school setting, and often, it is necessary to draw upon community resources as well.

■ Effects of Drug Abuse on Youth

Frequently, drug misuse and abuse negatively affects the physical and the mental health of young people and commonly results in social, academic, and legal problems (CDC, 2019d; Substance Abuse and Mental Health Services Administration [SAMHSA], 2019). The consequences of drug use can be viewed in developmental, health status, and environmental context.

■ Development: Drug use can be particularly damaging to the young person because their bodies are still growing and developing. In particular, the effects of drug use on the development of the adolescent brain are increasingly better understood. During adolescence, the prefrontal cortex and the outer mantle of the brain continue to develop. As these areas are responsible for reasoning, information processing, attention, perception, and impulse control, drug use during this period can be harmful in both the present and future (SAMHSA, 2019)

■ Health status: Judgment and inhibition are often impaired by drug use. Therefore, substance use increases risky behavior among many youth, putting them at greater risk for sexually transmitted infections, interpersonal violence, and unintentional injury. Drug use during youth and adolescence is associated with the development of health problems later in life, including sleep disorders, cardiovascular disease, and high blood pressure. Furthermore, use of drugs at a young age can increase the chance that a substance use disorder will develop in later adolescence or adulthood (CDC, 2019d)

■ Environment: Drug use frequently puts young people at odds with their environment. Drug use can result in a variety of social problems. This can include difficulties within the family unit, peer group, or with individuals of institutions of authority, such as law enforcement (NIDA, 2014)

■ Common Drugs Used by Youth

It is important for those working in the school setting to understand the range of drugs commonly used by youth, as well as the health-related consequences of their use. It is equally important for the school nurse to understand trends in drug use and emerging drugs of abuse.

Alcohol and marijuana are the most commonly used drugs among adolescents today and national data indicates that these substances have been the most used by young people for the past several decades. While tobacco use rates have declined, the emergence of e-cigarettes is increasing the number of youth consuming nicotine. Other drugs commonly used by youth often differ between age groups. Younger students report greater use of inhalants while use of synthetic marijuana is more likely to be used by older teens (NIDA, 2014). Table 14.2 provides the street names of some of the most common drugs used by youth.

During this past decade, prescription drug misuse, particularly prescription pain-killers, has increased substantially among teens (SAMHSA, 2019). Indeed, data from the Monitoring the Future Study suggests that misuse of prescription and OTC medications account for a large proportion of the drugs used by 12th grade students (NIDA, 2014). While it is not possible to review every drug used by young people today, the sections that follow provide a data snapshot for each of the drugs most commonly used by youth and adolescents in the United States:

TABLE 14.2 STREET NAMES OF DRUGS COMMONLY USED BY YOUTH

Alcohol	Booze, Brew, Liquor
Anabolic steroids	Gym Candy, Juice, Roids
Bath Salts	Bloom, Cloud Nine, Vanilla Sky, White Lightening
Cocaine	Blow, Bump, C, Coke, Coca, Flake, Rock, Snow, Toot
Cough and cold medicine	Candy, Dex, Drank, Robo, Skittles, Triple C, Tussin, Velvet
Ecstasy (MDMA)	Adam, Beans, Clarity, Hug, Love Drug, E, XTC
Heroin	Black Tar, Brown Sugar, H, Horse, Smack, Junk, Ska
Inhalants	Bold, Laughing Gas, Poppers, Snappers, Whippets
Marijuana	Grass, Herb, Mary Jane, Reefer, Hash, Pot, Weed, Skunk
Methamphetamine	Meth, Crank, Crystal, Speed
Salvia	Magic Mint, Sally-D, Ska Pastora, Maria Pastora
Spice	Fake Weed, K2, Skunk, Yucatan Fire
Tobacco	Chew, Cigs, Dip, Snuff

SOURCE: National Institute on Drug Abuse. (2019, October 30). *Teens: Drug facts.* Retrieved from https://teens.drugabuse.gov/teens/drug-facts

TABLE 14.3 TRENDS IN PREVALENCE OF ADOLESCENT ALCOHOL USE. NATIONAL YRBSS DATA: 1991 TO 2017

PERCENTAGES														TREND FROM 1991 TO 2017A	CHANGE FROM 2015 TO 2017B
1991	1993	1995	1997	1999	2001	2003	2005	2007	2009	2011	2013	2015	2017		
EVER DRANK ALCOHOL (at least one drink of alcohol on at least 1 day during their life)															
81.6	80.9	80.4	79.1	81.0	78.2	74.9	74.3	75.0	72.5	70.8	66.2	63.2	60.4	Decreased 1991–2017 Decreased 1991–2007 Decreased 2007–2017	No change
DRANK ALCOHOL BEFORE AGE 13 YEARS (had their first drink other than a few sips)															
32.7	32.9	32.4	31.1	32.2	29.1	27.8	25.6	23.8	21.1	20.5	18.6	17.2	15.5	Decreased 1991–2017 No change 1991–1999 Decreased 1999–2017	No change
CURRENT ALCOHOL USE (at least one drink of alcohol on at least 1 day during the 30 days before the survey)															
50.8	48.0	51.6	50.8	50.0	47.1	44.9	43.3	44.7	41.8	38.7	34.9	32.8	29.8	Decreased 1991–2017 Decreased 1991–2007 Decreased 2007–2017	No change

[a]Based on linear and quadratic trend analyses using logistic regression models controlling for sex, race/ethnicity, and grade, $p < .05$. Significant linear trends (if present) across all available years are described first followed by linear changes in each segment of significant quadratic trends (if present).
[b]Based on t-test analysis, $p < .05$.
SOURCE: Centers for Disease Control and Prevention. (2018, June 14). *Youth risk behavior surveillance system (YRBSS)* overview. Retrieved from https://www .cdc.gov/healthyyouth/data/yrbs/overview.htm

Alcohol

Youth alcohol use presents a serious public health concern, as it is associated with morbidity and mortality related to alcohol poisoning, motor vehicle accidents, unintentional injury, suicide, sexual assault, and high-risk sexual behavior. More than 4,300 youth die each year because of excessive use of alcohol. Alcohol use among youth is also associated with impaired judgment, memory problems, academic and social difficulties at school, abuse of other drugs, and legal problems (CDC, 2018b; U.S. Department of Health and Human Services [HHS], 2019).

National data reveal that alcohol is the most commonly used substance among adolescents. The most recently available YRBSS data indicate that in 2017:

- 60.4% of ninth to 12th graders surveyed indicated that they had consumed at least one drink of alcohol during their lifetime;
- 15.5% of those surveyed reported that they consumed their first alcoholic drink before the age of 13; and
- 29.8% of those surveyed reported that in the 30 days before completing the survey, that they had consumed at least one drink of alcohol (CDC, 2018a).

Table 14.3 displays these data in historical context. While youth alcohol use remains high, as shown in the table, for each of these three indicators of alcohol use, the proportion of adolescents reporting use has decreased dramatically. However, this trend seems to be leveling off, as there is no statistically significant difference in use between 2015 and 2017.

Participation in risky behavior is often associated with alcohol use among adolescents. YRBSS data reveal that, in the past 30 days, 14% of high school students engaged in binge drinking, 17% were a passenger in a car with a driver who had been drinking alcohol, and 6% drove after drinking alcohol (CDC, 2018b). The danger associated with alcohol use significantly increases when alcohol is mixed with other drugs, including many prescription and OTC drugs (Calhoun, 2017).

Tobacco

As stated in Healthy People 2020, "tobacco use is the single most preventable cause of disease, disability, and death in the United States" (Office of Disease Prevention and Health Promotion, 2019). Tobacco use has long been a concern for public health officials not only because of the highly addictive nature of nicotine, but also because of the many toxic chemicals produced by smoking tobacco, including tar, carbon monoxide, and the nitrosamines (NIDA, 2019c).

The proportion of youth who report using tobacco has declined steadily over the past 25 years:

- In 1991, 70.1% of ninth to 12th graders surveyed reported that they had ever tried cigarette smoking. In 2017, this proportion decreased to 28.9% (a difference of 41.2%),

- 27.5% of students surveyed in 1991 indicated that they had smoked at least one cigarette in the past 30 days. In 2017, only 8.8% reported current cigarette use (an 18.7% decline),

- Current frequent cigarette use, defined as smoking on 20 or more days during the 30-day period before the survey, was reported by 12.7% of the students in 1991 and 2.6% of the students in 2017 (a 10.1% decline), and

- Current daily cigarette use was reported by 9.8% of the students in 1991 and 2.0% in 2017 (a 7.8% decline). For complete data, see Table 14.4.

While use of tobacco has declined over the past several decades, because of the serious long-term consequences related to tobacco and the increasing availability of e-cigarettes and similar products used by young people, use of products containing tobacco remain a significant concern in the school setting.

Marijuana

Marijuana (cannabis) is classified by the federal government as a Schedule I substance under the Controlled Substances Act, therefore making its distribution illegal. This means it has no accepted medical use and has a high potential for dependency (National Conference of State Legislatures, 2019). However, with growing cultural acceptance of marijuana use in the United States, new formulations and higher potencies of the drug, and an increasing number of states that have legalized the use of marijuana for medical and/or recreational purposes, the school nurse must recognize the effect that this changing cannabis landscape has on youth use and the perceptions of the harm related to use.

Marijuana use among ninth to 12th graders has increased in the past several decades:

- The proportion of high school students who reported ever using marijuana in 1991 was 31.3%. In 2017, 35.6% of respondents indicated lifetime marijuana use (+4.3% difference).

- The proportion of high school students reporting current marijuana use during the past 30 days before the survey rose 5.1%, from 14.7% in 1991 to 19.8% in 2017 (CDC, 2018a).

Tetrahydrocannabinol (THC) is the psychotropic ingredient in marijuana and is responsible for many of the mind-altering effects that users seek. THC concentrations in marijuana today are much stronger than in the early 1990s, particularly when users consume cannabis extracts and resins. These extracts, sometimes called hash oil, budder, wax, or shatter, are several times more potent than the psychoactive ingredient found in the cannabis plant (NIDA, 2019c).

Synthetic marijuana, also called "K2" or "spice," is a designer drug that does not come from the cannabis plant, but is designed to mimic the effects of THC. Widely available in convenience stores beginning in the mid-2000s, K2 became a popular drug among youth. While sale of synthetic cannabinoids are now largely prohibited, new formulations being sold as "incense" or "potpourri" are not yet regulated and

TABLE 14.4 TRENDS IN PREVALENCE OF ADOLESCENT TOBACCO USE.NATIONAL YRBSS DATA: 1991 TO 2017

	1991	1993	1995	1997	1999	2001	2003	2005	2007	2009	2011	2013	2015	2017	TREND FROM 1991 TO 2017A	CHANGE FROM 2015 TO 2017B
PERCENTAGES																
EVER TRIED CIGARETTE SMOKING (even one or two puffs)																
	70.1	69.5	71.3	70.2	70.4	63.9	58.4	54.3	50.3	46.3	44.7	41.1	32.3	28.9	Decreased 1991–2017 No change 1991–1997 Decreased 1999–2017	No change
CURRENT CIGARETTE USE (on at least 1 day during the 30 days before the survey)																
	27.5	30.5	34.8	36.4	34.8	28.5	21.9	23.0	20.0	19.5	18.1	15.7	10.8	8.8	Decreased 1991–2017 Increased 1991–1999 Decreased 1999–2017	No change
CURRENT FREQUENT CIGARETTE USE (on 20 or more days during the 30 days before the survey)																
	12.7	13.8	16.1	16.7	16.8	13.8	9.7	9.4	8.1	7.3	6.4	5.6	3.4	2.6	Decreased 1991–2017 Increased 1991–1999 Decreased 1999–2017	Na change
CURRENT DAILY CIGARETTE USE (on all 30 days during the 30 days before the survey)																
	9.8	10.0	12.2	12.2	12.8	10.3	7.6	7.2	6.1	5.3	4.8	4.0	2.3	2.0	Decreased 1991–2017 Increased 1991–1999 Decreased 1999–2017	No change

SOURCE: Centers for Disease Control and Prevention. (2018, June 14). *Youth risk behavior surveillance system (YRBSS) overview.* Retrieved from https://www .cdc.gov/healthyyouth/data/yrbs/overview.htm

continue to appear in retail establishments (DEA, 2017). Data from the *Monitoring the Future* study indicate that 3.5% of 12th graders have used a synthetic cannabinoid in the past year (NIDA, 2019b).

Opioids

Opioids are a classification of drugs that include opium, opium derivatives, and their semi-synthetic substitutes. These drugs act on pain receptors in the body to dull the senses and relieve physical pain. As such, many opioid formulations are used in pharmaceutical drugs (e.g., morphine, methadone, OxyContin, Vicodin, and fentanyl). Heroin is an illicit opioid drug (DEA, 2017).

The YRBSS first collected data about the use of heroin among ninth to 12th graders in 1999; however, it wasn't until 2017 that the YRBSS collected data about the misuse of prescription opioids. During the period between 1999 and 2017, youth lifetime use of heroin remained low, with 2.4% reporting use in 1999 and 1.7% reporting use in 2017. However, youth misuse of prescription opioids is much higher, with 14.0 of respondents indicating lifetime use in 2017. While not statistically significant, female students (14.4%) were slightly more likely than male students (13.4%) to misuse a prescription opioid medication. Misuse of prescription opioids was highest among Hispanic students (15.1%), followed by White students (13.5%) and Black students (12.3%; CDC, 2018a).

Opioid use among youth presents a unique challenge to the school nurse. As many opioids are legally prescribed medications, it can be difficult to know which students are using the drug under a doctor's order and which are not. However, as the nation is in the midst of an opioid crisis largely fueled by the misuse of prescription opioids, it is important for the school nurse to remain involved in bringing greater awareness about the dangers of prescription opioid misuse in the school setting.

Inhalants

Inhalants represent a wide variety of invisible, volatile substances which, when inhaled, result in psychoactive or mid altering effects. Many commonly available household items are inhaled by youth, including dry erase markers, correction fluid, paint thinner, spray paint, glue, butane, air freshener, and cooking spray. Inhalants may be sniffed directly from their original container, but are more commonly used by "bagging" (inhaling the fumes from a substance placed in a plastic or paper bag) or "huffing" (inhaling the fumes from an inhalant-soaked rag that is stuffed in the mouth).

An inhalant is frequently the first drug used by a young person, and it is reported that one in five children has used an inhalant by the eighth grade (DEA, 2017). Therefore, assessing for use of inhalants may be particularly important for the nurse who works with younger students.

Current Issues in Drug Use

As mentioned in the opening paragraphs, drug trends change over time, reflecting societal influences and the preferences of the consumer. While there are always new and emerging issues related to youth substance abuse, several current issues are particularly relevant for the school nurse to understand.

Prescription Drug Misuse

Prescription drug misuse, most notably misuse of prescription opioid medications, is one of the fastest emerging drug problems in the United States. In 2018, 15.5% of high school seniors reported misusing a prescription drug at some point in their life. Among this same group, 9.9% reported past year use and 4.2% reported past month use (NIDA, 2019b).

Many young people believe that use of prescription drugs is safer, or at least less harmful to one's health, than the use of other drugs. However, misuse of prescription drugs has been associated with a number of short- and long-term health outcomes. Prescription drugs used by youth are often selected because of their resultant effects on the body (see Table 14.5). Prescription drugs are often more accessible to young people, as these drugs are frequently diverted from their intended purpose, usually when a young person accesses a family member's medications for their own use or to distribute to their peers.

Drug diversion is defined as the "illegal distribution or abuse of prescription drugs or their use for unintended purposes" (Centers for Medicare & Medicaid Services [CMS], 2014). Common classifications of prescription drugs that are frequently diverted and misused by youth include stimulants, depressants, and opioids (SAMHSA, 2019).

Prescription stimulants used to treat attention deficit hyperactivity disorder (ADHD) and narcolepsy (Ritalin and Adderall) are sometimes misused by young

TABLE 14.5 PHYSICAL HEALTH EFFECTS OF COMMON SUBSTANCES USED BY YOUNGPEOPLE

DEPRESSANTS	STIMULANTS	OPIOIDS
Slurred speech	Paranoia	Drowsiness
Shallow breathing	Dangerously high body temperature	Nausea
Fatigue	Irregular heartbeat	Constipation
Disorientation	Excitation	Slowed respiration
Lack of coordination	Insomnia	

SOURCE: Substance Abuse and Mental Health Services Administration. (2019, August 2). *Rise in prescription drug misuse and abuse impacting teens.* Retrieved from https://www.samhsa.gov/homelessness-programs-resources/hpr-resources/teen-prescription-drug-misuse-abuse

people because they believe the drug will improve their mental functioning and boost their academic performance (NIDA, 2018). Past year misuse of Ritalin among high school seniors in 2018 was less than 1%, representing a significant decrease in use since 2015. Likewise, past year use of Adderall decreased from 7.5% in 2015 to 4.6% in 2018 among high school seniors (NIDA, 2019b).

While the large majority of teens do not report prescription depressant use, they are misused by some teens to get "high," to counteract the effect of other drugs, or to induce sleep. In 2018, lifetime use of prescription tranquilizers was 3.5% among eighth graders, 6.0% among 10th graders, and 6.6% among 12th graders (NIDA, 2019c).

Of all the prescription drugs that are misused, perhaps the most concerning are the prescription opioids due to their highly sought-after pain relieving effects and great potential for abuse and addiction. Until recent legislation in many jurisdictions restricted the amount of prescription opioid that could be prescribed in the health-care setting, access to these medications was widespread, particularly among youth with sports-related injuries or those recovering from recent surgery. In part due to new prescribing guidelines and other prevention initiatives, misuse of prescription opioids like Vicodin and OxyContin has declined steadily among youth since 2009 (NIDA, 2019c).

■ The Opioid Crisis

Drug overdose deaths continue to rise in the United States, largely fueled by the misuse and abuse of prescription and illicit opioid drugs. Between 1999 and 2017, nearly 400,000 Americans (adults and youth) died from an opioid drug overdose. Figure 14.1 illustrates three distinct "waves" in opioid overdose deaths during this time, including:

- First wave: Beginning in 1999, opioid overdose deaths largely involved the use of prescription opioids (both natural and semi-synthetic).

- Second wave: Beginning in 2010, there was a rapid increase in opioid overdose deaths involving heroin.d

- Third wave: Beginning in 2013, opioid overdose deaths increasingly involved illicitly manufactured synthetic opioids, such as fentanyl (IMF). IMF was also found to be combined with other drugs, such as heroin and cocaine (CDC, 2018c).

Early in the opioid crisis, efforts by public health officials focused on decreasing public access to prescription opioid medications and increasing access to naloxone (Narcan, Evzio), an opioid antagonist medication designed to rapidly reverse an opioid overdose. Programs to monitor rates of physician prescribing were initiated and physicians found to be overprescribing opioids or operating "pill mills" faced professional and legal consequences. In recognition of the significant risks to youth related to the diversion of prescription opioids, programs to raise awareness about the dangers of keeping unused prescription medications in the household began to surface at both the state and federal levels. To assist those individuals already using opioids, efforts were increased to provide greater access to Medication Assisted Treatment (MAT).

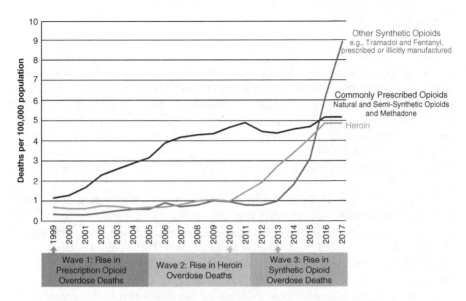

FIGURE 14.1 U.S. mortality data related to opioid drugs, 1999-2017.

SOURCE: Centers for Disease Control and Prevention. (2020). *Understanding the epidemic. Opioid overdose.* Retrieved from https://www.cdc.gov/drugoverdose/epidemic/index.html

In 2017, the White House declared the opioid crisis a public health emergency. Concurrently, several federal initiatives were put in place to combat this crisis. That same year, the HHS (2018) unveiled a five-point strategy to combat the opioid crisis that includes:

- Improved access to opioid prevention, treatment, and recovery services;
- Collecting more timely and specific public health data related to the opioid crisis;
- Promoting health and evidence-based methods of pain management, including the development of alternative, non-addictive approaches to pain management;
- Improved targeting of overdose-reversing drugs and better access to naloxone at the community level;
- Better research on pain and addiction (HHS, 2018).

Youth use of heroin remains relatively low and use of prescription opioids is currently in decline among adolescents in the United States (CDC, 2018a). However as teens leave school and enter adulthood, the likelihood that they may use a prescription or illicit opioid drug increases. Past year use data indicates that young adults aged 18 to 24 are the most likely age group to engage in the non medical use of opioids (National Academies of Sciences, Engineering, and Medicine, 2017). Therefore, schools must prepare students through education and prevention initiatives with the knowledge and skills needed to refrain from opioid drug misuse while enrolled in school and thereafter.

▨ Vaping

Perhaps one of the most concerning drug trends seen in recent years among youth is that of vaping. Vaping is the inhalation of vapor through the mouth from an electronic device that heats up and turns a liquid or solid substance into an aerosol that can be inhaled into the lungs (Loschiavo, 2020). These electronic devices have a variety of common names, including "e-cigs," "vapes," "mods," "e-hookahs," "vape pens," and "electronic nicotine delivery systems (ENDS)." E-cigarettes come in a variety of shapes. Some look like cigarettes, cigars, or pipes; others are attached to small tanks; while others may look like everyday items, such as pens or USB flash drives (CDC, 2019b).

This particular issue is of paramount importance in the school setting. Driven by widespread availability and the belief that they are safer than cigarette's, the use of e-cigarette's and related products has increased significantly among adolescents since they were first introduced in the United States in 2006 (Partnership for Drug-Free Kids, 2018b). Indeed, among youth, e-cigarettes are now the most commonly used tobacco product.

Use of e-cigarettes in youth may increase the likelihood that young people will smoke cigarettes later in life (CDC, 2019b). This is troubling as a recent study of U.S. middle and high schools students found that 3.6 million youth reported use of e-cigarettes in the past 30 days, including 4.9% of students in middle school and 20.8% of students in high school (Cullen et al., 2018).

E-cigarettes and other forms of vaping products are used by young adults to deliver a variety of substances. While many youth use these products to consume tobacco, these systems are also used to deliver marijuana (hash oil or other THC-rich extracts) and other drugs (Partnership for Drug-Free Kids, 2018b). Many of these products contain fruit or candy flavoring, and youth often report these flavorings as the primary reason why they use e-cigarettes. While the long-term health effects of vaping are not fully understood, recent national reports warn of significant serious health issues associated with the use of vaping products, including lung injury and death (CDC, 2019b).

▨ The Role of the School Nurse

On issues related to substance abuse the school nurse wears many hats. From administering the school's drug-testing program to the early identification of students who may have substance use disorders, the school nurse is a central figure in providing substance use and abuse services in the school setting. It often falls to the school nurse to be the gatekeeper of school drug policies as well as the person who raises the alarm when new drug trends emerge within the school setting.

The school nurse is also someone who is sought out by other school personnel for questions related to student substance abuse. As such, the school nurse is responsible for maintaining an accurate and current working knowledge of issues related to substance use as well as acting as an advocate for youth. Therefore, there are several things the school nurse can do to ensure the provision of high-quality care.

Recognize That Easy Access Facilitates Substance Use

Drug use occurs in an environment where there is ready access to the substance. The school nurse must understand that for many youth, substances of abuse are readily accessible in their homes, work settings, and community. According to a 2017 national survey of high school students, the school environment itself often provides access to illegal drugs. When asked if ever offered, sold, or given an illegal drug on school property in the 12 months before the survey, 19.8% responded "yes" (CDC, 2018a). Working with school officials and local substance abuse prevention organizations, the school nurse can be part of a team effort in bringing about community awareness about the local conditions that facilitate youth access to drugs.

Identify Vulnerable Students

Several factors can make a student more vulnerable to drug abuse than their peers. It is important for the school nurse to recognize the various factors that might be associated with drug use as the presence of these factors might put a student at higher risk. It is equally important to note that the presence of one or more of these characteristics does not mean that a student will use drugs.

One group of high-risk students are those who experience major life transitions while in school. Changes in the school of enrollment, the home environment, or health status can all cause upset and disruption such that the young person seeks out substances for relief or escape. Other major life changes that may put a young person at greater risk for substance abuse include parental divorce, loss of a loved one, sudden illness of a family member, or experiences with bullying (Loschiavo, 2020). Young people who have experienced a traumatic life event, such as being involved in a natural disaster or witnessing violence or a fatal accident, are known to be at higher risk for substance abuse later in life (Partnership for Drug-Free Kids, 2018a).

A young person's social environment may also increase their likelihood of using a drug. In one large-scale study, marijuana use was associated with living in a rough neighborhood, associating with drug-using peers, lack of participation in religious activities, and having parents who do not seem to care. This same study found that students who perform poorly in school, who steal, or who get into fights were also more likely to report use (Hart & Ksir, 2018). This is particularly true for teens who have impulse control problems or who frequently take risks (Partnership for Drug-Free Kids, 2018a).

Biological factors that may put some students at higher risk include mental health or behavioral issues that affect a young person's ability to regulate emotions and thoughts, such as anxiety, depression, or ADHD. Family history of drug use can also place a student at greater risk, particularly when the child's parents have substance abuse problems (Partnership for Drug-Free Kids, 2018a).

Students returning to school after a medical illness or injury may be a higher risk for substance use. For example, when a student athlete returns to school after treatment for a sports-related injury the school nurse should question the student concerning what pain medication they are is taking (Loschiavo, 2020). If the school nurse learns that the student is prescribed a prescription opioid, it can be used as an opportunity to educate the student about the dangers associated with misuse.

Ensure Evidence-Based Substance Abuse Policy Development

As the medical professional in the school setting, the school nurse should be active in an advisory capacity to school administrators when drafting new or revising existing policies that relate to student substance use, misuse, and abuse. This can be a challenging role for the school nurse as the number of substance-related issues has significantly increased in the past several decade. Schools commonly have policies related to drug-testing, tobacco use, and alcohol use on school grounds. With recent emerging drugs trends, schools have had to consider policies about vaping and the use of e-cigarettes among youth, naloxone access in schools, and the medical use of cannabis on school grounds. The school nurse can provide the necessary medical and health promotion information needed for effective policy development.

Encourage School-Wide Prevention Programming

While it may not be the primary role of the school nurse when providing health care to students in the school setting, the school nurse can team up with other specialized support staff in the school to initiate and promote substance abuse prevention programming. Prevention programming is most effective when offered at each level of prevention:

- Primary prevention programs targeted specifically at students who have not yet begun to misuse or abuse substances
- Secondary prevention programs aimed at identifying students who use substances and may have experienced negative consequences related to their use, but who have not yet developed a substance use disorder
- Tertiary prevention programs to identify and assist students who require professional treatment for a substance use disorder

Programs can also target parents by providing them important information about drug abuse and trends. Recent studies have shown that the presence of a caring adult (a parent or a guardian) who speaks with their child regularly about substance abuse and other issues of concern can lower rates of substance abuse among children (National Center on Addiction and Substance Abuse, 2010). In support of this, the school nurse promote the use established national campaigns, including the *Stop Medicine Abuse* and *Talk, They Hear You* prevention programs.

The school nurse may also be directly involved in the school health curriculum in several ways, including the development of substance abuse lesson plans, providing health teachers with updated content and instructional material, or connecting the school curriculum to substance abuse prevention resources in the community. When appropriate, the school nurse can make time in their busy schedule to teach in the classroom setting or provide guest lectures (Loschiavo, 2020).

Enhance Perceptions of School Connectedness

Another important protective factor against youth substance abuse is the concept of **school connectedness**, which is "the belief held by students that adults and peers in the school care about their learning as well as about them as individuals" (CDC, 2018d, p. 1). Students who feel a sense of connectedness to their school are more likely to regularly attend school, remain enrolled, and experience higher grades and exam scores. Furthermore, these same students are less likely to carry weapons, be involved in violence, or engage in risky activities, such as drinking and driving. School nurses can enhance the sense of school connectedness among students by encouraging students to reaffirm their commitment to their education and encourage membership in positive peer groups. Furthermore, in the role of trusted adult, the school nurse can offer a safe and welcoming environment for students in times of need or crisis.

Conclusion

In summary, it should be emphasized that the prevention of substance abuse and the identification and treatment of students who are using and abusing drugs is not the sole responsibility of the school nurse. It must be a team effort involving school administrators, counselors, support staff, parents, and, of course, the students. The school nurse provides many services in the school setting and, in doing so, may be one of the first individuals to learn of a student's drug use. The school nurse can provide the necessary healthcare for the student, while simultaneously acting as a student advocate, a liaison with the parents, and a source of important health information for colleagues within the school.

References

Calhoun, N. (2017). *The dangers of prescription drug abuse*. Santa Cruz, CA: Journeyworks Publishing.

Centers for Disease Control and Prevention. (2018a, June 14). *Youth risk behavior surveillance system (YRBSS) overview*. Retrieved from https://www.cdc.gov/healthyyouth/data/yrbs/overview.htm

Centers for Disease Control and Prevention. (2018b, August 2). *Fact sheets—Underage drinking*. Retrieved from https://www.cdc.gov/alcohol/fact-sheets/underage-drinking.htm

Centers for Disease Control and Prevention. (2018c, December 19). *Opioid basics*. Retrieved from https://www.cdc.gov/alcohol/fact-sheets/underage-drinking.htm

Centers for Disease Control and Prevention. (2018d, August 7). *School connectedness*. Retrieved from https://www.cdc.gov/healthyyouth/protective/school_connectedness.htm

Centers for Disease Control and Prevention. (2019a, January 11). *CDC's response to the opioid overdose epidemic.* Retrieved from https://www.cdc.gov/opioids/strategy.html

Centers for Disease Control and Prevention. (2019b, March 11). *Electronic cigarettes.* Retrieved from https://www.cdc.gov/tobacco/basic_information/e-cigarettes/index.htm

Centers for Disease Control and Prevention. (2019c, May 7). *School health policies and practices study (SHPPS).* Retrieved from https://www.cdc.gov/healthyyouth/data/shpps/index.htm

Centers for Disease Control and Prevention. (2019d, April 1). *Teen substance use and risks.* Retrieved from https://www.cdc.gov/features/teen-substance-use/index.html

Centers for Disease Control and Prevention. (2020). *Understanding the epidemic. Opioid overdose.* Retrieved from https://www.cdc.gov/drugoverdose/epidemic/index.html

Centers for Medicare & Medicaid Services. (2014, January). *What is a prescriber's role in preventing the diversion of prescription drugs?.* Retrieved from https://www.pharmacy.umn.edu/sites/pharmacy.umn.edu/files/prescriber_role_in_preventing_diversion.pdf

Cullen, K. A., Ambrose, B. K., Gentzke, A. S., Apelberg, B. J., Jamal, A., & King, B. A. (2018). Notes from the field: Use of electronic cigarettes and any tobacco product among middle and high school students—United States, 2011–2018. *Morbidity and Mortality Weekly Report, 67*(45), 1276. doi: 10.15585/mmwr.mm6745a5

Food and Drug Administration. (2017, November 14). *Drugs@FDA glossary of terms.* Retrieved from https://www.fda.gov/drugs/drug-approvals-and-databases/drugsfda-glossary-terms

Hart, C., & Ksir, C. (2018). *Drugs, society and human behavior.* Boston, MA: McGraw-Hill.

Loschiavo, J. (2020). *Fast facts for the school nurse: School nursing in a nutshell* (3rd ed.). New York, NY: Springer Publishing Company.

Musto, D. F. (1996). Drug abuse research in historical perspective. In Committee on Opportunities in Drug Abuse Research (Ed.), *Pathways of addiction: Opportunities in drug abuse research* (pp. 284–294). Washington, DC: National Academies Press.

National Academies of Sciences, Engineering, and Medicine. (2017). *Pain management and the opioid epidemic: Balancing societal and individual benefits and risks of prescription opioid use.* Washington, DC: National Academies Press.

National Center on Addiction and Substance Abuse. (2010, August). *National survey of American attitudes on substance abuse XV: Teens and parents.* New York, NY: Columbia University.

National Conference of State Legislatures. (2019, October 16). *State medical marijuana laws.* Retrieved from http://www.ncsl.org/research/health/state-medical-marijuana-laws.aspx

National Institute of Justice. (2011, June 3). *Program profile: Drug abuse resistance education (DARE).* Retrieved from https://www.crimesolutions.gov/ProgramDetails.aspx?ID=99

National Institute on Drug Abuse. (2014, January). *Principles of adolescent substance use disorder treatment: A research-based guide.* Retrieved from https://www.drugabuse.gov/publications/principles-adolescent-substance-use-disorder-treatment-research-based-guide/introduction

National Institute on Drug Abuse. (2018, June). *Prescription stimulants.* Retrieved from https://www.drugabuse.gov/publications/drugfacts/prescription-stimulants

National Institute on Drug Abuse. (2019a, August). *Monitoring the future.* Retrieved from https://www.drugabuse.gov/related-topics/trends-statistics/monitoring-future

National Institute on Drug Abuse. (2019b, January). *Opioid overdose crisis.* Retrieved from https://www.drugabuse.gov/drugs-abuse/opioids/opioid-overdose-crisis

National Institute on Drug Abuse. (2019c, October 30). *Teens: Drug facts*. Retrieved from https://teens.drugabuse.gov/teens/drug-facts

Partnership for Drug-Free Kids. (2018a). *All About the teen years*. Retrieved from https://drugfree.org/landing-page/learn/all-about-the-teen-years/

Partnership for Drug-Free Kids. (2018b, August 15). *E-cigarettes/vaping*. Retrieved from https://drugfree.org/drug/e-cigarettes-vaping/

Office of Disease Prevention and Health Promotion. (2019, November 1). *Tobacco*. Retrieved from https://www.healthypeople.gov/2020/leading-health-indicators/2020-lhi-topics/Tobacco

Substance Abuse and Mental Health Services Administration. (2019, August 2). *Rise in prescription drug misuse and abuse impacting teens*. Retrieved from https://www.samhsa.gov/homelessness-programs-resources/hpr-resources/teen-prescription-drug-misuse-abuse

U.S. Drug Enforcement Administration. (2017). *Drugs of abuse: A DEA resource guide*. Retrieved from https://www.dea.gov/sites/default/files/drug_of_abuse.pdf

U.S. Department of Health and Human Services. (2018, August 7). *5-point strategy to combat the opioid crisis*. Retrieved from https://www.hhs.gov/opioids/about-the-epidemic/hhs-response/index.html

U.S. Department of Health and Human Services. (2019, March 29). *Risks of adolescent alcohol use*. Retrieved from https://www.hhs.gov/ash/oah/adolescent-development/substance-use/alcohol/risks/index.html

Online Resources

National Association of School Nurses. https://www.nasn.org/nasn-resources/practice-topics/drugs-abuse

National Institute on Drug Abuse for Teens. https://teens.drugabuse.gov/teens

Partnership for Drug-Free Teens. https://drugfree.org/landing-page/learn/all-about-the-teen-years/

Smart Moves Smart Choices Toolkit. https://smartmovessmartchoices.org/school-tool-kit

Stop Medicine Abuse. https://stopmedicineabuse.org/

Substance Use Screening and Intervention Implementation Guide. https://www.aap.org/en-us/Documents/substance_use_screening_implementation.pdf

Talk, They Hear You. https://www.samhsa.gov/underage-drinking

Further Readings

Contreras, R. (2013). *The stickup kids: Race, drugs, violence, and the American dream*. Berkeley: University of California Press.

Courtwright, D. T. (2009). *Forces of habit*. Cambridge, MA: Harvard University Press.

Quinones, S. (2015). *Dreamland: The true tale of America's opiate epidemic*. London, UK: Bloomsbury Publishing.

15

GENDER IDENTITY: SUPPORTING NONBINARY AND TRANSGENDER STUDENTS IN THE SCHOOL SETTING

SEAN LARE

LEARNING OBJECTIVES

- Describe transgender, nonbinary related terminology.
- Recognize the importance of proper language use for transgender, nonbinary people.
- Increase understanding of what it is like to be a school-aged transgender or nonbinary person.
- Identify at least three strategies the school nurse can employ to support nonbinary and transgender students.

▧ Introduction

Schools play a key role in every aspect of students' lives, including their physical and mental health. It is the place where students gain knowledge and develop social skills. Schools can nurture young people as their identities emerge. In recent years, more and more of these young people are sharing with others that they identify as transgender. A recent study estimates that over 0.7% of youth are transgender (Herman, Flores, Brown, Wilson, & Conron, 2017), and this number may be an underestimate (Transathlete, n.d.) given the many systemic barriers to collecting information on transgender youth (e.g., a lack of data collection forms that include questions about gender identity; challenges related to obtaining parental consent from youth who may not be able to safely tell guardians they are transgender). What we do know is that the need for transgender-affirmative school environments is increasing. More individuals are able to live their lives as their affirmed gender, more families accept their transgender loved ones, and more school administrators are being contacted by students and families seeking support and affirmation for students. School nurses are often brought into these conversations, as many schools offer a bathroom in the nurse's office for transgender students to use. This chapter provides these nurses with the language, information, and guidance to increase confidence and competence when asked to support transgender and nonbinary students in schools.

Terminology and Language: What the Words Mean

Nurses working with people who identify as transgender or nonbinary need an understanding of the language used to discuss aspects of gender and provide affirming care. This language is always evolving and may vary regionally or by culture, age, or other factors, and there are many other terms that nonbinary and transgender youth may use to describe their identities and experiences. Of course, school personnel should give preference to the terms transgender or nonbinary students use to describe themselves and they should avoid terms that make the students uncomfortable (GLSEN, formerly Gay, Lesbian, and Straight Education Network and the National Center for Transgender Equality, n.d.). The following are definitions of some of the terms frequently used to support transgender and nonbinary students in schools or health settings at the time of this publication (Green & Maurer, 2015).

- **Biological Sex**: A designation determined by a combination of chromosomes, hormones, genitalia, and reproductive organs.
- **Sex Assigned at Birth**: The "male" or "female" label used at birth and placed on a baby's birth certificate; the label is usually based on visual assessment of genitalia at birth (or in ultra-sound when in utero).
- **Gender Identity**: A person's intrinsic view of the gendered way they see themselves, such as "male," "female," "nonbinary," or any other affirming gender term.
- **Gender Expression**: The way in which a person may convey their gender outwardly to other people through signals such as clothing, hair style, make-up, fingernail style, mannerisms, jewelry, language use, and voice inflection.
- **Cisgender**: A word used to describe a person whose gender identity does align with their sex assigned at birth.
- **Transgender**: A word used to describe a person whose gender identity does not align with the sex assigned at birth.
- **Nonbinary**: A word used to describe a person whose gender identity is within a continuum or spectrum and cannot be categorized as wholly "male" or wholly "female." Individuals who identify as nonbinary reject the concept that gender identity is strictly male or female based on sex assigned at birth.

■ **Gender Dysphoria**: A medical diagnosis defined in the American Psychiatric Association's (APA) *Diagnostic and Statistical Manual of Mental Disorders, Fifth Edition (DSM-5)* (APA, 2013), used by mental health and medical professionals to indicate a person's experienced incongruence between gender identity and sex assigned at birth. This diagnosis is used to justify the need for medical transition care services (e.g., puberty blockers, hormone therapy, or gender-affirming surgeries).

■ **Transition**: The process(es) transgender or nonbinary individuals may take to align their gender identities with their bodies or to influence how other people see them or interact with them. Three primary types of transition include:

   ● **Social transition**: The process of signaling a new gender identity to others. This can include changes in names and pronouns, changes in choice of single-sex bathroom, and changes in gender expression.

   ● **Medical transition**: The process of using one or more medical interventions to align the body with gender identity. Available medical interventions include hormone treatments (e.g., puberty blockers, hormone therapy) and gender affirming surgeries.

   ● **Legal transition**: The process of changing legal documentation to reflect a different gender identity. This can include legal changes to names, gender markers, or other identifiers on birth certificate, school records, state IDs, and passports.

■ **Sexual Orientation**: Identity determined by physical, psychological, romantic, and/or sexual attraction to other people (e.g., heterosexual, gay, lesbian, bisexual). Sexual orientation is distinct from gender identity, which is the focus of this chapter.

Notably, everyone has a biological sex, a sex assigned at birth, a gender identity, a gender expression, and a sexual orientation. Gender identities and gender expressions may be fluid or rigid, but they cannot be changed, including through the so-called "conversion therapies" that attempt to change them. Most professional organizations (including the American Academy of Child and Adolescent Psychiatry, American Academy of Family Physicians, American Academy of Nursing, American Academy of Pediatrics, American Medical Association, APA, American Psychological Association, American School Counselor Association, National Association of School Psychologists, Substance Abuse and Mental Health Services Administration) have specifically banned the use of conversion therapy for an individual who is transgender, nonbinary, or gender nonconforming (Ashley, 2018). Nonaffirming language used for transgender and nonbinary individuals ranges from intentionally transphobic comments to microaggressions.

In 2006 to 2007, GLSEN surveyed 6,209 students for their fifth National School Climate Survey. GLSEN was formed by educators in 1990, in acknowledgment of the key role educators play in LGBTQ students' lives. Through research (i.e., the biennial

National School Climate Survey), advocacy, and resources, they support students, educators, and school administrators in creating an affirming school climate toward improving LGBTQ students' ability to learn. In 2009 GLSEN published the Harsh Realities report (Greytak, Kosciw, & Diaz, 2009). This report specifically looked at the experiences of the 295 students in the survey who identified as transgender, and found that:

- Ninety percent of transgender students reported hearing derogatory re- marks such as "dyke" or "faggot" sometimes, often, or frequently in school.

- Ninety percent of transgender students reported hearing negative remarks about someone's gender expression sometimes, often, or frequently in school. Students more frequently heard remarks about students not acting "masculine" enough than remarks about students not acting "feminine" enough (82% vs. 77% hearing remarks sometimes, often, or frequently).

- Approximately one third of transgender students reported each of the fol- lowing occurred sometimes, often, or frequently in the past year: hearing school staff make homophobic remarks (32%), hearing them make sexist remarks (39%), and hearing negative comments about someone's gender expression (39%).

When people within schools hear such derogatory language, they must intervene to let students and colleagues know that such language is not tolerated. The cumu- lative effects of hearing these negative comments throughout the school day include deteriorating academics, increased somatic symptoms, and poor mental health, as discussed in the next section.

Statistics: The Importance of Affirmation and Support at School

Schools need to support youth who identify as transgender or nonbinary and who want to live their lives according to their gender identities instead of their sex as- signed at birth. In recent years, researchers have studied the effects of negative expe- riences (e.g., individual and systemic discrimination; harassment; lack of affirmation from families, schools, and professionals) on transgender or nonbinary young people in the areas of mental health, education, and other life domains. These studies illus- trate strongly the importance of affirming school climates, so that transgender and nonbinary students may be more likely to reach their academic and social-emotional potential.

A 2018 report by the Human Rights Campaign revealed important challenges in school for the 4,132 youth who identified as transgender in a survey of 12,000 LGBTQ youth, aged 13 to 17 (Human Rights Campaign, 2018). Slightly less than half (49%) of the transgender or nonbinary students reported they could not use the facilities that aligned with their gender identities. Only 31% were able to present in school in a manner consistent with their gender identity. Just one third were able to use their affirming names in school, and only one fifth reported they were consistently referenced using their affirming pronouns. Statements from transgender and nonbinary students revealed additional challenges and the need for specific supports for these students:

> Despite how confident I feel in my gender identity, I'm afraid of being judged and mistreated because I am still in the early stages of transitioning, particularly because my parents don't allow me to present as a female when it comes to dress and makeup. (Human Rights Campaign, 2018)

In 2017, the Centers for Disease Control and Prevention's (DC) Youth Risk Behavior Survey (YRBS), a biennial survey of U.S. high school students in grades 9 to 12, piloted questions related to gender identity in 10 states and 9 urban school districts in order to better understand the numbers and experiences of transgender students in the United States (Johns et al., 2019). Among the 131,901 students who took the survey with the pilot questions on gender identity, almost 2% identified as transgender, a rate more than double the previously estimated rate of 0.7% (Herman et al., 2017). Notably, the survey questions did not provide options for other noncisgender identities sometimes claimed by youth (e.g., nonbinary, gender fluid, agender); therefore, the percentage of gender diverse survey respondents is likely an underestimate. A comparison of responses from transgender students and cisgender students revealed significantly higher rates of negative outcomes for transgender students (Table 15.1). Many students who identified as transgender had experienced physical and sexual

TABLE 15.1 HIGHLIGHTS FROM 2017 PILOT YRBS AMONG STUDENTS WHO IDENTIFIED AS TRANSGENDER

DOMAIN	OUTCOMES FOR TRANSGENDER STUDENTS
Violence victimization	■ Over one third (35%) reported experiencing bullying at school; 30% electronically. ■ Almost one quarter (24%) reported they had experienced physical or sexual violence or threats or injury involving a weapon. ■ Over one quarter (27%) reported feeling unsafe traveling to/from school.
Substance use	■ One third (33%) reported cigarette use. ■ 70% reported alcohol use. ■ Over one quarter (25%–31%, depending on substance) reported using cocaine, heroin, methamphetamines, ecstasy, and/or inhalants (a rate more than 5–6 times that of their cisgender peers). ■ Over a one third reported prescription opioid misuse (a rate more than 3 times that of their cisgender peers).
Suicide risk	■ Over half (53%) reported feeling sad or hopeless. ■ 44% had considered attempting suicide and 39% had made a suicide plan (approximately 4 times that of their cisgender peers). ■ Over one third reported they had attempted suicide (a rate more than 6 times that of their cisgender peers).

(continued)

TABLE 15.1 HIGHLIGHTS FROM 2017 PILOT YRBS AMONG STUDENTS WHO
IDENTIFIED AS TRANSGENDER (*CONTINUED*)

DOMAIN	OUTCOMES FOR TRANSGENDER STUDENTS
Sexual risk	■ 16% reported having sexual intercourse with more than 4 partners in the past 12 months (compared to 9% of their cisgender peers). ■ Almost two thirds (64%) reported they did not use condoms during their last sexual intercourse (compared to 38% of their cisgender peers). ■ 30% reported they drank alcohol or used drugs before their last sexual intercourse (compared to 19% of their cisgender peers).

YRBS, Youth Risk Behavior Survey.

violence or other forms of victimization. These students were more likely than their cisgender peers to use substances or engage in risky sexual behavior, and they were more likely to consider or attempt suicide.

Another study that examines the experiences of LGBTQ students in the United States is GLSEN's biennial National School Climate Survey, which has identified and documented the challenges and supports experienced by LGBTQ students in the United States since 1999. The 2017 National School Climate Survey included 23,001 students between the ages of 13 and 21 (grades 6–12), with the largest numbers in grades 9, 10, and 11; 42% identified as gay or lesbian; 25% identified as transgender or nonbinary, 11% identified as "Genderqueer," 8% identified as "Another Nonbinary Identity (e.g. agender, genderfluid)," and 2% identified their gender as "Questioning or Unsure" (Kosciw, Greytak, Zongrone, Clark, & Truong, 2018). Compared to their cisgender LGBQ peers, students who identified as transgender most often reported negative experiences. They were more likely to report difficulties resulting from discriminatory policies and practices related to names, clothing, and facilities use. Such policies required students to use only their legal names and associated pronouns instead of affirming names and pronouns in the classroom, on school identification cards, or in the school yearbook. They regulated gendered attire for school concerts, dances, and graduation according to legal gender or sex assigned at birth, and they required all students to use the bathrooms, locker rooms, and other gender-segregated spaces specified by their legal gender or sex assigned at birth.

Not surprisingly, then, transgender students were more likely to report feeling unsafe and avoiding bathrooms, locker rooms, and physical education classes. They were less likely to participate in after school or extracurricular activities or clubs. They reported experiencing the highest levels of victimization, including harassment and assault, discrimination concerning facilities use, and name and pronoun discrimination. They reported they were more likely to miss school or change schools, and they were four times more likely than cisgender LGBQ students to report they were unsure they would complete high school or they did not plan to complete high school; other noncisgender students reported similar levels of concern about their abilities to complete high school. Quotes in this survey from transgender and nonbinary students emphasized these challenges:

> I was barred from using the boys' bathroom and when forced to use the girls' I experienced frequent harassment and physical assault. I frequently went a whole day without using the bathrooms, and this has led to severe health complications. (GLSEN, 2018)

Clearly, transgender and other noncisgender students continue to experience difficulties. Comparing the 2017 National School Climate Survey data to data from previous years reveals downward trends in harassment, assault, and other negative school climate experiences for LGBQ students, but increases for nonbinary and transgender students. Although more schools have implemented supportive policies and resources for LGBTQ students, nonbinary and transgender students indicated they had experienced more enforcement of discriminatory policies related to name use, pronoun use, and facilities access.

To combat these trends, based on information the survey collected related to school-based resources and supports, the survey report authors suggested that concerned stakeholders focus on building supportive school environments for nonbinary and transgender students. These supports may include: transgender and nonbinary student clubs, transgender competency training for all school staff, additions to the curriculum focused on transgender history and people, and the inclusion of transgender-affirmative resources in school libraries and media centers (Kosciw et al., 2018). Perhaps the most effective efforts would focus on increasing the number of schools that adopt and enforce affirmative policies, as discussed in the next section.

■ Improving School Climate: A Brief Review of How Some Schools Navigate Supporting Transgender Students

Schools are always working to meet the unique and varied needs of all their students (e.g., students who are gifted and talented, students with learning and behavior differences or physical challenges, students who speak English as a second language). Administrators have a duty to meet these needs so that all students, including transgender and nonbinary students, are supported in their learning. Although the needs of transgender students vary, all students have the right to be in a safe and supportive environment that supports their learning and provides equal opportunities. All students should be surrounded by adults who are committed to their safety, well-being, and learning (Shumer, 2018).

Students in a hostile school environment may experience negative life-long consequences. When a student cannot pay attention in class, have equal access to facilities, or do their best work, they are not able to succeed. As shown in the 2015 U.S. Transgender Survey, when a person cannot successfully attend school due to mistreatment and a hostile school climate, they become at risk for reduced job opportunities, lower income, unstable housing, increased mental health challenges and suicidality, and disparities (James et al., 2016).

On the other hand, for transgender students, schools can also play a crucial role as one of few spaces where a student feels accepted and affirmed, where they may fully be themselves. If a student is not accepted or supported at home for who they are regarding their gender identity and/or gender expression, it becomes even more important that the school is a safe place where their identity is respected and they have access to services and resources (e.g., a transgender peer affinity club, inclusive curriculum, supportive teachers and counselors). For these instances, it is vital that policies created do not require a caregiver's approval in order for a student's gender identity (including name and pronoun use) to be respected at school (GLSEN and the National Center for Transgender Equality, n.d.).

Given the unique needs and the statistics related to transgender and nonbinary students, and as more students are identifying as transgender and nonbinary, more schools are discovering they need to update their policies and procedures to provide these students with the needed support. These policy updates focus on several areas affecting both students and staff, including nondiscrimination, bullying, and harassment; facilities use; club and activity access (including sports participation); and dress code. These policy changes have the added benefit of helping all students avoid the negative effects of sex and gender stereotypes that prevent people from reaching their full potentials. Creating an inclusive school environment, climate, and culture benefits all students (Shumer, 2018).

Some state and local laws protect transgender people, and schools should be aware of such laws affecting their jurisdictions. Additionally, courts have upheld that Title IX, a federal law banning sex discrimination, includes protections for transgender students based on their gender identity and regardless of their gender expression. Title IX applies to all schools (including both K–12 schools and colleges) that get federal money. Although the Department of Education rolled back a guidance document promoting protection of transgender students in 2017, courts have continued through the time of this publication to interpret Title IX as banning anti-transgender discrimination. Plus, some courts have held that the Equal Protection Clause of the Constitution protects transgender students from discrimination (National Center for Transgender Equality, n.d.). As of October 2019, 17 states plus the District of Columbia had rules, policies, or guidance on supporting transgender students in schools. Additionally, it is estimated that hundreds of schools and school districts in other states have also provided guidance; and there are an increasing number of private schools who are also updating their policies according to many other models cited here in support of transgender students (Sherouse, n.d.).

The existing policies include statistics about the importance of supporting transgender students toward improved educational outcomes within a framework that may honor the individual needs of the student. They also provide guidance on a range of topics (e.g., language use and terms; privacy; facilities use; bullying and harassment). They remind readers that a student's gender identity cannot be confirmed by any medical tests, psychological tests, or treatment protocols; therefore, no legal documentation should be required for the school administration to proceed in supporting the student's transition. Accordingly, student education records (e.g., class rosters, school IDs, online student platform logins and emails, and names listed in yearbooks and on diplomas) should list the names used by students, not students' legal names.

To accommodate students experiencing varied levels of support or rejection at home, administrators should meet with transgender and nonbinary students to discuss communication with guardians. During these meetings, administrators can discuss with students the form of school–guardian communication, the identifying information that communication may contain, and any alterations that can be made to that communication. For example, a transgender or nonbinary student may use a new affirming name different than the legal name at school, but safety concerns may have prevented the student from informing guardians of the new name. The school would then ensure all teachers, class rosters, and other materials seen by the student and peers use the affirming name, while report cards and other home communication would continue using the student's legal name (U.S. Department of Education, 2016).

Affirming policies also include language regarding facility use. These policies state that students may use facilities according to their gender identity and do not require use of an alternative facility. As explained in the Oregon policy, "Many students seek additional privacy in school restrooms and locker rooms. Some schools have provided students increased privacy by making adjustments to sex-segregated facilities or providing all students with access to alternative facilities" (U.S. Department of Education, 2016). Possible accommodations for facilities use include bathroom passes allowing students to access bathrooms during less crowded times, privacy curtains in locker rooms, or separate changing schedules for gym class.

Facility-related issues are also addressed in connection to overnight school trips, since students have traditionally been separated or grouped according to sex assigned at birth during these trips. Inclusive policies update this practice by allowing students to be grouped according to their gender identity. For example, guidelines for Colorado's Boulder Valley School District provide that schools planning overnight accommodations for a transgender student should consider "the goals of maximizing the student's social integration and equal opportunity to participate in overnight activity and athletic trips, ensuring the [transgender] student's safety and comfort, and minimizing stigmatization of the student" (Boulder Valley School District [CO], 2016). The Chicago Guidelines remind school staff, "In no case should a transgender student be denied the right to participate in an overnight field trip because of the student's transgender status". (Chicago Public Schools [IL], 2016).

In addition to referring to any local or state laws, some state athletic leagues or associations may have their own rules regarding transgender athletes and access to facilities. As of September 2019, 17 state high school athletic associations plus DC have inclusive and affirming policies for transgender athletes, while other states have policies that require certain medical procedures and/or specified documentation (U.S. Department of Education, Office of Elementary and Secondary Education, Office of Safe and Healthy Students, 2016).

Schools often include updates to bullying and harassment policies and nondiscrimination statements in their policy updates related to the treatment of transgender and nonbinary students. These policies specifically address bullying and harassment of both students and staff based on gender identity and gender expression. Inclusive policies highlight language-related examples of bullying or harassment such as intentional use of the wrong name and/or pronouns, as well as harassment related to personal questions about bodies, body histories, and medical information. The best inclusive policies for students and staff also address electronic bullying and harassment on social media and other forums.

Lastly, to create an inclusive school climate, many school districts have reconsidered the purpose and necessity of the traditional practice of grouping students by gender. For example, the Maryland State Department of Education issued guidelines for elementary students that include an example of how to eliminate gender-based sorting of students: "Old Practice: boys line up over here." New Practice: birthdays between January and June; everybody who is wearing something green, so forth (Maryland State Department of Education, 2015). Other jurisdictions have updated policies to no longer separate by gender such as: dress codes (e.g., changing language regarding "girls shirts may not be off the shoulder" to "shirts may not be off the shoulder"); different colored gowns for graduation or other ceremonies based on gender; field trips, clubs and activity participation that presumed interest by gender. Like many of the changes made to accommodate transgender and nonbinary students, these updates help all students by eliminating the previous acceptance of sometimes harmful sex stereotypes (U.S. Department of Education, 2016).

▣ Role of the School Nurse: How the School Nurse May Help

School nurses have many opportunities to support transgender and nonbinary students. They may advocate with their school administrators or district school boards for updated policies and procedures that affirm and support transgender and nonbinary students, and reference the statistics discussed earlier in this chapter; they may practice using affirming language and continue in their learning about the experiences of transgender and nonbinary youth; and they may ensure that practices within their job and the health room follow an affirming approach.

Frequently, schools without affirming policies require that transgender and nonbinary students must go to an alternative facility such as a bathroom in the nurse's office to use the restroom or to change for activities. In these schools, nurses can speak to administrators about creating supportive, affirming, and inclusive policies for all students. When schools have affirming policies permitting students to use facilities according to their gender identities, some students may request a more private, alternative space and look to the nurse's office. For these students, nurses can advocate for schools to identify safe, single use facilities outside of the health room, so that healthy transgender and nonbinary students are not exposed to sick students visiting the nurse.

Nurses might also have more interactions with transgender and nonbinary students who are avoiding or experiencing discrimination. For example, transgender and nonbinary students may go to the nurse's office stating they are sick in order to avoid certain people (e.g., nonaffirming teachers or peers) or subjects (e.g., health class or gym) that bring attention to their gender identities or gender expressions in a negative way. Additionally, some students experiencing distress related to lack of acceptance of their gender may experience an increase in somatic symptoms (e.g., headaches and stomachaches) that contribute to visits to the school nurse. School health professionals in these situations should be mindful of the challenges experienced by transgender and nonbinary students, provide empathy and support, and look for opportunities to speak with school administrators and advocate for change on behalf of these marginalized students.

School nurses must strive to maintain the privacy of transgender and nonbinary students. These nurses may have access to students' medical records, including the legal identifying information that differs from the names used by students and the genders with which they identify. Disclosure of this private information may be a violation of privacy laws, including the federal Family Educational Rights and Privacy Act (FERPA). Additionally, school nurses should discuss names and pronoun use with transgender and nonbinary students prior to any calls to guardians. To ensure the safety of these students at home, the school nurse needs to avoid disclosing that they are transgender or nonbinary if the students have not done so. Students must provide explicit permission to share information about their transgender or nonbinary gender identities with others, even if they have already shared information about their gender identities with some of their peers or school staff (GLSEN and the National Center for Transgender Equality, 2014).

School nurses can also support transgender and nonbinary students by ensuring their spaces, forms, and health interactions checklists are as affirming as possible. A safe and welcoming space includes images, resource materials, and other décor that are inclusive of transgender youth, families, and lives. If the office offers health-related supplies, ensure that they are offered in a gender-neutral way that does not presume who will need or use them. For example, bandages should be fun or plain instead of obviously gendered (e.g., pink with dolls or blue with cars). Menstrual supplies are not in "pink" boxes, since students who are nonbinary or transmasculine may have a uterus and benefit from these supplies; they may feel uncomfortable requesting them, and that could be heightened if the supplies are clearly marked for "girls." Health inventory or intake forms should include questions about gender identity, name use (instead of only legal name), "sex assigned at birth" (instead of only "sex"), and "parent/guardian" (instead of "mother" and "father"). These forms should also include options for all body parts and all health concerns for all students regardless of gender identity—versus separate "boy" and "girl" inventories.

When interacting with transgender or nonbinary students, promoting a safe and trusting environment and showing empathy are key. School nurses can ask open-ended questions, avoid making assumptions, and explain the necessity of the questions they are asking (Eckstrand & Ehrenfeld, 2016). If students say they use names or pronouns that are different from those in their medical records, or if they share terms that they would rather use for their body parts, school nurses can increase trust by using those affirming words (Poretsky & Hembree, 2019).

In conclusion, as noted and as exemplified throughout this chapter, in the school setting, when working with transgender and nonbinary students, it is key that the school nurse and other staff believe them, validate and empathize.

Use affirming name and pronouns. Help connect to support and resources. Advocate and be proactive for all students, especially those who are transgender or nonbinary (National Center for Transgender Equality, 2017).

All of this strategies help a young person feel seen, heard, and understood. They will most likely reduce some of the negative statistics reviewed earlier and combat a potentially hostile environment.

Initialed by the school nurse, with the support of other staff and educated students, the transgender and nonbinary student can feel safe and be their very best selves at school.

References

American Psychiatric Association. (2013). *Diagnostic and statistical manual of mental disorders* (*DSM-5*®). Arlington, VA: American Psychiatric Publishing.

Ashley, F. (2018, October 4). *List of professional organizations opposing conversion or reparative therapy targeting transgender and gender non-conforming individuals*. Retrieved from https://medium.com/@florence.ashley/list-of-professional-organisations-opposing-conversion-or-reparative-therapy-targeting-transgender-f700b4e02c4e

Boulder Valley School District (CO). (2016). *Guidelines regarding the support of students and staff who are transgender and/or gender nonconforming*. Retrieved from https://www.bvsd.org/about/board-of-education/policies/policy/~board/a-policies/post/guidelines-regarding-the-support-of-students-and-staff-who-are-transgender-andor-gender-nonconforming-exhibit

Chicago Public Schools (IL). (2016). *Guidelines regarding the support of transgender and gender nonconforming students*. Retrieved from cps.edu/SiteCollectionDocuments/TL_TransGenderNonconformingStudents_Guidelines.pdf

Eckstrand, K. L., & Ehrenfeld, J. M. (2016). *Lesbian, gay, bisexual, and transgender healthcare*. Cham, Switzerland: Springer International Publishing.

GLSEN and the National Center for Transgender Equality. (2014). *Model district policy on transgender and gender non-conforming students*. Retrieved from trans_school_district_model_policy_FINAL.pdf

GLSEN and the National Center for Transgender Equality. (n.d.). *The 2018 model school district policy on transgender and gender nonconforming students*. Retrieved from https://transequality.org/sites/default/files/images/resources/trans_school_district_model_policy_FINAL.pdf\

Green, E. R., & Maurer, L. M. (2015). *The teaching transgender toolkit: A facilitator's guide to increasing knowledge, decreasing prejudice & building skills*. Ithaca, NY: Planned Parenthood of the Southern Finger Lakes: Out for Health.

Greytak, E. A., Kosciw, J. G., & Diaz, E. M. (2009). *Harsh realities: The experiences of transgender youth in our nation's schools*. New York, NY: GLSEN.

Herman, J. L., Flores, A. R., Brown, T. N. T., Wilson, B. D. M., & Conron, K. J. (2017). *Age of individuals who identify as transgender in the United States*. Los Angeles, CA: The Williams Institute.

Human Rights Campaign. (2018). *LGBTQ youth report* (2018). Retrieved from https://assets2.hrc.org/files/assets/resources/2018-YouthReport-NoVid.pdf?_ga=2.35147236.458806514.1572582730-1698477667.1510238605

James, S. E., Herman, J. L., Rankin, S., Keisling, M., Mottet, L., & Ana, M. (2016). *The report of the 2015 U.S. transgender survey*. Washington, DC: National Center for Transgender Equality.

Johns, M. M., Lowry, R., Andrzejewski, J., Barrios, L. C., Demissie, Z., McManus, T., … Underwood, M. J. (2019). Transgender identity and experiences of violence victimization, substance use, suicide risk, and sexual risk behaviors among high school students—19 states and large urban school districts, 2017. *Morbidity and Mortality Weekly Report, 68*, 67–71. doi:10.15585/mmwr.mm6803a3

Kosciw, J. G., Greytak, E. A., Zongrone, A. D., Clark, C. M., & Truong, N. L. (2018). *The 2017 National School Climate Survey: The experiences of lesbian, gay, bisexual, transgender, and queer youth in our nation's schools*. New York, NY: GLSEN.

Maryland State Department of Education. (2015). *Providing safe spaces for transgender and gender non-conforming youth: Guidelines for gender identity non-discrimination*. Retrieved from http://marylandpublicschools.org/about/Documents/DSFSS/SSSP/ProvidingSafeSpacesTransgendergenderNonConformingYouth012016.pdf

National Center for Transgender Equality. (2017, February 21). *FAQ on the withdrawal of federal guidance on transgender students*. Retrieved from https://transequality.org/issues/resources/faq-on-the-withdrawal-of-federal-guidance-on-transgender-students

National Center for Transgender Equality. (n.d.). *School action center*. Retrieved from https://transequality.org/schoolaction

Sherouse, B. (n.d.). *Schools in transition: A guide for supporting transgender students in K-12 schools*. Retrieved from https://assets2.hrc.org/files/assets/resources/Schools-In-Transition.pdf?_ga=2.5687030.458806514.1572582730-1698477667.1510238605

Shumer, D. (2018). Health disparities facing transgender and gender nonconforming youth are not inevitable. *Pediatrics, 141*(3), e20174079. doi:10.1542/peds.2017-4079

Transathlete. (n.d.). Retrieved from https://www.transathlete.com/k-12

U.S. Department of Education, Office of Elementary and Secondary Education, Office of Safe and Healthy Students. (2016, May). *Examples of policies and emerging practices for supporting transgender students*. Retrieved from https://eric.ed.gov/?id=ED572043

▇ Online Resources

GLAAD and Movement Advancement Project (MAP). *An ally's guide to terminology: Talking about LGBT people & equality*. Retrieved from https://www.glaad.org/sites/default/files/allys-guide-to-terminology_1.pdf

GLSEN. *A U.S. national organization focused on supporting K-12 LGBTQ students through programs, resources, and research; the site includes helpful information for developing policy, inclusive curriculum, and an affirming school climate*. Retrieved from https://www.glsen.org

National LGBT Health Education Center, A Program of the Fenway Institute. *Glossary of LGBT terms for health care teams*. Retrieved from https://www.lgbthealtheducation.org/wp-content/uploads/LGBT-Glossary_March2016.pdf

▪ Further Readings

Bongiovanni, A., & Jimerson, T. (2018). *A quick and easy guide to they/them pronouns.* Portland, OR: Limerence Press, Inc.

Brill, S., & Kenney, L. (2016). *The transgender teen: A handbook for parents and professionals supporting transgender and non-binary teens.* Jersey City, NJ: Cleis Press.

Brill, S., & Pepper, R. (2008). *The transgender child: A handbook for families & professionals.* San Francisco, CA: Cleis Press.

Eckstrand, K., & Ehrenfeld, J. M. (Eds.). (2016). *Lesbian, gay, bisexual, and transgender healthcare: A clinical guide to preventive, primary, and specialist care.* Cham, Switzerland: Springer International Publishing.

Ehrensaft, D. (2011). *Gender born, gender made: Raising healthy gender non-conforming children.* New York, NY: The Experiment Press.

Erickson-Scroth, L. (Ed.). (2014). *Trans bodies, trans selves: A resource for the transgender community.* New York, NY: Oxford University Press.

Ettner, R., Monstrey, S., & Coleman, E. (Eds.). (2016). *Principles of transgender medicine and surgery* (2nd ed.). New York, NY: Routledge.

GLSEN & Harris Interactive. (2012). *Playgrounds and prejudice: Elementary schools climate in the United States, a survey of students and teachers.* New York, NY: GLSEN.

Hubbard, E., & Whitley, C. (Eds.). (2012). *Trans-Kin: A guide for family and friends of transgender people.* Boulder, CO: Bolder Press.

Keo-Meier, C., & Ehrensaft, D. (Eds.). (2018). *The gender affirmative model: An interdisciplinary approach to supporting transgender and gender expansive children (perspectives on sexual orientation and diversity)* (1st ed.). Washington, DC: American Psychological Association.

Poretsky, L., & Hembree, W. C. (Eds.). (2019). *Transgender medicine: A multidisciplinary approach.* Cham, Switzerland: Humana Press.

Stryker, S. (2017). *Transgender history, (2nd ed.): The roots of today's revolution* (2nd ed.). New York, NY: Seal Press.

16

EATING DISORDERS AND OBESITY

LAURA A. GUERRA

LEARNING OBJECTIVES

- Describe the common behavioral and physical signs of anorexia, bulimia, binge eating, and obesity.
- Compare the biological, psychological, and behavioral risk factors associated with anorexia, bulimia, binge eating, and obesity.
- Describe the potential health consequences of anorexia, bulimia, binge eating, and obesity.
- Identify resources for anorexia, bulimia, binge eating, and obesity where students and their families can learn more about these disorders and potential treatments.

■ Introduction

The passage from childhood into and through adolescence includes a set of biological, cognitive, social, and emotional transitions that unfold gradually and touch upon many aspects of the individual's behavior, development, and relationships. Shifts in eating patterns resulting from these significant changes are not uncommon. Research also suggests a dose-effect relationship between childhood trauma and eating disorders (Guillaume et al., 2016). Prevalence rates of eating disorders and obesity vary significantly by gender and race (Allen, Byrne, Oddy, & Crosby, 2013). Early intervention is critical for recovery, yet weight-related problems are underdiagnosed and often left untreated (Campbell & Peebles, 2014; Hart, Granillo, Jorm, & Paxton, 2011).

With access and the ability to monitor student well-being, school nurses can play a key role in identifying potential weight-related problems. Understanding the risk factors and signs associated with weight-related problems may increase the identification of an issue and the referral to appropriate resources for treatment. This chapter provides diagnostic criteria, symptoms, and informational resources for various weight-related problems.

Eating Disorders

The Nature of the Problem

The *Diagnostic and Statistical Manual of Mental Disorders, Fifth Edition* (*DSM-5*; American Psychiatric Association [APA], 2013) characterizes an "eating disorder" (ED) as an ongoing disruption in eating behavior such that the consumption and absorption of food are altered, and physical or psychological function is impaired. EDs include anorexia nervosa (AN), bulimia nervosa (BN), and binge-eating disorder (BED; APA, 2013). While AN, BN and BED share some common psychological and behavioral features, the *DSM-5* notes that significant differences in clinical course, outcome, and treatment call for specific diagnostic criteria to ensure practitioners have classification criteria that force a mutually exclusive diagnosis and, ideally, intervention and treatment (APA, 2013). Unfortunately the majority of EDs are undiagnosed and left untreated (Campbell & Peebles, 2014; Hart et al., 2011), and there are well-documented negative impacts on healthy childhood and adolescent development arising from the cardiovascular, gastrointestinal, musculoskeletal, endocrine, reproductive and dermatological complications associated with EDs (Campbell & Peebles, 2014; Westmoreland, Krantz, & Mehler, 2016). Among psychiatric illnesses, EDs have the highest mortality rate (Arcelus, Mitchell, Wales, & Nielsen, 2011).

The Prevalence of Eating Disorders

Broadly defined, EDs affect slightly more than 15% of female adolescents and just under 3% of male adolescents. Recent efforts to understand the prevalence of EDs have begun to take an intersectional approach, seeking to understand how health outcomes associated with particular intersecting identities differ when characteristics such as gender and race or ethnicity are considered in light of one another. Using this approach, Beccia et al. found that, compared to White boys, girls of all racial and ethnic identities and racial and ethnic minority boys had a higher risk of disordered eating. They also found a positive interaction between gender and race and ethnicity for Hispanic girls resulting in an excess risk of disordered eating (Beccia et al., 2019). Their findings suggest that school nurses and other health professionals must consider the effects of multiple social identities simultaneously, and not solely student gender. It is also important to note that identifying adolescents or youths with an ED may be difficult because they may try to hide their behaviors or may appear to be "normal weight." As a result, it is critical to understand the specific warning signs of each ED and its respective diagnostic criteria.

Anorexia Nervosa

AN is a serious psychiatric disorder characterized by extreme dissatisfaction with one's body that results in food aversion and a phobia of weight gain. Typically, highly restrictive diets and/or excessive exercise are used to achieve and maintain a reduced body weight. Some persons affected with AN may see themselves as overweight, even when they are starved or are clearly malnourished, while others may recognize that they are extremely thin but find it attractive.

There are three main diagnostic criteria for AN. The first is a restriction of food intake relative to the amount that is required given a person's age, sex, developmental trajectory, and physical health. The second criterion is an intense fear of gaining weight despite an already low body weight, and the third is lack of recognition or understanding of one's shape or of the consequences of the person's low body weight (APA, 2013).

Symptoms include:

- Extremely restricted eating;
- Extreme thinness (emaciation), unwillingness to maintain a normal or healthy weight, and a relentless pursuit of thinness;
- Intense fear of gaining weight;
- Distorted body image; self-esteem is heavily influenced by perceptions of body weight and shape;
- Osteopenia or osteoporosis;
- Muscle wasting and weakness and mild anemia;
- Brittle hair and nails;
- Dry and yellowish skin;
- Lanugo, or the growth of fine hair all over the body;
- Severe constipation;
- Low blood pressure and slowed breathing and pulse;
- Damage to the structure and function of the heart;
- Drop in internal body temperature, causing a person to feel cold all the time; and
- Lethargy, sluggishness, or feeling tired all the time.

Bulimia Nervosa

BN is characterized by eating large amounts of food in a relatively short period of time, along with the sense of a loss of control, followed by a type of behavior that compensates for the excessive eating such as vomiting, excessive use of laxatives, or diuretics, fasting, and/or excessive exercise. Like those with AN, people with BN often fear gaining weight, want desperately to lose weight, and are intensely unhappy with their body size and shape. Unlike AN, however, those with BN can fall within the normal range for their weight.

There are five diagnostic criteria for BN. These include repeated occurrences of binge eating which is typically accompanied by compensatory behavior to prevent weight gain; for example, self-induced vomiting; fasting; excessive exercise; or misuse of diuretics, laxatives, or other medications. Both the binge eating and inappropriate compensatory behaviors occur an average of at least once a week for 3 months. For BN, self-evaluation is disproportionately influenced by weight and body shape; and importantly the disturbance does not occur exclusively during AN episodes (APA, 2013).

Symptoms include:

- Chronically inflamed and sore throat;
- Swollen salivary glands in the neck and jaw area;
- Worn tooth enamel and increasingly sensitive and decaying teeth due to exposure to stomach acid;
- Acid reflux disorder and other gastrointestinal problems;
- Intestinal distress and irritation from laxative abuse;
- Severe dehydration from purging of fluids; and
- Electrolyte imbalance.

Binge-Eating Disorder

The *DSM-5* characterizes BED as recurrent episodes of eating larger amounts of food in a shorter period of time than most people would eat under similar circumstances and where a person feels a loss of control or marked distress over their eating. Unlike BN, BED episodes are not followed by purging, excessive exercise, or fasting. The most common of the eating disorders, those with BED are often overweight or obese.

Binge eating disorder also has a number of specific diagnostic criteria. These include recurrent episodes of binge eating (at least once a week for 3 months), which occur in a discrete period of time and are accompanied by a lack of control over the amount eaten. Episodes of binge-eating are associated with three (or more) of the following: eating alone, eating much more rapidly than normal, eating larger amounts of food than is necessary, eating until feeling uncomfortably full, and feelings of disgust with oneself or of guilt. Other diagnostic criteria include feeling marked distress regarding binge eating. Finally it should be noted that binge eating is not associated with the recurrence of inappropriate compensatory behavior as exhibited in BN. Binge eating does not occur exclusively during episodes of BN or AN (APA, 2013).

Symptoms include:

- Eating unusually large amounts of food in a specific amount of time, such as a 2-hour period
- Eating even when full or not hungry
- Eating fast during binge episodes
- Eating until uncomfortably full
- Eating alone or in secret to avoid embarrassment
- Feeling distressed, ashamed, or guilty about such eating
- Frequently dieting, possibly without weight loss

The Population at Risk for Eating Disorders

While the vast majority of eating disorders present in the late teens, behaviors and other symptoms are also common in pre- and early adolescence (Micali et al., 2015). During this developmental period, youth experience numerous biological, cognitive, social, and emotional transitions that unfold gradually and touch upon many aspects of the individual's behavior, development, and relationships. While such changes may also occur at other ages, and while it is not uncommon for shifts in eating patterns to result, it's important to note that the higher volume of such changes in pre- and early adolescence may make such youths more susceptible.

School nurses may also wish to pay particular attention to adolescent athletes or students involved in the arts, such as dance. Among these groups, thinness is often considered optimal for performance and may go underreported as disordered eating because it is not associated with a general dissatisfaction with their shape or weight (Martinsen & Sundgot-Borgen, 2013). Athletes and artists are a unique subgroup because their psychological profiles have a number of factors in common with EDs such as AN: perfectionism, high self-expectations, competitiveness, hyperactivity, repetitive exercise routines, compulsiveness, and drive. There are also distinct advantages and disadvantages to working with this population. An advantage may be a higher likelihood of positive outcomes in treatment, as members of this group are used to conforming to the expectations of coaching and training programs. Disadvantages may include limited psychological mindedness, limited social experiences from immersion in a narrow athlete or artist subculture, and parents who focus primarily on their children's competitive success rather than emotional balance or health.

The Risk Factors for an Eating Disorder

Biological Risk Factors

Gender and race or ethnicity: Female teens, especially females of racial and ethnic minorities, are more likely than White boys to have EDs. In addition, racial and ethnic minority boys are more likely to have disordered eating than their White peers.

Age—Although eating disorders can occur at any age, their highest incident rate is during the teens and early 20s.

Genetics, Family History—Transgenerational and twin studies show that EDs run in families. There is a 5 to 6 times greater chance of developing an ED if an immediate relative has an ED.

Type 1 (Insulin-Dependent) Diabetes—Current studies show approximately one quarter of women diagnosed with type 1 diabetes will develop an ED. The most common pattern is skipping insulin injections, known as diabulimia, which can be fatal.

Psychological Risk Factors

- **Perfectionism:** Research indicates a significant indirect (mediating) relationship between perfectionism and ED symptoms via depression, as well as a significant direct relationship between perfectionism and eating disorders symptoms. Taken together, these findings suggests that higher perfectionism is associated with more severe ED symptoms directly, and indirectly because of the association perfectionism has with depression (Drieberg, McEvoy, Hoiles, Shu, & Egan, 2019).

- **Control**—Adolescence and young adulthood is a time of change, and changes can bring emotional stress and may increase the risk of disordered eating during attempts to bring order to one's life (Nicholls & Barrett, 2015).

- **Self-Worth**—Cultural norms of beauty and the emphasis on thinness in the media may impact youths' attitudes toward themselves. While body dissatisfaction or low body self-worth is often presented as a risk factor, research examining preadolescent populations suggest it may develop alongside ED symptoms (Evans et al., 2017). Children who experience bullying are at increased risk for EDs (Copeland et al., 2015).

- **Negative Family Patterns**—Parents who stress fitness or athleticism to an unhealthy degree, or have unrealistic expectations for their children, can contribute to eating problems.

Behavioral Risk Factors

Dieting—People who lose weight are often reinforced by positive comments from others and by their changing appearance. This may cause some people to take dieting too far, leading to an ED.

Sports, Work, and Artistic Activities—Athletes, actors, dancers, and models are at higher risk of EDs. Coaches, instructors, and parents may unwittingly contribute to EDs by encouraging young athletes and performers to lose weight (Martinsen & Sundgot-Borgen, 2013).

Environmental Risk Factors

There is growing evidence that a person's immediate social environment, including family (Allen, Byrne, & Crosby, 2015), friends, and media (Micali et al., 2015) can amplify the importance of thinness and weight control. For example, regular discussion of weight and dieting may normalize societal pressure to be thin. Weight-related teasing by peers and family is often related to low self-esteem and eating disturbances in young girls. Studies have shown that girls who live in families that tend to be strict and that place strong emphasis on physical attractiveness and weight control are at an increased risk for destructive eating behaviors.

Getting Treatment for Eating Disorders

Treatment for EDs is determined on a case-by-case basis and may require a multidisciplinary team approach, including a physician, psychiatrist, psychologist, and dietitian. Treatment may include a combination of behavior modification, nutritional rehabilitation, and some form of psychotherapy, such as individual therapy, cognitive-based therapy, and family-based therapy. Among those with AN, research indicates family-based treatment to be the most effective treatment in adolescents and young adults; the Maudsley model, for example, has a strong evidence base and is empirically supported. In family-based therapy, the main role of bringing a child back to health is given to the family and the therapists and medical providers act as treatment consultants to the family (Sorrell & Sorrell, 2017). A specific treatment plan will depend on the person's age, overall health, medical history, symptoms, tolerance for specific medications, procedures or therapies, expectations for the course of the condition, and opinion or preference.

Early diagnosis and treatment can improve the overall prognosis for an individual with an ED. Many individuals require ongoing treatment over several years, as persistence varies by the type and severity of the ED (Kessler et al., 2013). The longer the disease goes on, the more difficult it is to treat.

The Health Consequences of Eating Disorders

Serious medical complications may result from an ED, including but not limited to the following:

- **Skeletal**: Low calcium intake and absorption causes an increased risk for skeletal fractures. Bone density is often found to be low in those with AN. When symptoms of AN occur before peak bone formation has been attained (usually mid to late teens), a greater risk of osteopenia (decreased bone tissue) or osteoporosis (bone loss) exists.

- **Cardiovascular**: Myocardial damage that can occur as a result of changes in the heartbeat, or repeated vomiting, may be life-threatening.

- **Hematological**: Mild anemia (low red blood cell count) and leukopenia (low white blood cell count) are commonly found.

- **Gastrointestinal**: Normal motility often slows down with very restricted eating and severe weight loss. Gaining weight, and some medications, may help to restore normal intestinal function.

- **Renal**: Dehydration results in highly concentrated urine. Polyuria (increased production of urine) may also develop when the kidney's ability to concentrate urine decreases. Renal changes usually return to normal with the restoration of normal weight.

- **Endocrine**: Amenorrhea is one of the hallmark symptoms of AN. Reduced levels of growth hormones are sometimes found in anorexic patients and may explain growth retardation sometimes seen in patients. Normal nutrition usually restores normal growth.

- **Suicide**: EDs in adolescents have been shown to be a risk factor for suicide later (Sorrell & Sorrell, 2017). Suicide is the second leading cause of death in patients with EDs.

- **Death**: Research indicates EDs are usually associated with an increased risk of premature death with a wide range of causes of mortality (Jáuregui-Garrido & Jáuregui-Lobera, 2012).

- **Obesity**

The Nature of the Problem

Childhood overweight and obesity can affect a child's immediate health and is associated with many negative long-term health consequences. Yet, despite obesity and weight-related behaviors being both a clinical and public health focus for over two decades, overweight and obesity prevalence remains high. According to recent data from the National Center for Health Statistics, which conducts the National Health and Nutrition Examination Survey (NHANES), 18.5% of the U.S. population aged 2 to 19 years are overweight and 7.9% are obese (Cockrell Skinner, Ravanbakht, Skelton, Perrin, & Armstrong, 2018).

Childhood overweight and obesity are typically measured using body mass index (BMI) which is calculated by dividing a person's weight in kilograms by the square of height in meters. BMI is not a measure of body fat, and therefore should not be used as a diagnostic tool. It is however correlated with more direct measures of body fat, such as skinfold thickness measurements, bioelectrical impedance, densitometry (underwater weighing), and dual energy x-ray absorptiometry (DXA). Since children's body composition varies by age and gender, a child's weight status is determined using an age- and sex-specific percentile for BMI, rather than the BMI categories used for adults. Table 16.1 provides the BMI-for-age weight status categories and corresponding percentiles.

The Prevalence of Obesity

Nationally representative data provided by the NHANES demonstrate that childhood overweight and obesity varies significantly by age and race. According to data from the 2015 to 2016 NHANES cycle, 18.5% of youth aged 2 to 19 years old are overweight, and 6.9% are obese (Cockrell-Skinner et al., 2018). Prevalence rates for overweight and obesity increased with age. Hispanic and non-Hispanic African American children had higher prevalence rates of overweight and obesity, compared to their White or Asian peers (Cockrell-Skinner et al., 2018; Ogden et al., 2016).

TABLE 16.1 BMI FOR AGE WEIGHT STATUS

WEIGHT STATUS CATEGORY	PERCENTILE RANGE
Underweight	Less than 5th percentile
Normal or healthy weight	5th percentile to less than 85th percentile
Overweight	85th to less than the 95th percentile
Obese—Class I	≥95th percentile
Obese—Class II	≥120% of the 95th percentile
Obese—Class III	≥140% of the 95th percentile

BMI, body mass index.

The Risk Factors for Obesity

Overweight and obesity are not caused by a single factor; many factors such as genetics, socioeconomic status, eating patterns, and environment work in combination along direct and indirect pathways to increase the risk of overweight and obesity. More specific to the audience, youth and adolescent overweight and obesity are widely recognized as having a multifactorial etiology where family, peers, school and community environments influence each other, and in turn, youth and adolescent health behaviors and status.

Biological Risk Factors

Genetics—Genetics are frequently implicated in fat accumulation and variation in obesity susceptibility. For example, a systematic review of twin studies on childhood and adolescent obesity found that genetic factors had a strong effect on BMI from early childhood through adulthood (Silventoinen, Rokholm, Kaprio, & Sørensen, 2010). Still, while body composition appears to be strongly influenced by genetics, research also demonstrates that genetic and environmental factors work synergistically rather than independently of one another (Fernandez, Klimentidis, Dulin-Keita, & Casazza, 2012; Silventoinen et al., 2010).

Race—Race is frequently used to categorize populations based on shared biological characteristics of genes, shared features, and skin color. Race, however, is a constantly evolving concept, with an increasing proportion of the population self-reporting as "mixed race" or "other." While prevalence is higher for non-White populations, it is likely that the differences among groups are attributable to a complex combination of genetics, socioeconomic status, culture, and environment.

Gut Microbiota—Research show differences in fecal microbiota composition in children may precede overweight development. According to one study, the genus Bifidobacterium, which affects both the quality and quantity of the microbiota a child has during their first year of life, was lower in children who developed overweight by age 7 years (Kalliomäki, Collado, Salminen, & Isolauri, 2008).

Physiological Risk Factors

Stress—Adolescence is one of the most dynamic and complex transitions in the lifespan. It can be a time of great stress; and in response to stress, a cascade of hormones is released that help the adolescent to react to, and cope with, the internal and external demands imposed by the stressful event. While these hormones can mediate a number of beneficial effects such as mobilization of needed energy stores, reduction of inflammation, enhanced immune activity, and memory formation, given prolonged exposure to these stress-related hormones, many negative effects on physiological and neurobehavioral function may emerge, including altered metabolism and development of psychiatric disorders. Research indicates that adolescent psychological health can impact weight gain and overweight, with disordered eating behaviors such as extreme dieting and binge eating leading to weight gain, impeding weight loss, and maintaining overweight status over time.

Behavioral Risk Factors

Eating Habits—Multiple studies indicate a bi-directional relationship between obesity development and eating behaviors. A number of aspects relating to youth and adolescent eating patterns have been identified as potential risk factors associated with increased risk of overweight and obesity, including speculation regarding frequency of meals. While research did not confirm that frequent meals increased the rate of obesity, skipping breakfast has been associated with obesity development in the majority of cross-sectional and longitudinal studies in children and adolescents (Elgar, Moore, Roberts, & Tudor-Smith, 2004; Wang et al., 2017). Sugar-sweetened beverage consumption is another often-cited risk factor for overweight and obesity. One prospective study examined the relationship between changes in sugar-sweetened beverage (SSB) intake and central adiposity in older children, and found that SSB intake has unique effects on adipose tissue distribution with a greater preference for central fat accumulation (Bigornia et al., 2015).

Inadequate Sleep—Shortened sleep and disrupted circadian rhythms due to electronic device use, or regular late night social activities, have been associated with increased weight gain as well as a barrier to weight loss (Covassin, Singh, & Somers, 2016; Fatima, Doi, & Mamun, 2015).

Increases in "Screen Time"—One study suggests a bi-directional relationship between TV viewing and increased BMI in children; general sedentariness may predispose children to higher BMIs, which in turn may lead to greater engagement in sedentary behaviors such as watching TV (Fuller-Tyszkiewicz, Skouteris, Hardy, & Halse, 2012). Research indicates that computer time and television's role in increasing the risk of obesity is significant, and may be explained by both direct and indirect pathways. Such pathways may include displacing time for physical activity, promoting poor diets, and giving more opportunities for unhealthy snacking (during TV viewing).

Decreased Physical Activity—According to the Youth Risk Behavior Surveillance study in 2017, only 46.5% of adolescents met the current recommendations for physical activity: increasing heart rate for at least 60 minutes a day on 5 of the past 7 days. While research indicates sedentary behaviors increase the risk of becoming obese, research also suggests that overweight or obesity may also lead to more sedentary behavior (Fuller-Tyszkiewicz et al., 2012). It is also important to note that physical activity behaviors are heavily influenced by surrounding social and environmental factors.

Environment Risk Factors

Built Environment—The term "built environment" refers to the human-made surroundings that provide the setting for human activity, ranging in scale from buildings and parks or green space to neighborhoods and cities, and can include their supporting infrastructure, such as water supply or energy networks. Research has uncovered many links between the built environment and physical activity, but there does not yet appear to be conclusive evidence that aspects of the built environment promote obesity. Several studies found a positive association between walkability of environment and minutes of moderate-to-vigorous physical activity, as well as between distance combined with more dangerous conditions and decreased walking and bike riding.

Another aspect of built environment is the presence of supermarkets, which is associated with a reduced prevalence of obesity. In low-income neighborhoods, supermarkets may be less accessible than small, independent grocery stores. These community grocery stores frequently allocate less shelf-space to "healthier" (low-fat and high-fiber) products and tend to charge higher prices than supermarkets. Reduced availability has been associated with lower consumption. The picture outside North America is different. Studies in the UK found no differences in food price, availability, and access to supermarkets by socioeconomic status. In a study in Eindhoven, The Netherlands, there was increased proximity to food stores rather than less for low-socioeconomic status families, and studies in Brisbane, Australia found no evidence of shopping differences in fruit and vegetable purchasing patterns between families in various socioeconomic status groups.

Family—Parents play a critical role in shaping their child's food experiences, which can be positive or negative. When children grow up in families with bad eating habits (e.g., skipping breakfast, high consumption of SSB) and sedentary lifestyles dominated by TV watching and video games, they are more likely to become overweight or obese as young adults (Harding, Teyhan, Maynard, & Cruickshank, 2008; Kirschenbaum, Germann, Rich, & Daniel, 2005; Kremers, van der Horst, & Brug, 2007; Lindsay, Sussner, Kim, & Gortmaker, 2006). Research supports that parents categorized as obese have relationships with their adolescents that have the potential to increase the adolescent's development of obesity (Kosti et al., 2008).

Peers—Adolescent peers are an important determinant of many health behaviors; in particular, they have been found to influence adolescent consumption of snack foods and foods high in saturated fat (de la Haye, Robins, Mohr, & Wilson, 2010; Wouters, Larsen, Kremers, Dagnelie, & Geenen, 2010). Another way in which peers may become a risk factor is related to how adolescents form social networks or cliques. Adolescents tend to bond with people who are similar to themselves; specifically, adolescent friendships cluster on the basis of weight status and physical activity (Koehly & Loscalzo, 2009).

Media—Adolescents are bombarded with advertising and promotional messages aimed at influencing their behavior. According to a recent report, the average adolescent sees approximately 3,500 ads per year, the majority of them for SSBs and fast food (UConn Rudd Center, 2018). Marion Nestle notes of the approximately $33 billion spent on food advertising annually, about 70% is for sweets and just 2% goes toward fruit and vegetable promotion. The food industry exerts an enormous influence on children through advertising on television and in the community. Children who watch an excess of television are exposed to advertisements for sweetened drinks, fast food restaurants, and high-calorie snacks. A 2006 Institute of Medicine report cited television advertising as influencing children and adolescents to adopt unhealthy lifestyle choices (Caprio et al., 2008).

Getting Treatment for Obesity

Treatment for obesity, like other adolescent chronic diseases, is determined on a case-by-case basis and guided by the patient's age and pubertal status, severity of obesity, psychosocial factors and comorbidities (Grossman et al., 2017). According to the U.S. Preventive Services Task Force, one form of successful treatment included intensive behavioral interventions that targeted both the parent and child (separately, together, or both). These interventions, which typically included both family and group sessions, provided information about healthy eating, reading food labels, and regular physical activity. They also sought to develop youth skills in the areas of stimulus control, such as limiting access to tempting foods and limiting screen time, goal setting, self-monitoring, and problem-solving. Other treatments include pharmacotherapy and bariatric surgery (Cardel, Jastreboff, & Kelly, 2019).

The Health Consequences of Obesity

Obesity in childhood can affect both a child's immediate and long-term health. Serious medical consequences may result from overweight and obesity. The systems affected include but are not limited to the following:

- Psychological: Obese children and adolescents are often stigmatized and frequently teased and bullied by their peers based on their weight.
- Cardiovascular: Childhood obesity is associated with adult hypertension and increased triglycerides, suggesting that childhood obesity is a risk factor for cardiovascular disease (Umer et al., 2017). The increased cardiovascular risk in adulthood was irrespective of adult risk factor status, indicating that permanent damage to the arterial wall may occur during childhood.
- Endocrine: Metabolic syndrome is an insulin-resistance–related set of clinical characteristics known to increase the risk of type 2 diabetes, cardiovascular disease, and death in adults. Obesity in childhood has been linked to a number of metabolic risk factors, including increased waist circumference, hypertension, hyperglycemia, low HDL cholesterol, and high triglycerides (Kelsey, Zaepfel, Bjornstad, & Nadeau, 2014; Pulgarón, 2013).
- Orthopedic: Taylor et al. (2006) found overweight children reported a greater prevalence of fractures and musculoskeletal discomfort than their nonoverweight peers. The most common self-reported joint complaint was knee pain; overweight children also reported greater difficulties in mobility (Taylor et al., 2006).
- Hepatic: Research indicates an increased risk of nonalcoholic fatty liver disease among children and adolescents with obesity (Fabbrini, Sullivan, & Klein, 2010).
- Pulmonary: Obesity is indicated as a risk for asthma (Pulgarón, 2013).

References

Allen, K. L., Byrne, S. M., & Crosby, R. D. (2015). Distinguishing between risk factors for bulimia nervosa, binge eating disorder, and purging disorder. *Journal of Youth and Adolescence, 44*(8), 1580–1591. doi:10.1007/s10964-014-0186-8

Allen, K. L., Byrne, S. M., Oddy, W. H., & Crosby, R. D. (2013). Early onset binge eating and purging eating disorders: Course and outcome in a population-based study of adolescents. *Journal of Abnormal Child Psychology, 41*(7), 1083–1096. doi:10.1007/s10802-013-9747-7

American Psychiatric Association. (2013). *Diagnostic and statistical manual of mental disorders* (5th ed.). Arlington, VA: American Psychiatric Publishing.

Arcelus, J., Mitchell, A. J., Wales, J., & Nielsen, S. (2011). Mortality rates in patients with anorexia nervosa and other eating disorders: A meta-analysis of 36 studies. *Archives of General Psychiatry, 68*(7), 724–731. doi:10.1001/archgenpsychiatry.2011.74

Beccia, A. L., Baek, J., Jesdale, W. M., Austin, S. B., Forrester, S., Curtin, C., & Lapane, K. L. (2019). Risk of disordered eating at the intersection of gender and racial/ethnic identity among U.S. high school students. *Eating Behaviors, 34*, 101299. doi:10.1016/j.eatbeh.2019.05.002

Bigornia, S. J., Lavalley, M. P., Noel, S. E., Moore, L. L., Ness, A. R., & Newby P. (2015). Sugar-sweetened beverage consumption and central and total adiposity in older children: A prospective study accounting for dietary reporting errors. *Public Health Nutrition, 18*(7), 1155–1163. doi:10.1017/S1368980014001700

Campbell, K., & Peebles, R. (2014). Eating disorders in children and adolescents: State of the art review. *Pediatrics, 134*(3), 582–592. doi:10.1542/peds.2014-0194

Caprio, S., Daniels, S. R., Drewnowski, A., Kaufman, F. R., Palinkas, L. A., Rosenbloom, A. L., & Schwimmer, J. B. (2008). Influence of race, ethnicity, and culture on childhood obesity: Implications for prevention and treatment: A consensus statement of Shaping America's Health and the Obesity Society. *Diabetes Care, 31*(11), 2211–2221. doi:10.2337/dc08-9024

Cardel, M. I., Jastreboff, A. M., & Kelly, A. S. (2019). Treatment of adolescent obesity in 2020. *JAMA, 27*(2), 190–204. doi:10.1002/oby.22385

Cockrell Skinner, A., Ravanbakht, S. N., Skelton, J. A., Perrin, E. M., & Armstrong, S. C. (2018). Prevalence of obesity and severe obesity in US children, 1999–2016. *Pediatrics, 141*(3), 11. doi:10.1542/peds. 2017-3459

Copeland, W., Bulik, C., Zucker, N., Wolke, D., Lereya, S. T., & Costello, E. J. (2015). Is childhood bullying involvement a precursor of eating disorder symptoms? A prospective analysis. *International Journal of Eating Disorders, 48*(8), 1141–1149. doi:10.1016/j.physbeh.2017.03.040

Covassin, N., Singh, P., & Somers, V. K. (2016). Keeping up with the clock: Circadian disruption and obesity risk. *Hypertension, 68*(5), 1081–1090. doi:10.1161/HYPERTENSIONAHA.116.06588

de la Haye, K., Robins, G., Mohr, P., & Wilson, C. (2010). Obesity-related behaviors in adolescent friendship networks. *Social Networks, 32*(3), 161–167. doi:10.1016/j.socnet.2009.09.001

Drieberg, H., McEvoy, P. M., Hoiles, K. J., Shu, C. Y., & Egan, S. J. (2019). An examination of direct, indirect and reciprocal relationships between perfectionism, eating disorder symptoms, anxiety, and depression in children and adolescents with eating disorders. *Eating Behaviors, 32*, 53–59. doi:10.1016/j.eatbeh.2018.12.002

Elgar, F. J., Moore, L., Roberts, C., & Tudor-Smith, C. (2004). Sedentary behaviour, physical activity and weight problems among adolescents in wales. *Psychology Health, 19*(Suppl. 1), 48–49. doi:10.1016/j.puhe.2004.10.011

Evans, E. H., Adamson, A. J., Basterfield, L., Le Couteur, A., Reilly, J. K., Reilly, J. J., & Parkinson, K. N. (2017). Risk factors for eating disorder symptoms at 12 years of age: A 6-year longitudinal cohort study. *Appetite, 108,* 12–20. doi:10.1016/j.appet.2016.09.005

Fabbrini, E., Sullivan, S., & Klein, S. (2010). Reply. *Hepatology, 51*(2), 679–689. doi:10.1097/IAE.0000000000002105

Fatima, Y., Doi, S. A. R., & Mamun, A. A. (2015). Longitudinal impact of sleep on overweight and obesity in children and adolescents: A systematic review and bias-adjusted meta-analysis. *Obesity Reviews, 16*(2), 137–149. doi:10.1111/obr.12245

Fernandez, J. R., Klimentidis, Y. C., Dulin-Keita, A., & Casazza, K. (2012). Genetic influences in childhood obesity: Recent progress and recommendations for experimental designs. *International Journal of Obesity, 36*(4), 479–484. doi:10.1038/ijo.2011.236

Fuller-Tyszkiewicz, M., Skouteris, H., Hardy, L. L., & Halse, C. (2012). The associations between TV viewing, food intake, and BMI. A prospective analysis of data from the Longitudinal Study of Australian Children. *Appetite, 59*(3), 945–948. doi:10.1016/j.appet.2012.09.009

Grossman, D., Bibbins-Domingo, K., Curry, S., Barry, M. J., Davidson, K. W., Doubeni, C. A., ... Tseng, C. W. (2017). Screening for obesity in children and adolescents: US preventive services task force recommendation statement. *JAMA, 317*(23), 2417–2426. doi:10.1001/jama.2017.6803

Guillaume, S., Jaussent, I., Maimoun, L., Ryst, A., Seneque, M., Villain, L., ... Courtet, P. H. (2016, October 6). Associations between adverse childhood experiences and clinical characteristics of eating disorders. *Scientific Reports,* 1–8. doi:10.1038/srep35761

Harding, S., Teyhan, A., Maynard, M. J., & Cruickshank, J. K. (2008). Ethnic differences in overweight and obesity in early adolescence in the MRC DASH study: The role of adolescent and parental lifestyle. *International Journal of Epidemiology, 37*(1), 162–172. doi:10.1093/ije/dym252

Hart, L. M., Granillo, M. T., Jorm, A. F., & Paxton, S. J. (2011). Unmet need for treatment in the eating disorders: A systematic review of eating disorder specific treatment seeking among community cases. *Clinical Psychology Review, 31*(5), 727–735. doi:10.1016/j.cpr.2011.03.004

Jáuregui-Garrido, B., & Jáuregui-Lobera, I. (2012). Sudden death in eating disorders. *Vascular Health and Risk Management, 8*(1), 91–98. doi:10.2147/VHRM.S28652

Kalliomäki, M., Collado, M. C., Salminen, S., & Isolauri, E. (2008). Early differences in fecal microbiota composition in children may predict overweight. *The American Journal of Clinical Nutrition, 87*(3), 534–538. doi:10.1093/ajcn/87.3.534

Kelsey, M. M., Zaepfel, A., Bjornstad, P., & Nadeau, K. J. (2014). Age-related consequences of childhood obesity. *Gerontology, 60*(3), 222–228. doi:10.1159/000356023

Kessler, R. C., Berglund, P. A., Chiu, W. T., Deitz, A. C., Hudson, J. I., Shahly, V., ... Xavier, M. (2013). The prevalence and correlates of binge eating disorder in the World Health Organization World Mental Health Surveys. *Biological Psychiatry, 73*(9), 904–914. doi:10.1016/j.biopsych.2012.11.020

Kirschenbaum, D. S., Germann, J. N., Rich, B. H., & Daniel, S. (2005). Treatment of morbid obesity in low-income adolescents: Effects of parental self-monitoring. *Obesity Research, 13*(9), 1527–1529. doi:10.1038/oby.2005.187

Koehly, L. M., & Loscalzo, A. (2009). Adolescent obesity and social networks. *Preventing Chronic Disease, 6*(3), A99. Retrieved from https://www.cdc.gov/pcd/issues/2009/Jul/08_0265.htm

Kosti, R. I., Panagiotakos, D. B., Tountas, Y., Mihas, C. C., Alevizos, A., Mariolis, T., ... Mariolis, A. (2008). Parental Body Mass Index in association with the prevalence of overweight/obesity among adolescents in Greece; dietary and lifestyle habits in the context of the family environment: The Vyronas study. *Appetite, 51*(1), 218–222. doi:10.1016/j.appet.2008.02.001

Kremers, S. P. J., van der Horst, K., & Brug, J. (2007). Adolescent screen-viewing behaviour is associated with consumption of sugar-sweetened beverages: The role of habit strength and perceived parental norms. *Appetite, 48*(3), 345–350. doi:10.1016/j.appet.2006.10.002

Lindsay, A. C., Sussner, K. M., Kim, J., & Gortmaker, S. L. (2006). The role of parents in preventing childhood obesity. *The Future of Children, 16*(1), 169–186. doi:10.1353/foc.2006.0006

Martinsen, M., & Sundgot-Borgen, J. (2013). Higher prevalence of eating disorders among adolescent elite athletes than controls. *Medicine and Science in Sports and Exercise, 45*(6), 1188–1197. doi:10.1249/MSS.0b013e318281a939

Micali, N., De Stavola, B., Ploubidis, G., Simonoff, E., Treasure, J., & Field, A. E. (2015). Adolescent eating disorder behaviours and cognitions: Gender-specific effects of child, maternal and family risk factors. *The British Journal of Psychiatry, 207*(4), 320–327. doi:10.1192/bjp.bp.114.152371

Nicholls, D., & Barrett, E. (2015). Eating disorders in children and adolescents. *BJPsych Advances, 21*, 206–216. doi:10.1017/CBO9780511543890

Ogden, C. L., Carroll, M. D., Lawman, H. G., Fryar, C. D., Kruszon-Moran, D., Kit, B. K., & Flegal, K. M. (2016). Trends in obesity prevalence among children and adolescents in the United States, 1988–1994 through 2013–2014. *JAMA, 315*(21), 2292–2299. doi:10.1001/jama.2016.6361

Pulgarón, E. R. (2013). Childhood obesity: A review of increased risk for physical and psychological comorbidities. *Clinical Therapeutics, 35*(1), A18–A32. doi:10.1016/j.clinthera.2012.12.014

Silventoinen, K., Rokholm, B., Kaprio, J., & Sørensen, T. I. A. (2010). The genetic and environmental influences on childhood obesity: A systematic review of twin and adoption studies. *International Journal of Obesity, 34*(1), 29–40. doi:10.1038/ijo.2009.177

Sorrell, S., & Sorrell, M. D. S. (2017). Is an eating disorder related to suicide? *International Journal of Child Health and Human Development, 10*(4), 339–343.

Taylor, E. D., Theim, K. R., Mirch, M. C., Ghorbani, S., Tanofsky-Kraff, M., Adler-Wailes, D. C., … Yanovski, J. A. (2006). Orthopedic complications of overweight in children and adolescents. *Pediatrics, 117*(6), 2167–2174. doi:10.1542/peds.2005-1832

UConn Rudd Center for Food Policy and Obesity. (2018). *Trends in television food advertising to young people: 2017 Update*. Retrieved from http://uconnruddcenter.org/files/Pdfs/TVAdTrends2018_Final.pdf

Umer, A., Kelley, G. A., Cottrell, L. E., Giacobbi, P., Innes, K. E., & Lilly, C. L. (2017). Childhood obesity and adult cardiovascular disease risk factors: A systematic review with meta-analysis. *BMC Public Health, 17*(1), 1–24. doi:10.1186/s12889-017-4691-z

Wang, S., Schwartz, M. B., Shebl, F. M., Read, M., Henderson, K. E., & Ickovics, J. R. (2017). School breakfast and body mass index: A longitudinal observational study of middle school students. *Pediatric Obesity, 12*(3), 213–220. doi:10.1111/ijpo.12127

Westmoreland, P., Krantz, M. J., & Mehler, P. S. (2016). Medical complications of anorexia nervosa and bulimia. *The American Journal of Medicine, 129*(1), 30–37. doi:10.1016/j.amjmed.2015.06.031

Wouters, E. J., Larsen, J. K., Kremers, S. P. J., Dagnelie, P. C., & Geenen, R. (2010). Peer influence on snacking behavior in adolescence. *Appetite, 55*(1), 11–17. doi:10.1016/j.appet.2010.03.002

Online Resources

Alliance for a Healthier Generation. (n.d.). *Professional site—The Alliance for a Healthier Generation and Voices for Healthy Kids works to elevate the importance of strong wellness policies in schools. School leaders, community members, and parents can visit WellnessWins. org to download resources, read success stories, and learn how to support and advance school wellness policies.* Retrieved from https://www.healthiergeneration.org

American Academy of Pediatrics. (n.d.). *Professional and consumer site—Contains family, community, and professional resources.* Retrieved from https://healthychildren.org

American Psychiatric Association. (n.d.). Retrieved from http://www.psych.org/

EAT-26 Self-Test. (n.d.). *Consumer site—Offers a screening measure to help determine if a person has an eating disorder that needs professional attention. The 26-item instrument is available with free, confidential feedback.* Retrieved from http://www.eat-26.com

Maudsley Parents. (n.d.). *Consumer site—Offers information on eating disorders and family-based treatment; family stories of recovery; supportive parent-to-parent advice; and treatment information for families that opt for family-based Maudsley treatment.* Retrieved from http://Maudsleyparents.org

National Association of Anorexia Nervosa & Associated Disorders, Inc®. (n.d.). *Consumer site—Offers information about eating disorders; insurance discrimination; referrals to hospitals, doctors, therapists, and support groups; opportunities to get involved; prevention programs for all ages; and educational materials.* Retrieved from http://www.anad.org

National Association of School Nurses. (n.d.). *Professional site—A position statement by the National Association of School Nurses (NASN) on childhood obesity.* Retrieved from https://www.nasn.org/nasn/advocacy/professional-practice-documents/position -statements/ps-overweight

National Eating Disorders Association (NEDA) Formerly EDAP & AABA. (n.d.). *Consumer site—Offers information about eating disorders and body image; referrals to treatment centers, doctors, therapists, and support groups; opportunities to get involved in prevention efforts; prevention programs for all ages; and educational materials.* Retrieved from http://www.nationaleatingdisorders.org

Nemours. (n.d.). *Consumer site—Offers information on developing health eating habits, sleep hygiene and being physical active.* Retrieved from https://healthykidshealthyfuture .org/resources-for-parents/

Stop Obesity Alliance. (n.d.). *Consumer site—Aimed at parents and caregivers; offers guidance on talking with children about weight and scenarios to help guide discussions for parents and children.* Retrieved from http://weighinguide.com

U.S. Department of Agriculture. (n.d.). *Professional site—USDA resource for wellness advocacy in schools and resources for families.* Retrieved from https://www.fns.usda .gov/tn

Further Readings

American Psychiatric Association. (2013). *Diagnostic and statistical manual of mental disorders* (5th ed.). Arlington, VA: American Psychiatric Publishing. The American Psychiatric Association's *Diagnostic and Statistical Manual of Mental Disorders (DSM-5)* is used by clinicians and researchers to diagnose and classify mental disorders. It includes concise and specific criteria to aid practitioners in an objective assessment of symptom presentations in a variety of clinical settings: inpatient, outpatient, partial hospital, consultation-liaison, clinical, private practice, and primary care.

Cash, T. F., & Smolak, L. (2011). *Body image: A handbook of science, practice, and prevention* (2nd ed.). New York, NY: Guilford Press. Considered a standard reference for practitioners, researchers, and students. It reviews established and emerging theories and findings; examines questions of culture, gender, health, and disorder; and presents evidence-based assessment, treatment, and prevention approaches for the full range of body image concerns.

Goldstein, D. J. (2005). *The management of eating disorders and obesity*. Totowa, NJ: Humana Press. A concise, practical, state-of-the-art review of obesity, eating disorders, and their management including treatment. The book reviews the history, diagnosis, prevalence, psychiatric comorbidity, and medical complications of each of these disorders, along with the scientific evidence for various pharmacologic therapies.

BULLYING IN THE SCHOOL SETTING

BRENDA MARSHALL | KATHERINE J. ROBERTS

▨ Introduction

A school's environment has a major impact on a child's ability to learn and thrive. A positive school climate ensures that students are safe, supported, challenged, and socially capable. Bullying interferes with all aspects of student development, from academic success to good health. The effects of bullying can include poor self-worth, psychiatric symptoms, psychosomatic symptoms, and social conduct. These responses from the child experiencing bullying often make them a frequent visitor to the nurse's office. The school nurse who is aware of the impact of bullying on child development engages in evidence-based nursing interventions. These interventions include, but are not limited to, rapid identification of symptoms and referrals to appropriate providers. The informed nurse can also be a key collaborator in creating a safe haven for the child while improving the overall school climate by engaging and educating school professionals. This chapter provides definitions, clear identification strategies for recognizing and reporting the discrimination and harassment of bullying, the laws that protect all of those in the school environment, and introduces some restorative practice approaches.

Legislation

There are no federal laws specifically addressing bullying. All 50 states, however, have passed some form of antibullying legislation. The first law passed in the state of Georgia (1999) defined bullying, mandated school policies prohibiting bullying and encoded it into school conduct handbooks (Barge, 2011). The U.S. Department of Education, in 2010, outlined critical components of strong state antibullying laws in response to requests for assistance by state and local officials (Duncan, 2010). Despite differences across state legislations, multiple common components include the definition of bullying, specific characteristics of bullying behavior, and requirements for school district policies.

Currently, each state has legislation requiring school districts to develop and implement a policy prohibiting bullying; however, not all states have developed standardized components like identifying protected groups or clear communication of policies (Laws, Policies & Regulations, 2018). The majority of states have procedures mandating prompt investigations responding to all reported incidents of bullying, require bullying prevention programs, the inclusion of bullying prevention in health education standards, and teacher professional development. State laws generally do not prescribe specific consequences for students who engage in bullying behavior; instead they suggest a graduated range of consequences.

Definitions

What Is Bullying?

Despite most people believing that they can identify bullying, actual definitions of bullying vary. The commonly cited Olweus Bullying Prevention Program states that: Bullying is negative behavior that (a) is intentional (those who bully know/understand that their behavior is unpleasant or hurtful to the target); (b) is usually repetitive; and (c) involves some degree of power imbalance between the targeted individual and the perpetrator(s) in favor of the latter (Olweus & Limber, 2019). The term "bullying" does not apply to conflict arising between two students who are considered equals (physically or cognitively), differentiating it from peer conflict. The criteria of repetitiveness imply a type of relationship, although unwanted, between the predator and the target (Olweus & Limber, 2019). Individuals, besides the persons either engaging in bullying or receiving the impact, are involved as observers who choose to do something or stay silent. Youth who witness bullying, called bystanders, often report increased feelings of guilt or helplessness for not stopping the bullying behavior. However, when bystanders choose to take action to stop bullying, they become upstanders (Padgett & Notar, 2013)

Harassment

The term "harassment," having an established history in civil rights law, is often used interchangeably with bullying (Cornell & Limber, 2015). Harassment can include actual or perceived negative actions that offend, ridicule, or demean another individual based on a protected class which include but are not limited to race, religion, religious practice, sex, age, color, disability, national origin, weight, sexual orientation, sex, and gender. Federal laws protect students from harassment including (a) Title VI of the Civil Rights Act of 1964 which prohibits discrimination on the basis of *race, color*, or *national origin*; (b) Title IX of the Education Amendments of 1972 which prohibits discrimination on the basis of *sex*, including sexual harassment and stereotyping; and (c) Section 504 of the Rehabilitation Act of 1973 and Title II of the Americans with Disabilities Act of 1990 prohibits discrimination on the basis of *disability* (Cornell & Limber, 2015). School districts violate these civil rights when harassment, based on one of these protected classes, is sufficiently serious. A hostile environment can develop when harassment is encouraged, tolerated, not adequately addressed, or ignored by school employees. "Intimidation" is often used interchangeably with harassment and bullying (Cascardi, Brown, Iannarone, & Cardona, 2014). However, the legal definition of intimidation, unlike harassment, is when a person feels that an action is intentional and seriously threatens their safety and well-being (U.S. Legal, n.d.). Intimidation subjects the individual to an intentional action that is meant to induce fear, a sense of inferiority, and results in a sense of being seriously threatened.

Types of Bullying

Bullying may be direct or indirect. Direct bullying includes physical assault and taunting as well as verbal teasing and inappropriate sexual language. The person who engages in direct bullying is known to the target. Indirect bullying is not face to face and often uses the tactic of rumors, spreading lies about another person, and social exclusion. Cyberbullying, or using electronic communication tools to harass, intimidate, or insult another can engage both direct and indirect methods of bullying behaviors (Box 17.1).

Prevalence

Prevalence rates identify the proportion of the population that has experienced bullying during a specific time period. Prevalence rates of bullying across studies vary as a result of differences in measurement and the operationalization of the bullying construct (Menesini & Salmivalli, 2017). Therefore, the actual prevalence of bullying is not well-known. Studies have suggested that the prevalence of bullying is highest in middle school years (i.e., 12–15 years old) and tends to decrease by the end of high school (Hymel & Swearer, 2015). Almost one fifth (19%) of high school students reported being bullied at school and an additional 15% were bullied electronically (Kann et al., 2018).

Cyberbullying

Cyberbullying includes all repeated deliberate acts of aggression that are intended to insult or cause harm and distress (Kowalski, Giumetti, Schroeder, & Lattanner, 2014). There is a high correlation between cyberbullying and traditional bullying, indicating that these are two different methods of enacting similar behavior (Modecki, Minchin,

---

BOX 17.1

TYPES OF BULLYING

Verbal (Direct)

- Name-calling
- Threats
- Sexual intimidation

Physical (Direct)

- Pushing
- Hitting
- Kicking

Psychological/Emotional/Social (Indirect)

- Spreading rumors
- Excluding the person from conversations/activities on purpose
- Mocking

Cyberbullying (Direct and Indirect)

- Harassment or threats made through electronic communication
  - Texting
  - Sexting
  - Posts meant to hurt or insult another

Harbaugh, Guerra, & Runions, 2014). As social media platforms increase in use by youth, the risk of cyberbullying also increases (Juvonen & Gross, 2008). Often it is not the physical, cognitive, or social power imbalances that underlie the bullying. Cyberbullying can also be reflective of imbalances in technological capacity (Whittaker & Kowalski, 2015).

Trends in Cyberbullying

Anyone who has used a cell phone or computer in the past decade is aware of how rapidly technology changes. As new modes of technology emerge, new means of cyberbullying appear. Texting remains dominant; however, social networking sites are common locations for cyberbullying. Some forms of social media provide an environment where a person can post anonymously, allowing the negative statement to appear without fear of personal identification. This level of anonymity is a factor that is highly conducive to cyberbullying. See Box 17.2 for examples of cyberbullying.

BOX 17.2

EXAMPLES OF CYBERBULLYING

- Happy slapping—recording video of harassing or bullying of an individual (often involving physical abuse), then circulating the video online

- Identity theft—stealing an individual's password and hijacking their online accounts, often in order to send humiliating information or images

- Photoshopping—doctoring digital images of a person with the goal of placing the subject in a compromising or embarrassing situation

- Physical threats—messages involving threats to an individual's physical safety

- Rumor spreading—disseminating gossip through email, text messages, and/or social media posts

- Trolling and flaming—posting or sending offensive or inflammatory messages

SOURCE: Adapted from Hinduja, S., & Patchin J. (2009). *Bullying beyond the schoolyard: Preventing and responding to cyberbullying.* Thousand Oaks, CA: Corwin Press.

Effects of Bullying

The effects of bullying on students have been widely reported. If bullying can be thought of as a disease, then the impact of bullying should be seen as the sequelae. As with any disease, treating the disease is only the first step. Just as important is to be aware of the signs and symptoms of the sequelae in order to engage in long-term treatment.

Physical: It is often the physical responses to bullying that brings the student to the health office. Some of the indicators of physical reaction to bullying include reporting or complaining of health problems (e.g., stomachaches, headaches), engaging in self-destructive behavior such as cutting, and exhaustion secondary to sleeplessness or frequent nightmares, and attempted suicide. These students might also present with unexplained bruises, eating disorders, and overall multiple somatic complaints.

Emotional: Students who are the target of bullying might present with symptoms of depression, anger, anxiety, and lowered self-worth. Suicidal ideation may be present and must be investigated for intention, plan, and access. They might have engaged in withdrawing from friends and family and other social activities secondary to emotional distress.

Academic: Students may avoid coming to school citing illnesses, health problems, or truancy, which in turn affects their academic performance. Persistent bullying can even lead to school withdrawal.

Subsequent outcomes: Left untreated, the student who experiences bullying may move on to engage in acts of violence and delinquency and is at increased risk for substance abuse and eating disorders (Copeland et al., 2015; Kowalski, & Limber, 2013).

▨ Assessing the Safety of the School Environment

A safe school environment is one where students are able to pursue their interests and studies without fear of violence or intimidation. The impact of a safe environment allows students to feel free to express themselves and to engage in respectful collaboration with peers and staff. The student is physically, emotionally, and socially safe during the hours of school attendance, which is reflected by meaningful connections, strong school bonds, positive peer relations, and effective and available supports.

Bullying that is allowed to exist in the school environment can remove a student's sense of environmental safety. When bullying is not immediately identified and addressed, it can send a signal to the students that they are not safe at school. The repetitive nature of bullying can often give way to the sense of "this is the way things are," which cannot be an acceptable climate for learning. In order to assess the safety of the school environment, there needs to be transparency and communication of expected civility norms. Establishing a safe and welcoming environment sets the foundation for allowing children to achieve their highest potential in a nurturing space.

The Role of the School Nurse in Assessing Bullying

School nurses are fundamental in the assessment and planning to establish a comprehensive healthy and safe school climate. Utilizing the nursing process, the school nurse can assess the situation from both the faculty/staff perspective as well as the student's view. Bullying is a public health concern and needs to be approached as such. Bullies thrive in the absence of adults, so being aware of those places in the school that lack adult supervision, like bathrooms, playgrounds, and cafeterias, and alerting others assists in the development of a school plan. In addition to identifying bullying from a public and personal health vantage point, the school nurse can also engage in risk management assessment.

In terms of risk management, schools should be proactive in preventing intimidation, harassment, and bullying to prevent the school from failing to provide a safe learning environment for their students. Schools must also address cyberbullying since it creates a risk of substantial disruption within the school environment. It is frequently the school nurse who will have the first indicators of a child being bullied in the environment. These indicators include a student who is making frequent visits with generalized somatic complaints or students with unexplained newly acquired bruises. In order to assess bullying, the school nurse needs to routinely ask school staff and students about their experiences and thoughts related to bullying. Administering a student survey can assist in determining the frequency and location of bullying behavior. There is a multitude of tools that can measure a range of bullying experiences from bullying to bystander experiences (Hamburger, Basile, & Vivolo, 2011). One of the school nurse's best tools, however, is to ask direct questions of the students.

MAX AND THE SCHOOL NURSE

Max, a third grader, was a frequent visitor to the nurse's office, usually right after lunch period. The nurse asked him why he was always coming after lunch even though he denied having any stomach problems. Max thoughtfully replied: "I don't like going on the playground after lunch." The nurse asked him why and he responded, "Well, there are three kinds of people on the playground. The runners, the chasers, and the heroes. The runners are the ones everybody knows are scaredy-cats, the chasers go after them for the whole time or unless another kid steps in—that's the group I call heroes. I used to be a runner, now I think I'm more like the heroes, but I'm afraid that I might get thrown back into the runner's group. I know I don't want to join the chasers ... so I'd rather visit with you." The nurse asked, "What about the adults on the playground, Max?" "Oh them," Max frowned, "they just stand there and watch."

Max, only 8 years old was able to identify bullying behaviors, recognize upstanding and bystanding behaviors in the playground. He believed that he had to join one of the existing groups. The school nurse allowed him to feel safe and tell someone what was going on so that the situation could be identified and rectified.

▪ Methods to Improve the School Environment

Evidence-based school-based programs appear in multiple ecological models, where individual relationships are examined in a broader context within schools, communities, and cultural settings. Effective multitiered systems include (a) universal programs for all youth within the school, (b) selective preventive interventions for youth at risk for being involved in bullying, and (c) indicated preventive intervention tailored for students already displaying bullying behavior or are being bullied (Bradshaw, 2015). The nurse is instrumental in identifying cases, explaining the standard treatment for the known disorders that can emerge from an environment of bullying, and work with parents and other healthcare professionals to ensure compliance with long-term treatment and aftercare. Health promotion and positive development interventions that reduce the risk of negative psychological and behavioral outcomes can fit under universal, selective, and indicated prevention programs. Social emotional learning programs which focus on health skills can be particularly helpful in reducing bullying and cyberbullying. Although cyberbullying requires interventions at multiple settings including the home and school, the school nurse can provide a bridge informing students, families, teachers, administrators, and school safety participants of the physical and psychological effects of bullying behaviors. Informational gatherings to explain symptoms that might be emerging secondary to an online bullying experience can empower the school community to early identification and intervention.

Embarking on a comprehensive approach, where the school is one of the settings within the youth's experience, helps to foster a more positive, healthy living environment. Other settings where bullying interventions should be implemented include the home, neighborhood agencies, primary care, outpatient mental health, day treatment programs, residential, and inpatient units.

Strategies for Reducing Risk, Combating Bullying, Buffering Negative Impacts

Comprehensive programs should include school-wide, classroom, and intervention components. A school-wide component includes training, awareness, monitoring, and assessment of bullying; a classroom component is focused on reinforcing school-wide rules and building social and emotional skills; and an intervention component is for students who engage or receive bullying behaviors. To enhance the prevention strategies and positive school climate approaches, the school nurse can support the development of social and emotional skills needed to recognize and manage emotions, demonstrate caring and concern for others, establish positive relationships, make responsible decisions, and handle challenging social situations constructively. Five categories of social and emotional skills identified by Ragozzino and O'Brien (2009) are presented in Table 17.1.

TABLE 17.1 FIVE CATEGORIES OF SOCIAL EMOTIONAL SKILLS

Self-awareness	The ability to honestly and correctly evaluate one's own feelings, values, abilities, strengths, and interests while also keeping a sense of balance and self-worth.
Self-management	The ability to self-regulate emotional responses to stress through responding with plans rather than impulse, engaging in goal setting and keeping the course even when there are barriers. Self-management includes the skills of self-monitoring progress and modulating emotional responses.
Social awareness	Holding an empathetic attitude toward others with the ability to demonstrate appreciation to others (groups and individuals) whether there are similarities or differences in opinion. Following rules and relying on the support of community, school, and family resources.
Relationship skills	The ability to connect and cooperate with others in order to participate in positive, healthy, and fulfilling relationships. Resist peer pressure, work through interpersonal conflicts, and find resources for help when needed.
Responsible decision-making	Using ethics and safety concerns to direct decision making. Taking into account the rights of others as well as probable consequences or outcomes of personal decisions on the lives of others in both academic and social situations. Being able to be a positive contributor to the healthy community atmosphere of the school.

SOURCE: Adapted from Ragozzino, K., & O'Brien, M. U. (2009). *Social and emotional learning and bullying prevention*. Retrieved from https://www.casel.org/wp-content/uploads/2016/01/3_SEL_and_Bullying _Prevention_2009.pdf

Emotional coping in the face of bullying behaviors supports student development for effectively dealing with the impact of the behaviors. Healthy strategies to combat all forms of bullying include recognizing that the behavior is unpleasant and unacceptable, choosing not to react to it, and instead to walk away or purposely ignore the online bullying. Through the lack of attention and response, negative bullying behaviors can be discouraged. In a study by Machackova, Cerna, Sevcikova, Dedkova, and Daneback (2013) purposeful ignoring was considered to be emotionally helpful by almost two thirds of those experiencing cyberbullying, and for half of them, it also helped stop the cyberbullying. Another strategy that the nurse can introduce to the student is understanding the impact of body language and helping the student appear physically more confident. The student can learn that by appearing more confident, they will be less likely to be vulnerable. Confident body language includes standing up straight, putting the shoulder back, and walking with a sure stride. One of the most important instructions to give a child is to tell a caring adult in the school about the situation.

Effective Strategies for Staff to Engage in When Confronted With Bullying Behaviors

Intervention strategies should be systematic and consistent in order to prevent disruptive behaviors. The types of activities that can reduce bullying behaviors include increased supervision and on-the-spot intervention that immediately enforce the school rules against bullying. Nurses can engage in on-the-spot interventions which takes minimal time yet communicates that bullying is not acceptable and will not be permitted. Steps include (a) remain calm and model respectful behavior to stop the bullying, (b) support the child who has been bullied, (c) name the bullying behavior and refer to school rules, (d) empower the bystander with information on how to act in the future, and (e) impose immediate consequences (Limber, 2011).

ON-THE-SPOT INTERVENTION BY THE SCHOOL NURSE

The nurse takes Max out to the playground and observes a child being chased. The nurse steps in and stops the child from chasing, standing between the chaser and the runner. Looking at the runner, the nurse says, "I'm sorry this happened to you, I am going to stop it now. If you would like, you can come inside with me."

Turning to the chaser the nurse states, "This kind of behavior is unacceptable. It is an act of bullying and is against school rules. You must stop now and sit with the lunch monitor."

The nurse notices the others watching (the bystanders) and says, "You might not have known what to do this time, but next time come and get someone to help." The nurse adds to the chaser, "I will be watching to make sure this behavior doesn't happen again. Please come and see me after school so we can talk about this."

The nurse reports the incident to the school bullying prevention coordinator or school administrator to enforce guidelines to prevent further bullying at recess.

Other aspects of improving school environments include involving families and communities by educating them about bullying and encouraging them to become involved in school-based prevention efforts. It takes a village to establish and maintain a safe environment in which a youth can learn and grow.

Collaborating With Other School Professionals to Reduce Bullying

The school nurse provides key leadership to promote and enhance student safety, wellness, engagement, and learning. The school nurse should collaborate with other staff in developing safe environment protocols. This also includes working with others in the school environment like aides, bus drivers, security, cafeteria workers, and librarians who might observe bullying in their practice environments and intervene. This way, students will receive similar and consistent messages from all school staff.

It is imperative that the school nurse is an active partner in antibullying initiatives in the school environment. As a key collaborator, the school nurse can share knowledge on the effects of bullying and can educate others against using labels like bully or victim and instead identify and name the behavior. It is well within the purview of the school nurse's role to be a participant on the school team working on the topic of bullying behaviors. The school nurse is also the professional voice who can share observations and assessments that identify students at high risk, or those who are exhibiting symptoms of being bullied. It is the office of the school nurse that provides a safe haven for many students who experience bullying, showing up with unexplained somatic complaints or stress-related emotional dysphoria. It is here that students should be able to verbalize their concerns about any problems that are bothering them and feel that they are being respected and heard (Selekman, Pelt, Garnier, & Baker, 2013). As a key figure in the school's response to bullying behaviors, the school nurse also provides the important role of bridging and strengthening relationships between school staff, administration, and families related to bullying concerns (Pigozi & Bartoli, 2016). Being prepared with assessment tools, collaborators, support through policies and evidence-based interventions can improve the school environment for all.

References

Barge, J. D. (2011). *Policy for prohibiting bullying, harassment and intimidation, Georgia Department of Education.* Retrieved from https://www.gadoe.org/schoolsafetyclimate/Documents/GaDOE%20Bullying%20Policy_August%202011.pdf

Bradshaw, C. P. (2015). Translating research to practice in bullying prevention. *American Psychologist, 70*(4), 322–332 doi:10.1037/a0039114

Cascardi, M., Brown, C., Iannarone, M., & Cardona, N. (2014). The problem with overly broad definitions of bullying: Implications for the schoolhouse, the statehouse, and the ivory tower. *Journal of School Violence, 13,* 253–276. doi:10.1080/15388220.2013.846861

Copeland, W. E., Bulik, C. M., Zucker, N., Wolke, D., Lereya, S. T., & Costello, E. J. (2015). Does childhood bullying predict eating disorder symptoms? A prospective, longitudinal analysis. *International Journal of Eating Disorders, 48*(8), 1141–1149. doi:10.1002/eat.22459

Cornell, D., & Limber, S. P. (2015). Law and policy on the concept of bullying at school. *American Psychologist, 70*(4), 333–343. doi:10.1037/a0038558

Duncan, A. (2010). *Key policy letters from the education secretary and deputy secretary.* Retrieved from https://www2.ed.gov/policy/gen/guid/secletter/101215.html

Hamburger, M. E., Basile, K. C., & Vivolo, A. M. (2011). *Measuring bullying victimization, perpetration, and bystander experiences: A compendium of assessment tools.* Atlanta, GA: Centers for Disease Control and Prevention, National Center for Injury Prevention and Control.

Hinduja, S., & Patchin J. (2009). *Bullying beyond the schoolyard: Preventing and responding to cyberbullying.* Thousand Oaks, CA: Corwin Press.

Hymel, S., & Swearer, S. M. (2015). Four decades of research on school bullying: An introduction. *American Psychologist, 70*(4), 293–299. doi:10.1037/a0038928

Juvonen, J., & Gross, E. F. (2008). Extending the school grounds? Bullying experiences in cyberspace. *Journal of School Health, 78*(9), 496–505. doi:10.1111/j.1746 -1561.2008.00335.x

Kann, L., McManus, T., Harris, W. A., Shanklin, S., Flint, K. H., Queen, B., … Ethier, K. A. (2018). Youth risk behavior surveillance—United States, 2017. *MMWR Surveillance Summaries, 67*(No. SS-8), 1–114. doi:10.15585/mmwr.ss6708a1

Kowalski, R. M., Giumetti, G. W., Schroeder, A. N., & Lattanner, M. R. (2014). Bullying in the digital age: A critical review and meta-analysis of cyberbullying research among youth. *Psychological Bulletin, 140*, 1073–1137. doi:10.1037/a0035618

Kowalski, R. M. & Limber, S. P. (2013). Psychological, physical, and academic correlates of cyberbullying and traditional bullying. *Journal of Adolescent Health, 53*(1),S13–S20. doi:10.1016/j.jadohealth.2012.09.018

Laws, Policies & Regulations. (2018). https://www.stopbullying.gov/resources/laws

Limber, S. P. (2011). Development, evaluation, and future directions of the Olweus Bullying Prevention Program. *Journal of School Violence, 10*, 71–87. doi:10.1080/15388220.2010 .519375

Machackova, H., Cerna, A., Sevcikova, A., Dedkova, L., & Daneback, K. (2013). Effectiveness of coping strategies for victims of cyberbullying. *Cyberpsychology: Journal of Psychosocial Research on Cyberspace, 7*(3), 5. doi:10.5817/CP2013-3-5

Menesini, E., & Salmivalli, C. (2017). Bullying in schools: The state of knowledge and effective interventions. *Psychology, Health & Medicine, 22*(1), 240–253. doi:10.1080/13 548506.2017.1279740

Modecki, K. L., Minchin, J., Harbaugh, A. G., Guerra, N. G., & Runions, K. C. (2014). Bullying prevalence across contexts: A meta-analysis measuring cyber and traditional bullying. *Journal of Adolescent Health, 55*, 602–611. doi:10.1016/j.jadohealth.2014.06.007

Olweus, D., & Limber, S. P. (2019). The Olweus bullying prevention program (OBPP) new evaluations and current status. In P. K. Smith (Ed.), *Making an impact on school bullying: Interventions and recommendations* (pp. 23–44). New York, NY: Routledge.

Padgett, M. S., & Notar, C. E. (2013). Bystanders are the key to stopping bullying. *Universal Journal of Educational Research, 1*(2), 33–41 doi:10.13189/ujer.2013.010201

Pigozi, P. L., & Jones Bartoli, A. (2016). School nurses' experiences in dealing with bullying situations among students. *The Journal of School Nursing, 32*, 177–185. doi:10.1177/1059840515613140

Ragozzino, K., & O'Brien, M. U. (2009). *Social and emotional learning and bullying prevention*. Retrieved from https://www.casel.org/wp-content/uploads/2016/01/3_SEL _and_Bullying_Prevention_2009.pdf

Selekman, J., Pelt, P., Garnier, S., & Baker, D. (2013). Youth violence. In J. Selekman (Ed.), *School nursing: A comprehensive text* (2nd ed., pp. 1087–1117). Philadelphia, PA: F.A. Davis.

USLegal. (n.d.). *Intimidation law and legal definition*. Retrieved from https://definitions .uslegal.com/i/intimidation/

Whittaker, E., & Kowalski, R. M. (2015). Cyberbullying via social media. *Journal of School Violence*, *14*, 11–29. doi:10.1080/15388220.2014.949377

Online Resources

StopBullying.gov provides information from various government agencies on what bullying is, what cyberbullying is, who is at risk, and how you can prevent and respond to bullying. https://www.stopbullying.gov

National Association of School Nurses. (2018). *Bullying and cyberbullying— Prevention in schools* (Position Statement). Silver Spring, MD: Author. Retrieved from https://www .nasn.org/advocacy/professional-practice-documents/position-statements/ps-bullying

American Psychological Association provides information on how to take action to address bullying, including cyberbullying. https://www.apa.org/topics/bullying/

Cyberbullying Research Center provides information about the nature, extent, causes, and consequences of cyberbullying among adolescents. https://cyberbullying.org

PACER's National Bullying Prevention Center provides resources designed to benefit all students, including those with disabilities. https://www.pacer.org

Further Readings

Patchin, J. W., & Hinduja, S. (2016). *Bullying today: Bullet points and best practices*. Thousand Oaks, CA: Corwin.

Swearer, S. M., Espelage, D. L., & Napolitano, S. A. (2009). *Bullying prevention and intervention: Realistic strategies for schools*. New York, NY: Guilford Press.

IV

FUTURE PERSPECTIVES FOR SCHOOL HEALTH PRACTICE

LEGAL ASPECTS OF SCHOOL NURSE PRACTICE

MARY ELLEN ULLMER BOLTON

LEARNING OBJECTIVES

- Describe the process by which an idea becomes legislation.
- Differentiate between statute, code, policy, and practice.
- Analyze the importance of malpractice insurance.
- Identify resources available to every school nurse to assist in the decision-making process.
- Examine, and where indicated, implement a change in practice to comply with statute and policy.

▨ Introduction

From the Declaration of Independence in 1776 and the adoption of the Constitution of the United States of America in 1789, our country has established basic rights and principles as a framework for Americans to live and work by. Planning that the Constitution would be a "living document" and adjust to change, the first 10 Amendments (commonly referred to as the Bill of Rights) were added with provisions to add additional amendments at a later date. State Constitutions were created to provide "We the People" with a detailed plan for local government and what some today refer to as "hometown rule." This chapter explores the process of creating a law (both federal and state), the difference between statute, code, policy, practice, and one's own liability according to those mandates. It cannot be emphasized enough that, although the federal government has a direct impact on all 50 states, each state may interrupt or create legislation, albeit compliant with federal laws, to fit the needs of their communities. Therefore, all legislation will not be the same in all states. What is mandated in Virginia may not be the same in Montana. Likewise, in most, but not all cases, the federal government primarily delegates matters of health and education to the states for creating laws that have a direct impact on the population it serves. This chapter is meant to be a guideline for practicing school nurses, with the recommendation to consistently refer back to the school board policy of their respective district as well as state code and statute.

■ Glossary of Terms for Legal Aspects in School Nursing

Common terminology in the field of education and legislation must be understood before entering into this chapter. Frequently, a term may have a different definition from the term customarily used in other venues. Table 18.1 includes an abbreviated list of terms for this chapter.

TABLE 18.1 GLOSSARY OF TERMS FOR LEGAL ASPECTS IN SCHOOL NURSING

TERM	DESCRIBED
ADA	Americans with Disabilities Act of 1990
ADAAA	Americans with Disabilities Act Amendments Act (effective 2009)
Assembly	The lower house of a legislature; representatives are elected by the populous; often referred to as Assemblywoman, Assemblyman, Assemblypersons.
Bill	a legislative proposal
BOE	The Board of Education, an elected or appointed apolitical body of citizens (depending upon the jurisdiction and or region) that determines educational policy for a regional area, such as a state, county, city, or town.
Case law	A law that has be decided by the outcome of a judicial decision.
Civil lawsuit	A legal action by which an individual or entity can hold another individual or entity liable for harm. If the court rules in favor of the plaintiff (the person or entity that filed the formal complaint), the other party (defendant) may be ordered to pay damages (monetary or punitive).
Certification	Although it is in the best interest of the school community to hire school nurses in possession of a state and/or National Association of School Nurses Certification, many states do not require certification. Readers are referred to the respective State Department of Education and National Association of School Nurses for certification requirements.
Code	The official compilation of a body of law. Codes may be considered regulations and at times are directed by a statute to be created. A code may direct the local Board of Education to create policy for compliance.
Congress	The Congress of the United States is the legislative branch of the federal government and it is a bicameral legislature, implying that it is made up of two chambers: The Senate and the House of Representatives.
Executive order	The President of the United States may issue directives to help officers and agencies of the executive branch within the federal government. Some presidents use more or less Executive Orders depending upon the ability of Congress to act in concert for the good of the public.
FAPE	Free appropriate public education is an educational right of all students in the United States that is guaranteed by the Rehabilitation Act of 1973 and the Individuals with Disabilities Education Act (IDEA; Wikipedia, n.d.-c).

(continued)

TABLE 18.1 GLOSSARY OF TERMS FOR LEGAL ASPECTS IN SCHOOL NURSING (*CONTINUED*)

TERM	DESCRIBED
FERPA	Family Education Rights and Privacy Act of 1974 gives parents access to their child's education records, an opportunity to seek to have the records amended, and some control over the disclosure of information from the records. With several exceptions, schools must have a student's consent prior to the disclosure of education records after that student is 18 years old.
Good Samaritan Act	A law that offers protection to civilians who help those who are or are believed to be injured or in peril. It also provides individuals the freedom to act without fear of a lawsuit.
HIPAA	Health Insurance Portability and Accountability Act is a U.S. law which took effect in 2009. It establishes policies and procedures for maintaining privacy standards for protecting patients' medical records and other health information made available to doctors, hospitals, and other health care providers and health plans.
House of Representatives	First known by this name in 1693, a group of elected officials with the responsibility of representing a portion of their state's population for legislative purposes.
IDEA	Individuals with Disabilities Act " is a four-part (A–D) piece of American legislation that ensures students with a disability are provided with free appropriate public education (FAPE) that is tailored to their individual needs" (Wikipedia, n.d.-d)
Legislation	A law that has been enacted by a governing body or other organization.
Licensure	Although each state may have separate and distinct requirements and criteria for governmental authorization to perform the functions of a registered nurse or as in some states called a professional registered nurse, in general, graduation from an accredited school of nursing and passing of the National Council on Licensure Examination-Registered Nurse (NCLEX-RN®) is required for licensure.
Malfeasance	Misconduct especially committed by a public official.
Malpractice	Professional negligence or incompetence that results in harm.
NCLB	The No Child Left Behind Act of 2001 "was in effect from 2002 to 2015. It was a version of the Elementary and Secondary Education Act. It was replaced by the Every Student Succeeds Act in 2015. When NCLB was the law, it affected every public school in the USA and held schools accountable for student success" (Understood, n.d.).
Nurse Practice Act	A law that establishes the scope of practice and responsibilities for nurses. All states and territories enact an NPA, which establishes a board of nursing (BON). The BON has the authority to develop rules or regulations that must be consistent with and stay within the parameters of the NPA.
Policy	A legal document, recommended by the school superintendent, read at two separate public BOE meetings. Depending upon the regulations set forth in a state, approval of a policy may require 33% to 66% affirmative votes by members of the board.

(continued)

TABLE 18.1 GLOSSARY OF TERMS FOR LEGAL ASPECTS IN SCHOOL NURSING (*CONTINUED*)

TERM	DESCRIBED
Practice	To do or to perform regularly and routinely, even customarily. This is not to be confused with a policy.
Procedure manual	A document created by the administration, with input from the nursing department, school physician, and the education association. This manual may memorialize the practices of district school nurses to be performed in a uniform fashion.
Section 504 of the Rehabilitation Act of 1973	"Section 504 is a federal law designed to protect the rights of individuals with disabilities in programs and activities that receive federal financial assistance from the U.S. Department of Education…. No otherwise qualified individual with a disability in the United States … shall, solely by reason of her or his disability, be excluded from the participation in, be denied the benefits of, or be subjected to discrimination under any program or activity receiving federal financial assistance" (U.S. Department of Education, 2020).
Senator	An elected official to a state or federal government position. The purpose of this prestigious position is to represent the voice of their constituents in the state capital or, on the federal level, in Washington, DC.
Statute	A law enacted by the legislative branch of a government; this requires the passage of both houses and a signature by the governor.

Federal Government

Our forefathers, having achieved independence from a monarchy form of government, penned the Constitution of the United States to establish a democracy, making all states equal and providing for the rights and privileges of all Americans. The Constitution begins with seven articles outlining the creation of the federal government as we know it, with three equal branches of government: executive, judicial, and legislative (Exhibit 18.1). It includes a system of checks and balances to ensure that no one branch of government dominates (U.S. National Archives and Records Administration, n.d.-a).

The Bill of Rights "guarantees civil rights and liberties to the individual—like freedom of speech, press, and religion. It sets rules for due process of law and reserves all powers not delegated to the federal government to the people or the states." The Constitution also states that "certain rights, shall not be construed to deny or disparage others retained by the people." (U.S. National Archives and Records Administration, 2016). Subsequent to the original 10 amendments, and over the past 230 years, there have been 17 additional amendments to the Constitution including but not limited to: abolishing slavery; providing the right to vote regardless of race, color or previous condition of servitude; prohibiting the right to vote on basis of gender; and lowering the voting age to 18 years of age.

EXHIBIT 18.1

THE THREE BRANCHES OF U.S. GOVERNMENT

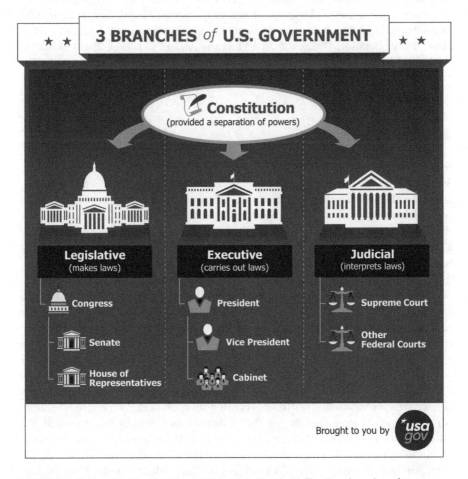

★ ★ **3 BRANCHES** *of* **U.S. GOVERNMENT** ★ ★

Constitution
(provided a separation of powers)

Legislative
(makes laws)

Executive
(carries out laws)

Judicial
(interprets laws)

Congress

President

Supreme Court

Senate

Vice President

Other
Federal Courts

House of
Representatives

Cabinet

Brought to you by *usa gov*

SOURCE: U.S. National Archives and Records Administration. (n.d.). The *three* branches of government. Retrieved from https://www.usa.gov/branches-of-government

▓ Executive Branch

The leader of the Executive Branch is the President of the United States of America, an elected political figure serving a 4-year term and is eligible for one additional term of office. The majority of work executed by this branch is accomplished by agencies, departments, and other ad hoc groups. In general, the role of the President is to communicate the presidential agenda, the federal budget, spearhead high priority issues, and function as the Commander in Chief of the United States military

To assist the President in the execution of duties is the Cabinet. The Cabinet is composed of department heads (secretaries) of the following departments: Agriculture, Commerce, Defense, Education, Energy, Health and Human Services, Homeland Security, Housing and Urban Development, Interior, Labor, State, Transportation, Treasury, and Veterans Affairs (usa.gov, 2019). Also included are an Attorney General, two directors (Central Intelligence and Office of Management and Budget), and one administrator of the Environment Protection Agency.

◾ Legislative Branch

In referencing Exhibit 18.2, note how a bill becomes a law. In most cases, United States citizens are reactionary. Reactionary responses to sentinel events, often extremely unfortunate or catastrophic in nature, spurs the community to advocate to the legislature to draft a bill. Families and/or advocacy groups make contact with their local legislator (Table 18.2) to express the concern, history, and benefit of action to be taken with legal intervention. If the legislator believes this is of benefit to the community, the concept will be sent to the Office of Legislative Affairs to draft a bill. Regardless of which chamber of Congress is involved, consideration of the bill begins in committee. The bill is discussed, researched, and amended; a second review with amendments is conducted. If it appears that this bill would be acceptable to the full chamber, it is sent for a vote. If affirmed, it is sent to the second chamber for a vote. Final legislative action taken by both the House and the Senate moves the bill to the President's desk for signature. The President may: (a) sign the bill and it becomes law, effective the date stated in the legislation; or (b) veto the bill and return it to the legislature. The Senate and House of Representatives may (a) override the veto with two-thirds vote in both chambers; (b) choose no action; (c) if Congress is in session during the 10 days of no action by the President, the bill automatically becomes law; or (d) pocket veto: If Congress goes out of session within the 10 days following the submission of the bill to the President's desk, the President may chose not to sign the bill and the bill is "dead," in other words, does not become law.

Although there are many federal laws that direct states to take action (ADA, IDEA, 504, NCLB, HIPAA, FERPA to name a few), the majority of legislation governing school districts throughout the country is enacted by the State Department of Health and Human Services and the State Department of Education. In many cases, school districts are geographically organized by counties; in other states school district may be structured according to municipalities.

EXHIBIT 18.2

HOW DOES A BILL BECOME A LAW?

1 EVERY LAW STARTS WITH AN IDEA

That idea can come from anyone, even you! Contact your elected officials to share your idea. If they want to try to make it a law, they will write a bill.

2 THE BILL IS INTRODUCED

A bill can start in either house of Congress when it's introduced by its primary sponsor, a Senator or a Representative. In the House of Representatives, bills are placed in a wooden box called "the hopper."

3 THE BILL GOES TO COMMITTEE

Representatives or Senators meet in a small group to research, talk about, and make changes to the bill. They vote to accept or reject the bill and its changes before sending it to:

the House or Senate floor for debate or to a subcommittee for further research.

Here, the bill is assigned a legislative number before the Speaker of the House sends it to a committee.

4 CONGRESS DEBATES AND VOTES

Members of the House or Senate can now debate the bill and propose changes or amendments before voting. If the majority vote for and pass the bill, it moves to the other house to go through a similar process of committees, debate, and voting. Both houses have to agree on the same version of the final bill before it goes to the President.

DID YOU KNOW?
The House uses an electronic voting system while the Senate typically votes by voice, saying "yay" or "nay."

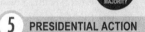

5 PRESIDENTIAL ACTION

When the bill reaches the President, he or she can:

✓ **APPROVE and PASS**
The President signs and approves the bill. The bill is law.

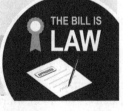

THE BILL IS LAW

The President can also:

Veto
The President rejects the bill and returns it to Congress with the reasons for the veto. Congress can override the veto with 2/3 vote of those present in both the House and the Senate and the bill will become law.

Choose no action
The President can decide to do nothing. If Congress is in session, after 10 days of no answer from the President, the bill then automatically becomes law.

Pocket veto
If Congress adjourns (goes out of session) within the 10-day period after giving the President the bill, the President can choose not to sign it and the bill will not become law.

Brought to you by

SOURCE: Orange County Virtual School. (2019, October 10). *How does a bill become a law?* Retrieved from http://ocvs.weebly.com/uploads/6/3/1/7/6317445/bill-to-law.png

TABLE 18.2 FEDERAL LEGISLATURE AND HOW THE MEMBERS ARE DETERMINED

CONGRESS	NUMBER OF MEMBERS	HOW THE NUMBERS ARE DETERMINED*
Senate	100	Two per state
House of Representatives	235	Proportional representation according to the population of the state

*Determined by United States Constitution.

The Judicial Branch

The Judicial Branch, whose members are nominated by the President to fill a vacancy and approved by the Senate with a simple majority of 51 affirmative votes, interprets the meaning of laws, how the meaning of the law impacts individual cases, and determines if any law violates the Constitution of the United States of America. The Judicial Branch is composed of the Supreme Court (a Chief Justice and eight Associate Justices, serving to death, retirement, or removal in exceptional cases) and other federal courts such as appeals to lower court decisions (Exhibit 18.3).

State and Local Governments

According to the 10th Amendment, the authority not granted to the federal government is governed by the states, counties, and municipalities. (USA.gov). The Constitution of the United States mandates all states operate under a republican form of government. All states conform to the concept of three branches of government (executive, legislative, and judicial) although the Constitution does not mandate this format. Most citizens have much more contact with municipal government than the state or federal government. The school nurse may have frequent contact with the local and county health department, police department, and even county and state hospitals. Every state has a written Constitution, which is more comprehensive than the Constitution of the United States. For example, Alabama's Constitution consists of approximately 310,300 words while the Constitution of the United States has an estimated 7,760 (Wikipedia, n.d.-a).

State Executive Branch

In all 50 States, the Governor is the duly elected head of the Executive Branch. In some cases, the Lieutenant Governor, Attorney General, Secretary of State, Auditor, Treasurer, and Commissioners are also duly elected by the registered voter, in other jurisdictions; these titles serve at the pleasure of the Governor.

State Legislative Branch

The legislature of all 50 states, comprised of elected officials, shoulder the responsibility of enacting statute and code, approving the state budget, the process of taxation

EXHIBIT 18.3

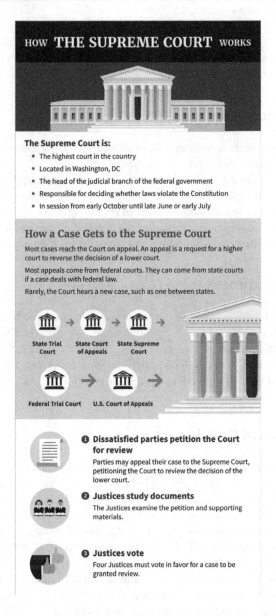

SOURCE: Rooster Today. (2019, October 10). *How the Supreme Court works.* Retrieved from http://
roostertoday.org/wp-content/uploads/2017/03/2017-03-03_13-32-52-Supreme-Court-top.png

imposed upon the citizens of each state, and exercises the responsibility of impeachment inquiries and articles of impeachment.

It should be noted that this branch of government is responsible for the statutes and codes that govern the role and function of the school nurse in the public, and at times non-public, school setting.

Forty-nine states have two chambers, similar if not identical to the federal government: A smaller upper house and a larger lower house. Together the two chambers make state laws and fulfill other governing responsibilities. The 50th state, Nebraska, has just one chamber in its legislature (Ballotpedia, n.d.).

State Judicial Branch

The State Supreme Court is generally responsible for hearing appeals from lower level state courts and leads this branch of government. A seat in the State Judiciary is outlined by each State Constitution and, depending upon the state, appointment is made by the governor and consent of the senate or election by the registered voters. The Supreme Court has the primary responsibility of reviewing decisions made in the lower courts, resulting in rulings that are usually binding. The appeal process would include a petition to the United States Supreme Court for a decision on constitutionality.

Local Government

Local governments may include two tiers: counties, also known as boroughs in Alaska and parishes in Louisiana, and municipalities, or cities/towns. Each state outlines the role and function of school district operations and funding. As legislation is passed by the state Senate and House of Representatives, these codes and statutes often direct the local Board of Education to craft and approve policy to be followed by the administration, faculty, and staff.

School Board Policies

Board policies "set forth the purposes and prescribe in general terms the organization and program of a school system." Board policies create a framework that "the superintendent and his/her staff can discharge their assigned duties with positive direction" (Oregon School Boards Association, n.d.). Policies are usually recommended by a Superintendent of Schools to the Board of Education. Discussion ensues and a vote for action or lack thereof is taken. Policies may be generated at the direction of state code or statutes that require a board policy to be in compliance with the legislation. The author of the policy may create a document that is broad enough to permit the administration the opportunity to interpret the document in the best way to serve the population and yet thorough enough to meet the intent of the legislature and give clear concise direction. Policies are not intended to be a procedure or a protocol. Policies do not dictate and provide templated forms. In many school districts, policies do not provide job descriptions; however, job description might be found in another location on the Board of Education website. In the day-to-day operation of a school district, it is important to have clear, consistent direction for the administration and faculty, as well as a ready reference to the public at large. Policies also provide legal documentation of compliance in meeting the elements of federal and state code and statute (Oregon School Boards Association, n.d.). It is highly recommended that the school nurse be extremely familiar with all code, statue, and policies that pertain to health education and health services.

An Example of Legislation on the Federal and State Level Resulting in School Board Policy

Consider the case of Sally, a child of 7, diagnosed with diabetes. What rights does Sally have, and her parents expect, for her care during school hours and school-sponsored activities?

Federal Legislation: As previously referenced in this chapter, Section 504 of the Rehabilitation Act of 1973, the IDEA, and ADA, all provide for the care of students, such as Sally, with diabetes (or any other disability). Sally may not be discriminated against due to her diagnosis by any school district that is in receipt of federal funding. She is entitled to a free, appropriate public education and shall enjoy all of the rights and privileges of other students. Due to these protections, Sally and her parents shall be afforded 504 accommodations. Sally's eligibility is determined by three important criteria: She (a) has a physical or mental impairment, which substantially limits one or more major life activities; (b) has a record of such impairment; and (c) is regarded as having such impairment. The ADA provides the same rights, as does the IDEA. These federal laws ensure that the parent and student will enjoy the appropriate health care needed as well as access to all curricular and extracurricular activities. The school will create a 504 plan to meet the individual needs of the student with any special accommodations specific to Sally's treatment plan. The plan will include, but not be limited to, the responsibilities of the school, the parent, and the student. For details on a 504 plan, please reference Chapter 11, The New Alphabet for School Personnel (Children with Diabetes, 2014).

State Legislation: Many states have enacted legislation specific to students with diabetes. It is suggested that the reader review the current statute in their state for direction. For example, New Jersey's response to the needs of children with diabetes resulted in the following legislation: N.J.S.A. 18A:40-12.3-12.6 addressing self-administration of insulin and other medications as well as the self-management and care of a student with diabetes. Likewise, N.J.S.A. 18A:40-12.11.c, 12.12, 12.13, and 12.15; and N.J.A.C. 6A:16-2.3(b) 3xii directed the creation of and IHP and ECP for students with chronic health conditions such as diabetes. These statutes paved the way for the New Jersey Department of Education to create *Guidelines for the Care of Students with Diabetes,* which includes but is not limited to: A *"PowerPoint: Care of Student with Diabetes in New Jersey Public Schools, FAQ, PowerPoint: Diabetes Care Tasks, Administering Glucagon, Quick Reference Emergency Plan for Student with Diabetes, Quick Reference (General) Acton Steps. Sample Diabetes Medical Management Plan, and IHP"* (New Jersey Department of Education, n.d.).

Board Policy: On the local level, Boards of Education have been directed to create policies to comply with the federal and state laws enacted. Those boards using an outside vendor have adopted Policy #5338: Management of Diabetes. Some policies are more or less comprehensive but in compliance with the state statute and providing the rights and privileges to all students with diabetes. In addition, each 504 coordinator shall create the 504 plan to meet the specific needs of the student with diabetes.

Legal Issues in Action

Unfortunately, rather than being proactive, our society and often our legislation is reactionary. Many of the statutes and codes are in response to sentinel events (Table 18.3).

Examples of Legislation in Response to Sentinel Events

Sam's Law (HB684) Texas

Samantha Watkins was an 18-year-old high school athlete and honor roll student diagnosed with a seizure disorder. Shortly following her diagnosis, Sam suffered a tonic clonic seizure resulting in her death. Sari Dudo, a retired teacher, advocate, and diagnosed with epilepsy herself, worked with the Epilepsy Foundation and Representative Travis Clardy to introduce Sam's Law to the legislature. HB 684 requires all Texas public school personnel, whose duties include regular contact with students, to receive training in seizure recognition and seizure first aid as well as a provision for

TABLE 18.3 SENTINEL EVENT

ESSENTIAL ELEMENTS	RESPONSE
Define sentinel event	In healthcare/school arena, a Sentinel Event is defined as an incident not anticipated as a natural result of the student/patient's initial diagnosis and results in catastrophic physical or psychological injury and at times fatal outcome.
Sentinel events in the school setting	Examples of Sentinel Events in the school setting might include but not be limited to: ■ Medication errors ■ Suicide ■ Injury or death by fall or armed intruder ■ Delayed or failure to provide appropriate care
Nursing action to be taken	Upon identification of a potential sentinel event, the School Nurse shall report such incident(s) to superior authorities, following the chain of command and complete the appropriate Accident/Incident Report according to School Board Policy and Procedures.

any equipment necessary to execute those first aid skills. In a cooperative venture, the two Epilepsy Foundation affiliates in Texas shall provide the free training (Sam's Law, n.d.). "Unfortunately, at this time we are not able to provide Texas Education Agency approved Epilepsy training … HB684 requires that the TEA approve on line training courses by December 1, 2019" (Sam's Law, n.d.).Therefore, many school districts do not have this policy in place at this writing.

Brown v. Board of Education of Topeka, 347 U.S. 483 (1954)

In 1951, Oliver Brown filed a class-action lawsuit against the Topeka Kansas Board of Education, claiming that his daughter, Linda, was denied entrance to an all-White elementary school citing the equal protection clause of the 14th Amendment to the United States Constitution. This case went through the United States District Court in Kansas and finally worked its way up to the Supreme Court in 1952. In Chief Justice Earl Warren's decision, issued on May 17, 1954, he wrote "in the field of public education the doctrine of 'separate but equal' has no place," because segregated schools are "inherently unequal." The Court ruled that the plaintiffs were being "deprived of the equal protection of the laws guaranteed by the 14th Amendment" (History, 2009).

Elijah's Law

Elijah Silvera, a 3-year-old New York City resident, was diagnosed with a severe dairy allergy and asthma. Being responsible parents, the instructions were communicated with the preschool staff in writing and verbally. Despite the diagnosis and instructions, Elijah was fed a grilled cheese sandwich. 911 was not called, epinephrine was not administered, and the child's parent transported him to the hospital where he died of anaphylaxis. Subsequently, Governor Andrew M. Cuomo signed legislation (S.218B/A.6971B) requiring all child daycare programs in New York to follow guidelines for preventing and responding to food allergy anaphylaxis. The legislation, which focuses on prevention, also requires preschools to follow state mandated food allergy guidelines and for faculty to identify signs and symptoms of anaphylaxis, set priorities, and implement the appropriate emergency care including but not limited to the administration of epinephrine auto-injector by trained staff. It must be noted that most preschools do not have full-time, if any, medical staff on site and most health care legislation is directed to the K–12 and university population (New York State, 2019).

Erin's Law

Erin's Law is named after Erin Merryn, herself a survivor of sexual assault. Erin spearheaded the legislation in her home state of Illinois, the need identified by the legislature and duplicated by 37 other states as of 2019. The law mandates prevention programming in child sexual abuse, age appropriate in grades prekindergarten to grade 12. The lessons include but are not limited to recognizing child sexual abuse and telling a trusted adult. In addition, school personnel shall participate in staff development on child sexual abuse and parents shall have programming on the warning signs of child sexual abuse and the need for resources and referrals to support victims. Access the following website for further information and to see if your state has adopted this legislation (Erin's Law, n.d.): http://www.erinslaw.org/erins-law/.

Marjory Stoneman Douglas Bill (Florida SB 7030)

In response to the mass shooting at Marjory Stoneman Douglas School in Parkland Florida on February 14, 2018 (ironically Valentine's Day) which left 17 dead and many more injured, the Florida legislature passed the Marjory Stoneman Douglas bill. This legislation authorizes classroom teachers to carry guns in school during the school day was passed in the Senate in April 2019 and the House of Representative the week of September 23, 2019. The law was signed by Governor Ron DeSantis on Wednesday, October 2, 2019. In the text of the legislation, it states that each school district shall approve or disapprove of this action, teachers shall volunteer for this responsibility, all volunteers must go through a background check and a psychiatric evaluation, as well as a gun safety course conducted by the County Sheriff's Department (Mettler, 2019).

Janet's Law (NJSA 18A:40-41a Through 41c)

On September 1, 2014, all school districts in the State of New Jersey were required to be compliant with the provisions of Janet's Law. Janet Zilinski was an 11-year-old cheerleader in Warren, New Jersey who died after a sudden cardiac arrest. Her tragic death led to the creation of Janet's Fund by her family with the express purpose of raising awareness and financial support for an automatic electronic defibrillator (AED) in every school in the state. As a result of the advocacy by the Zilinski Family and many others, Janet's Law was passed unanimously. The provisions include but are not limited to: All public and non-public schools must have an AED placed within a reasonable location to the gym and/or athletic field; the AED must be stored in a safe, secure but unlocked location and available during the school day as well as after school activities; each AED shall have identifying signage; each building shall have at least five trained members; trained personnel must be available for all school-sponsored activities before, during, and after school; and each school district shall create an emergency action plan (State of New Jersey, n.d.). Policy #5300 covers the implementation of Janet's Law in New Jersey school districts utilizing outside vendors to write policy for approval by the Board of Education. Other school districts may use the National School Board Association or write their own policy with other number designations. New Jersey is also in the process of implementing CPR and AED training as a high school graduation requirement.

Kevin and Avonte's Law

Kevin Curtis Willis, a 9 year old child diagnosed with autism, wandered from home, fell into the Raccoon River in Iowa, and perished in 2008. Avonte Oquendo, a 14-year-old boy wandered from a New York City school and drowned in the East River in 2014. As a result of these two sentinel events, and many others, autism advocacy groups were successful in the passage of Kevin and Avonte's Law which permits Justice Department grants to be used by law enforcement agencies and nonprofit groups for programs that provide training for school personnel and first responders, and GPS devices for individuals known to wander from school or caretakers.

On March 23, 2018, President Trump signed the Omnibus Bill providing final appropriations for Fiscal Year 2018 which includes Kevin and Avonte's Law (H.R. 4421 and S. 2070; Autism Society, 2018).

■ Frequently Asked Questions

1. Certification Versus Non-Certification:

Question: I am currently a pediatric nurse and think that I would be a good school nurse. Do I have to go back to school and take additional courses to apply for this position?

Answer: This is certainly a frequently asked question. There is no federal requirement that can provide you with a universal response. This is a topic governed by each state. Contact the county or state Department of Education for a clear and accurate response, or contact the county or state School Nurse Association. For example: Some states require a state certification as a certified school nurse-instructional or non-instructional, while other states require certification by the National Association of School Nurses, yet others require a current license as a registered nurse and a bachelor's degree in nursing.

2. Charter Schools and Private Schools

Question: My children go to a private school; are they required to have a Certified School Nurse? What about a charter school?

Answer: Charter schools are part of the public school system in most States. Therefore, they receive state and local funding and must provide health services in compliance with all of the statutes and codes established by the state legislature. Therefore, yes, charter schools must hire a school nurse. However, private schools fall into two categories: non-approved and parochial. They are not required to hire a certified school nurse. However, it is highly recommended that they do what is in the best interest and safety of their school community.

3. Civil Rights

Question: I heard that an employee may be dismissed for being part of the LGBT community. How can this happen?

Answer: The United States Supreme Court agreed to hear the Stephens case on October 8, 2019, to determine if the Federal Civil Rights Law, which protects against discrimination by virtue of sex, applies to the LGBTQ community. It is interesting to note that approximately 28 states do not prohibit discrimination by gender identity or sexual orientation in blatant disregard of the federal decision in 2015 to declare same-sex marriage legal in all 50 States. In a historic decision, the Supreme Court Justices voted on June 15, 2020, in a 6-3 decision to protect the rights of the LGBTQ employees against termination due to sexual orientation (npr.org, 2020, June 15).

4. Confidential List

Question: As a new school nurse, I have been assigned to work with a senior Certified School Nurse. I noticed that she distributes confidential lists of students and diagnoses to all faculty members. This makes me feel uncomfortable and appears to breach the federal laws of confidentiality.

Answer: You are correct. This practice is not acceptable and may violate confidentiality. Parental consent is required to provide medical information to those individuals with a "need to know." You may wish to share this information verbally with the individuals having direct contact with the student. Please reference the section on HIPAA and FERPA.

5. Continuing Education

Question: Are there continuing education requirements for certified school nurses?

Answer: This is controlled by the individual states. For example, in New Jersey, a Professional Registered Nurse must earn 30 continuing education contact hours every 2 year to maintain their license. In addition, a Certified School Nurse, considered teaching faculty, must accrue 20 hours of staff/professional development every year to maintain certification. To see the requirements to maintain licensure in your state visit www.4medtrainingcenter.com/rn-lpn-requirements

6. Fees

Questions: Are there any fees to become a school nurse?

Answer: The cost for processing the certification for school nursing would be dependent upon the authorizing agency. In the case of a state certification, the applicant applies directly to the State Department of Education or in some cases, the certification process is completed by the university you have attended for your required courses. National certification for school nursing is governed by the National Board for Certification of School Nurses (NBCSN). For detailed information, access the following website for exam requirements and fees: www.nasn.org/nasn/nasn-resources/professional-topics/certification

7. Field Trips

Question: In planning for a field trip, I was told to check the list of students needing medications and call the parent to attend the field trip to administer the medication ordered for the child by the primary care physician. If the parent could not attend, the child cannot attend the field trip. Is this common practice?

Answer: Every child is entitled to a free, appropriate public education. To exclude a child from a field trip, which has been carefully planned by the faculty and augments the core curriculum standards for that particular subject, is illegal and denying the child their rights, Many school districts train volunteer staff members to be delegates (for those medications that your state designates appropriate to delegate). Some medications, such as asthma MDI and epinephrine auto-injector may be approved by the primary care physician to be self-administered by the student, if appropriate. It is the school nurse's responsibility to be compliant with the state's statutes, codes, and school board policy. One state may authorize the delegation of glucagon and EpiPen, while another state may authorize the delegation of diazepam and nebulizer treatments.

8. Good Samaritan Law

Question: As a school nurse, am I protected by the Good Samaritan Law?

Answer: Generally, Good Samaritan laws do not extend to individuals providing "medical care or treatment in the course of their employment." For example, as "a nurse who works in a medical center, any action [taken] in an emergency would not be covered" (LawInfo, n.d.).

9. HIPAA Versus FERPA

Question: Would you outline the differences between HIPAA and FERPA?

Answer: HIPAA (Health Insurance Portability and Accountability Act) of 1996 with the HIPAA Privacy Rule effective 2003 is a federal act which protects the confidentiality of health records generated or in the possession of health care providers. HIPAA protects medical records identifying the patient by name whether stored/filed or transmitted in any format. FERPA (Family Educational Rights and Privacy Act; Wikipedia, n.d.-b) is a federal law enacted in 1974, which protects student records in educational institutions that receive funds from the U.S. Department of Education.

10. Immunizations

Question: I understand that review and documentation of immunizations is a major school nurse function. What agency or department dictates the requirements and exemptions?

Answer: Although recommendations come from the Centers for Disease Control and Prevention, there is no federal vaccination law. Mandatory vaccinations began approximately 70 years ago with BCG, polio, diphtheria, and tetanus. These requirements have broadened over the years and are enforced by the State Department of Health and Human Services and State Department of Education (for schools). For example, in June, 2019, the California Legislature passed a law which eliminated the personal belief exemption for required vaccinations. The previous practice permitted a parent to declare, in writing, that the administration of one or more immunizations was counter to their personal/religious beliefs. Today, California only permits medical exemptions, in which the treating physician declares that the immunization would be contraindicated due to the student's state of health. New York followed suit. The State of New Jersey is currently positioned to pass the same type of legislation. The New Jersey Chapter of the American Association of Pediatrics (NJAAP) petitioned the House of Representatives and Senate following an outbreak of measles in the United States. NJAAP supports A3818 and S2173 which would abolish religious exemptions for mandatory immunizations and support medical exemption for required immunizations. Contact the local, county or state health department for the required immunization schedule for pre-Kindergarten to grade 12. States have the prerogative of passing and enforcing legislation that has a direct impact on the responsibilities of the school nurse.

11. Making Change

Question: I am a new school nurse. How do I go about making changes to some of the previous practices?

Answer: This question will be addressed on two levels: Personal preference and district practice/policy. It is suggested that a list be created of the changes needed. Divide the list into two columns: Preference and practice/policy. Those things that are preferred may be accomplished without consultation or input from others. For example: If it is believed the placement of the desk needs adjustment to readily identify students as they enter the health office and the current configuration has the back of the school nurse facing the door, move the desk. However, if moving the desk requires moving telephone and computer lines, this now requires contacting the immediate supervisor, as the change to be made requires additional resources. It is recommended that the school nurse do research to support the need for change (find out what the other school nurses in the district do) and discuss the value of facing the students as they enter the health office. The school nurse must be patient as change does not happen quickly. But, if the change was to deny a child the right to attend a field trip because the parent could not attend for the sole purpose of medication administration, the school nurse must bring this to the attention of the administration. Once again, research the FAPE and ADA. Bring the research and concerns to the immediate supervisor according to the table or organization. A smart and successful change agent not only identifies the problem but is part of the solution. Therefore, one needs to include an action plan in any proposal for change and follow the chain of command. Often, the most powerful voices are the members of the PTO, PTA, or HSO, the local education association, or the county and state school nurses association.

12. Malpractice Insurance

Question: Do I really need malpractice insurance? My district is insured and has an attorney on retainer.

Answer: School districts do have insurance for a multitude of reasons and have a school attorney. However, with the litigious nature of our society, anyone can be sued for anything—both as the "school nurse" and as an individual. It is not required, but it is highly recommended that all school nurses have personal malpractice insurance.

13. Salary for a School Nurse

Question: How does the salary for a school nurse compare with working in an acute care facility?

Answer: In most states, the school nurse is certificated staff and paid according to the identical salary guide as any other teacher. The contract and salary guide is negotiated by the Board of Education and the local education association. Non-certified school nurses may be paid at the discretion of the superintendent and Board of Education. Contact the local or county Board or the teachers association requesting a salary guide to review.

14. School Nurse/Student Ratio

Question: I work in a large high school with 1,400 students. The health office is very busy and the student population is transient, resulting in daily transfers and paperwork. Is there any federal law that dictates a school nurse/student ratio?

Answer: Unfortunately, there is no federal or state legislation that mandates the school nurse/student ratio. Certainly, the number of students, the level of your students' health, as well as state mandates for screening must be taken into consideration in the determination of staffing levels in the health office. It should be noted that the National Association of School Nurses recommends "school nurse to student ratios based on student populations. For general populations, they recommend one nurse per 750 students. For populations with complex health care needs, they suggest at least one nurse to 125 students, depending on severity of student needs" (AAP, 2008; ANA/NASN, 2011)

15. Travel Out of State With a Field Trip

Question: A field trip to Washington, DC, is planned. I am not licensed in DC Should I be concerned?

Answer: The National Council of State Boards of Nursing (NCSBN) established the Nurse Licensure Compact, "an agreement between specific states to recognize nursing licenses without having to apply separately for licensure in another state" (Registered Nursing, 2020). Determine if you currently work in a compact state; if not, it is recommended that you contact your supervisor for permission to speak with the school attorney and/or your state board of nursing.

16. School Physician Orders

Question: Is the school nurse obligated to follow the school physician orders or are they recommendations for care in the health office?

Answer: School physician's orders are binding orders just as any other physician's authorized to write prescriptions in your state. Depending upon the authority granted by legislation and Board of Education policy, and, of course the style of the physician, the orders maybe extremely comprehensive (including routine first aid as well as medications such as but not limited to acetaminophen, antacid, antihistamines, inhalers). In other settings, they may be very brief and only include orders for Mantoux testing, epinephrine administration according to the state legislation. The orders are to be followed and no substitutions or additions may be made at the discretion of the school nurse.

References

4Med. (n.d.). *Continuing education requirements*. Retrieved from https://www.4med trainingcenter.com/rn-lpn-requirements/

Autism Society. (2018). *Kevin and Avonte's law*. Retrieved from https://www.autism -society.org/?s=Kevin+and+Avonte+law

Ballotpedia. (n.d.). *Composition of the state legislature*. Retrieved from https://ballotpedia .org/State_legislature

Children with Diabetes. (2014). *Care of students with diabetes*. Retrieved from https:// archive.childrenwithdiabetes.com/d_0q_600.htm

Erin's Law. (n.d.). *What is Erin's law?* Retrieved from http://www.erinslaw.org/erins-law/

History. (2009). *Brown v. Board of Education of Topeka, Kansas*. Retrieved from https:// www.history.com/topics/black-history/brown-v-board-of-education-of-topeka

LawInfo. (n.d.) *What are Good Samaritan laws?* Retrieved from https://resources.lawinfo .com/personal-injury/what-are-good-samaritan-laws.html

Mettler, K. (2019). *It's the law now: In Florida, teachers can carry guns at school*. Retrieved from https://www.washingtonpost.com/education/2019/05/09/its-law-now-florida-teachers -can-carry-guns-school/

National Association of School Nurses. (n.d.). *Fees for national certification*. Retrieved from https://www.nasn.org/nasn/nasn-resources/professional-topics/certification

New Jersey Department of Education. (n.d.). *Guidelines for the care of students with diabetes in the school setting*. Retrieved from https://www.state.nj.us/education/edsupport/ diabetes

New York State. (2019). *Governor Cuomo signs "Elijah's Law" requiring child care providers to follow guidelines for preventing and responding to food allergy anaphylaxis*. Retrieved from https://www.governor.ny.gov/news/governor-cuomo-signs-elijahs-law-requiring -child-care-providers-follow-guidelines-preventing

NPR.org. (2020, June 15). Supreme Court delivers major victory to LGBTQ employees. Retrieved from https://www.npr.org/2020/06/15/863498848/supreme-court-delivers -major-victory-to-lgbtq-employees

Orange County Virtual School. (2019). *How does a bill become a law?*. Retrieved from http://ocvs.weebly.com/uploads/6/3/1/7/6317445/bill-to-law.png

Oregon School Boards Association. (n.d.). *School board policies*. Retrieved from http:// www.osba.org/Resources/Article/Board_Policy/Policy_Definition.aspx

Registered Nursing. (2020). *Travel outside of state*. Retrieved from https://www .registerednursing.org/answers/nursing-licenses-valid-traveling-working-other-states/

Rooster Today. (2019). *How the supreme court works*. Retrieved from http://roostertoday .org/wp-content/uploads/2017/03/2017-03-03_13-32-52-Supreme-Court-top.png

Sam's Law. (n.d.). Retrieved from https://www.samslaw.org

State of New Jersey. (n.d.). *Janet's law*. Retrieved from https://www.state.nj.us/education/ students/safety/health/legislation/JanetsLawFAQ.pdf

Understood. (n.d.). *NCLB defined*. Retrieved from https://www.britannica.com/topic /No-Child-Left-Behind-Act

U.S. Department of Education. (2020). *Protecting students with disabilities*. Retrieved from http://www2.ed.gov/about/offices/list/ocr/504faq.html

U.S. National Archives and Records Administration. (2016). *The bill of rights: What does it say?* Retrieved from https://www.archives.gov/founding-docs/bill-of-rights/what-does-it-say

U.S. National Archives and Records Administration. (n.d.-a). *Federal government, a historical perspective*. Retrieved from https://www.usa.gov/history#item-37587

U.S. National Archives and Records Administration. (n.d.-b). *The three branches of government*. Retrieved from https://www.usa.gov/history#item-37587

usa.gov. (2019). *Composition of the president's cabinet*. Retrieved from www.usa.gov

The White House: President Barack Obama. (n.d.). *State and local government*. Retrieved from https://obamawhitehouse.archives.gov/1600/state-and-local-government

Wikipedia. (n.d.-a). *Constitution of Alabama*. Retrieved from https://en.wikipedia.org/wiki/Constitution_of_Alabama

Wikipedia. (n.d.-b). *Family educational rights and privacy act*. Retrieved from https://en.wikipedia.org/wiki/Family_Educational_Rights_and_Privacy_Act

Wikipedia. (n.d.-c). *Free appropriate public education*. Retrieved from https://en.wikipedia.org/wiki/Free_Appropriate_Public_Education

Wikipedia. (n.d.-d). *Individuals with Disabilities Education Act*. Retrieved from https://en.wikipedia.org/wiki/Individuals_with_Disabilities_Education_Act

SCHOOL-BASED HEALTH CLINICS

LUCILLE A. JOEL

LEARNING OBJECTIVES

- Understand the varied forms of school-based health clinics (SBHCs).
- Appreciate the benefits which SBHCs bring to individuals and communities.
- Identify the process for establishing an SBHC.
- Evaluate the success of SBHCs

▮ Introduction

School-based health centers (SBHCs) are health facilities based on elementary and high school campuses in the United States. Most SBHCs provide a combination of primary care, management of stabilized chronic disease, emergency response, mental health care, substance abuse counseling, case management, dental health, nutrition education, health education, and health promotion services. An emphasis is placed on prevention and early intervention. SBHCs generally operate as a partnership between the school district and a community health organization, such as a community health center, hospital, or the local health department.

SBHCs are a logical response to the challenges that youth face in healthcare access and use, and aim to place the learner in optimal physical and mental status to learn. SBHCs fortify kids by providing comprehensive care, building on strengths and protective factors, and establishing connections with trusted adults. This creates a safe "haven" where providers can help students gain the confidence and skills they need to maximize their learning, successfully navigate school, and understand that they have what it takes to reach their full potential.

Schools provide a space for the centers to operate, and depending on the organizational structure, local health care organizations can bring an array of services delivered by a multidisciplinary team. In addition to students in the school, there could be out-reach to school staff members, students' families, and others within the community. The market for the SBHC is only limited by our lack of creativity, vision, and leadership.

The History of SBHCs

The origins of school-based health can actually be traced back to the early 1900s with the public health nursing movement. At that time, student absenteeism rates were high because of communicable disease such as measles, scarlet fever, whooping cough, and tuberculosis. In an attempt to contain contagious illnesses, the Board of Health in New York City instituted a rule to exclude children with contagious disease from the classroom, sending them home without any treatment or plan of care. Many of these children received no medical attention, and without education, continued to play with other healthy children, thus spreading disease. In 1902, the first "school nurse," Lina Rogers, was brought in to help with these issues and she soon began creating treatment protocols and providing care to children who were unnecessarily being excluded from school. In addition, she and other nurses began conducting home visits to provide families with health education about hygiene and other methods to control the spread of disease. Within 1 year, the rates of absenteeism in the city had decreased by almost 90%, and the need for school nurses became nationally recognized. Over the next 50 years, the role of the school nurse continued to focus on health education, but also expanded to emphasize aspects of primary health care, including immunizations, health screenings, and referrals (Brodeurk, 1986; Vessey & McGowan, 2006).

President Lyndon Johnson's War on Poverty in the mid-1960s is credited with bringing into focus the significance of health issues among impoverished school-aged children. The enactment of Medicaid in 1965 was indicative of a perception in the public policy community that there was a need to develop programs in the service of better health care for low-income individuals (Lear, 1996). The nation was also experiencing a growing shortage of primary care physicians. This may well have been precipitated by the new demands of Medicaid. In response, the pediatric nurse practitioner was proposed and well accepted to fill many of these primary care gaps for well children.

By the mid-1970s, in response to public dissatisfaction with the limited role of the traditional school nurse, the recognized need for school health, and the proven efficacy of school-based health services, the state of Colorado initiated certification for a School Nurse Practitioner. This geographic site was no surprise since Loretta Ford, a nurse, partnering with pediatrician, Henry Silver, developed the first Pediatric Nurse Practitioner program in the country at the University of Colorado. And today, the majority of primary health care providers in SBHCs are either nurse practitioners or physician assistants (Brom, Salsberry, & Graham, 2018). This has become a well-established pattern of appropriate and effective workforce utilization.

In 1967, Philip J. Porter, head of pediatrics at Cambridge City Hospital in Massachusetts and director of Maternal and Child Health for the city's Health Department, began to address this issue. He assigned a nurse practitioner to work on site in an elementary school to deliver primary medical care to students. Four additional health clinics were opened in Cambridge schools in the years that followed (Porter, Avery, & Fellows, 1974).

The first recognized SBHCs opened in Cambridge, Massachusetts (1967), Dallas, Texas (1970), and St. Paul, Minnesota (1973). The first two were launched because their founders believed that school-based health care could provide accessible, affordable health care to poor children. In 1970, the West Dallas Youth Center at Pinkston High School was opened as an outreach center for a federally funded Children and Youth Program based at the University of Texas Health Sciences Center Pediatrics Department. Pinkston High School was the nation's first high school to offer comprehensive care provided by nurse practitioners, physicians, social workers, nutritionists, and health educators. These early centers demonstrated that they were effective in increasing young people's access to care (Ramos, Sebastian, Stumbo, McGrath, & Fairbrother, 2017).

Demographics

SBHCs are the obvious answer to the out-cry for universal access to health care services for children and youth. SBHCs bring critical, developmentally appropriate services to children and adolescents where they spend most of their waking hours: at school. Data collection accomplished in 2016 to 2017 identified 2,584 SBHCs in 48 of 50 states, the District of Columbia, and Puerto Rico. The National School-Based Health Care Census is a survey conducted by the School-Based Health Alliance, collecting this information about SBHCs every 3 years since 1998. The Alliance amasses descriptive information, but does not measure quality. It is currently in the process of extending its data collection into the realm of quality, and will have such information sometime in 2020. This work is being done through a joint initiative with the Center for School Mental Health Programs (CSMHPs) funded by a grant from the Health Resources and Services Administration (HRSA).

Over the past 20 years, the number of SBHCs in this country has more than doubled, being located in all states with the exception of North Dakota and Wisconsin, and growing from 1,135 SBHCs in 1998. The number of SBHCs range from a low of New Hampshire (1), Montana (2), and South Dakota (3) to a high of Texas (201), California (199), and New York (196; National School-Based Health Care Census, 2019).

SBHCs provided services to 6,344,907 students in 10,629 schools, or 13% of school-aged youth in approximately 10% of U.S. public schools. Forty percent of the centers provide access to elementary school-aged children, 30% to middle or high schoo aged youth, and 30% to youth in all other grade combinations (Love, Schlitt, Soleimanpour, Panchal, & Behr, 2019). Of the SBHCs in the United States in 2019, 57% of these serve urban areas, 27% are rural, and 16% are in suburban settings (National Research Council, Institute of Medicine, 2009).

Several factors explain this rapid two-decade expansion of SBHCs. The nation's pre-eminent health philanthropy, the Robert Wood Johnson Foundation, invested in SBHCs through multi-year, multi-site initiatives. Since 1987 the Foundation has invested over $40 million to demonstrate the efficacy and test the sustainability of SBHCs (Kanaan, 2007). Simultaneously, state governments began establishing their own demonstrations. By 1998, 38 states were allocating funds for SBHCs. Although many never ventured past the pilot phase, several states continued to expand their SBHC investments, and their grant programs remain operational. Medicaid expansion in the 1990s also contributed to a sustainable SBHC business model by guaranteeing health insurance coverage to a population of low-income children who historically had limited ability to pay for services. The economic status of these children is verified since most SBHCs report that the majority of their student population is eligible for the National School Lunch Program, a common indicator of low socio-economic status (Gunderson, 2019).

Contemporary SBHC Models

Early versions of SBHCs were focused on a traditional model of school healthcare—one in which a health center and healthcare providers were physically located in the school. With time, growth of technology and comfort in delivering an expanded range of services, four distinct delivery models emerged. In traditional SBHCs, students access care at a fixed site on school grounds or in a school building, and providers are physically on site. In school-linked centers, students access care at a fixed site near the school campus through formal or informal connections with the school. Providers are physically on-site or may be accessed remotely. In mobile centers, students access care at a specially equipped van or bus parked on or near a school campus. Here, providers may be physically on site or accessed remotely. In telehealth-exclusive centers, patients access care at a fixed site on a school campus, and providers are available remotely through telehealth for primary care services. Other services such as behavioral health and addiction services, reproductive health, case management, oral healthcare, nutrition, vision services, social services and health education may be available physically on site or remotely (Young & Ireson, 2003). In the midst of initial controversy over services associated with reproductive health and parental rights, SBHCs continued to grow rapidly in the 1990s.

Range of Services

Schools provide a space for the centers to operate, and local healthcare organizations bring an array of services delivered by a multidisciplinary team. SBHCs are most often sponsored or operated by a local healthcare organization such as a community health center (28%), hospital (25%), or local health department (15%). In addition, approximately one of 10 (12%) of SBHCs nationwide are sponsored by the school system it serves (Department of Education, 2019). Other sponsoring agencies include nonprofit organizations, universities, and mental health agencies. These lead agencies are typically charged with the administrative operations of the SBHCs and partner with other local community health and wellness practitioners to provide services outside of their usual scope of activities. For example, an SBHC that is operated by a medical lead organization may contract with a local mental health agency to provide on-site mental health services. In other models (e.g., "school-linked" services), a provider may come to the school periodically to conduct screenings and educational sessions, with any required follow-up occurring in their usual clinic or office setting.

Only 13% of public school students nationally have access to SBHC services (Department of Education, 2019). Clearly, this represents a small proportion of all schools currently operating in the United States. Nevertheless, SBHCs are a model that can inform the linkage between health and education systems through improving preventive and primary care. Health providers and school educators and administrators share mutual goals of ensuring that students are both healthy and ready to learn and thrive. This is a particularly timely moment to address the health needs of students as future members of the nation's workforce. With budget shortfalls in education and in health, collaboration across these two systems is needed to ensure that available resources can be used effectively and efficiently. Together, schools and health entities are investing in a healthy and productive future for the nation's children.

SBHCs may provide an entry point and source of primary care, with ongoing connections to a "medical home" for children who do not otherwise have access to consistent care. They may also provide additional needed care for those youth who already have primary pediatric providers. For example, mental health counseling is a service that may not be available within a traditional community-based primary care setting, but it could be provided at a youth's SBHC. A health educator working as part of the SBHC can also provide valuable reinforcement of health education messages delivered by the clinician and can, for example, continue to help in monitoring ongoing compliance with recommended medications. An example of this collaborative relationship is the implementation of a coordinated plan of care between an SBHC and primary care providers to manage chronic diseases in students, such as diabetes and asthma. In these examples, the SBHC can serve as an extension of youth's providers, as well as serve as the primary source of care if their families have no other resources.

SBHCs are a logical response to the challenges that underserved youth face in health care access and use. The centers represent a shared commitment by a community's schools and healthcare organizations to address healthcare access and use among the nation's underserved communities and aim to support children's and adolescents' health, well-being, and academic success. The centers help youth and their families overcome access barriers—including transportation, time, costs, and lack of continuity of care—that may prevent them from receiving needed health care services. Care is provided during and after school hours and ideally during the summer.

Funding

The growth of SBHCs sponsored by Federally Qualified Health Centers (FQHCs) reflects a promising opportunity, yet neither the importance of the sponsorship for SBHCs nor the significance of the SBHC as a delivery model for FQHCs has been fully described in the literature. Data show that FQHCs have recently become the dominant sponsor for SBHCs. In 2016 there were 1,367 FQHCs (Bureau of Primary Health Care, 2016). Thus, with 272 FQHCs sponsoring a total of 1,181 SBHCs in 2016 to 2017, 80% of FQHCs do not have SBHCs—leaving tremendous opportunity for partnership and growth. The Federal Torts Claims Act, the enabling legislation for FQHCs, updated in July 2014, makes specific mention of funding school-linked health facilities offering primary and preventive services at a location in a school, on school grounds, or not located on school grounds but servicing students, each entity having a written affiliation agreement with the other (U.S. Department of Health and Human Services [DHHS], 2014).

There are clear advantages for SBHCs sponsored by FQHCs. They receive better reimbursement rates from Medicaid and have avenues for funding through federal and state safety-net grant programs, thus improving their sustainability. But it is also likely that FQHCs will establish school sites as a way to reach underserved children and increase community engagement and buy-in to serve broader populations (Council on School Health, 2012). These services may be offered on a fee-for-service basis, as part of a managed care arrangement, or funded by philanthropy and grants where government dollars are not applicable. More than two thirds of SBHCs nationwide reported providing services to individuals beyond the student population at the sites in which they are located. These individuals include students from other schools in the community (58%); out-of-school youth (34%); faculty and school personnel (42%); family members of students (42%); and other community members (24%; Keeton, Soleimanpour, et al., 2012). Recently, the number of SBHCs that serve non-student populations nationwide has increased. Contributing factors may include families' loss of employer-sponsored health insurance coverage, increasing family financial strains, and a greater call for affordable health care delivery in the community due to an enlightenment about healthy living.

The Patient Protection and Affordable Care Act of 2010 (ACA) made provision for the establishment of Accountable Care Organizations (ACOs), an integrated model including the principle of shared risk. It is possible that SBHCs may qualify for this status. Expanding the population served would also open more payment streams. The social and health care services offered by the SBHCs and the population served would make it likely that every available route for financial coverage in this program be investigated and eventually tapped.

Over time, SBHCs' fiscal sustainability has improved through a diverse portfolio of reimbursement and funding sources including state and federal governments, private foundations, partner organizations, schools or school districts, the local community, and public and private insurance. This complex financial modeling justifies the need for sources with business acumen and public policy and reimbursement experience to be involved with the SBHC in some capacity, either as staff or consultants.

Since 2011, the HRSA has appropriated nearly $200 million to address the expansion and improvement of SBHC services. Part of this was the $11 million of funding awarded in February of 2019 by HRSA and the DHHS to 120 SBHCs to increase access to mental health, substance abuse, and childhood obesity-related services. To qualify for funding, these centers must have been operational and apply for dollars for minor alteration/renovation projects and/or the purchase of moveable equipment, including telehealth equipment (HRSA, 2019). The future of telehealth deserves careful evaluation in regard to both its economies and efficacy.

Outcomes

Physical Health

Physical health includes medical, vision, and dental health. SBHCs are defined first by their ability to provide medical care. SBHC services that improve physical health include preventive care (e.g., administering immunizations, screening), managing and coordinating care of chronic illnesses (e.g., asthma and obesity), and decreasing health-risk behaviors (e.g., tobacco, drug, and alcohol use). More than 83% of SBHCs provide treatment and management of chronic health conditions. Students with chronic health conditions may suffer academic setbacks, increased disability, fewer job opportunities, and limited community interactions as they enter adulthood. There is documented success of the SBHCs having had success treating many pediatric chronic conditions including asthma, obesity, children with special healthcare needs, and substance abuse (Leroy, Wallin, & Lee, 2017).

SBHCs have also improved prenatal care. For example, Barnet et al. showed that teens who received prenatal care at an SBHC comprehensive adolescent pregnancy prevention program (CAPP) had lower odds of delivering a low-birth weight baby than those who received CAPP at a hospital-based setting. They also provide reproductive health services that address issues such as "safe sex" and sexually transmitted infections. The biggest strength of on-site reproductive health is being able to provide care when students decide they want or need such a service.

Vision screening is provided by 84% of SBHCs (School Based Health Alliance, 2017). Some offer full vision services, including provision of eyeglasses. In addition, nearly 18% of SBHCs have oral health providers as a member of staff, and 20% provide oral health exams by a visiting dentist or dental hygienist on-site. Poor access to oral healthcare remains one of the most persistent health disparities in the United States and is one of the largest causes of chronic disease and absenteeism. SBHCs solve this problem by bringing dental services to children in school.

Mental Health

Confronted with the large and persistent unmet mental health needs of children and youth, schools in the United States have become the most common provider of children's mental health services. However, they have neither the resources nor the expertise to do so. Nearly one in five U.S. children have a mental, emotional, or behavioral disorder, such as anxiety, depression, or attention deficit hyperactivity disorder (Atkins, Capella, et al., 2017). Early diagnosis and treatment are critical, but access to mental health care can be a challenge due to shortages in the availability and affordability of child psychiatrists, psychologists, or behavior therapists. Minority racial/ethnic pediatric populations, as well as those living in poverty, are more likely to lack access to mental health resources (Atkins, Capella, et al., 2017). In either case, whether the barriers are cultural or economic, the school may represent the venue to move beyond these issues by providing accessible services or the attention of nurturing adults.

SBHCs are in a unique position not only to identify mental health problems among children and adolescents but also to provide treatment or links to appropriate services. Evidence shows students with either public or no health insurance are more likely to access SBHC mental health services. Nearly 70% of SBHCs offer mental health care services through licensed clinical social workers, psychologists, and/or substance abuse counselors. Services most often addressed include substance use counseling, violence prevention, suicide prevention, dating violence, mental health diagnoses, grief and loss therapy, crisis intervention, and medication management or administration. In addition, they often treat depression, anxiety, social conflict, sequelae of toxic stress, and attention disorders (Larsen, Chapman, Spetz, & Brindis, 2017).

Ultimately there remains a large need for school-based mental health services that effectively partner with families, schools, and other community systems. For example, mental health has been implicated as a top risk factor for mass school shootings (i.e., "rampage shootings"). The American Public Health Association (APHA) has endorsed SBHCs as a key mechanism through which gun violence prevention, intervention, and emergency preparedness can occur. Early identification of suicidal youth in schools and other settings could lend to a program of defense against school shooters. In addition, preventing the more common urban "street" (i.e., nonrampage) youth gun violence involves making mental health resources available in schools at all times (APHA, 2018).

Children exposed to adverse childhood experience (ACE) events have a greater risk for mental health disorders and school failure. ACEs are becoming a research priority across the country and are defined as childhood abuse, neglect, or dysfunction in the household (e.g., domestic violence, parental mental illness, or parental substance abuse). The effects of ACE exposure extend well beyond the immediate act of harm and include severe mental, physical, and behavioral health disorders across the life span. These include all forms of child maltreatment and exposure to stressful situations characterized by violence and anti-social behavior. Ultimately, the annual U.S. economic burden for childhood maltreatment (i.e., ACEs) is $124 billion. Associated costs to society include health care, productivity losses, child welfare costs, violence/crime costs, special education costs, and suicide death costs. Recently, a 4-year national effort culminated during which stakeholders engaged in creating a comprehensive national research and action agenda on ACEs. Research now prioritizes relationship-centered healthcare as well as family and community engagement in order to mitigate the effect of ACE-related stress and trauma, establish resilience, promote positive health skills, and improve child health and well-being. While SBHCs have engaged in trauma-informed care, research that has measured or evaluated this effectiveness is lacking. Future research ought to focus on whether young people with high ACE scores receiving trauma-informed care experience better outcomes in schools with SBHCs compared to those without. Intervening early with a child experiencing chronic trauma is critical but mental health services are often inaccessible, especially for children and adolescents of minority racial/ethnic groups and those living in poverty. SBHCs may have a unique role to play in improving screening, treatment, and prevention of ACEs (Larsen et al., 2017).

Education

The CDC considers academic success both a strong indicator and outcome of the overall health and well-being of a child. Children must learn how to be healthy and must be healthy to learn. Academic success is a social determinant of pediatric and adult health. For example, it has been shown that chronic health conditions decrease academic achievement, and safe school environments improve health behaviors and academic performance.

The evidence linking SBHC presence to educational outcomes, however, is still limited and mixed. The link between SBHC services and academic performance is indirect and intangible. For example, in a 2011 study, the authors reported that SBHC use decreased dropout rates. However, after the methodological concerns about the study were brought to their attention, the authors reanalyzed their data and retracted their results, finding no statistical relationship between SBHC use and dropout rates (Kerns et al., 2012).

Compared with other industrialized countries, the United States is not performing as well in math, science, and reading, even though the United States ranks fifth in spending per student. In response to these reports, there have been many efforts over the past few decades to reform education in the United States, focusing on instructional practices, teacher preparation programs, and education standards meant to ensure students are learning and to hold schools accountable (Runton & Hudak, 2016).

Despite these efforts, there has been minimal improvement in student achievement. One reason might be that these education-specific approaches are not addressing health-related barriers to learning. Basch argues that health-related problems greatly limit students' motivation and ability to learn. Furthermore, health problems (e.g., asthma and poor vision) and poor health behaviors (e.g., physical inactivity and poor nutrition) are linked to educational outcomes through five causal pathways: sensory perceptions, cognition, connectedness and engagement with school, absenteeism, and dropping out (Basch, 2011). In support of this conclusion, specific health-related problems and behaviors including vision, asthma, teen pregnancy, aggression and violence, physical activity, breakfast consumption, and inattention and hyperactivity have been shown to have an impact on learning. This important connection between health and education supports the need for a comprehensive school health approach that is strategic, high quality, and coordinated, which is the essence of the SBHC.

The SBHC been associated with improved academic outcomes, such as improved GPAs, attendance, grade promotion, college preparation, and reduced rates of suspensions. These rates may not have been statistically significant, but are promising enough to warrant renewed research activity. The APHA (2018) supports SBHCs because they foster school-wide programs that address bullying, violence, anger, depression and other social and emotional issues that are predictive to impede academic achievement. Additionally, a growing body of evidence suggests that SBHCs improve academic performance indirectly by increasing school connectedness, particularly in lower income youth populations. The CDC defines school connectedness as "the belief held by students that adults and peers in the school care about their learning as well as about them as individuals" (CDC, 2009). In one study, SBHC usage was significantly associated with school connection (bonding, attachment, and commitment), which was positively related to GPA and promotion to the next grade level (Bersamin, Coulter, et al., 2019).

More methodologically robust design and analysis is required in researching the outcomes of SBHCs on education. For example, there would be merit in linking educational data to health records. However, there remain large legal barriers to negotiating exchange of information about students. And we should not undermine that guarantees of confidentiality are significant with students in developing and maintaining connectedness with teachers and other school personnel. Finally, most studies on the benefits of SBHCs have chosen to focus on onsite SBHCs with minority populations, low-income schools, urban settings, and older groups of students. Further research should look at the sustainability of SBHCs in atypical environments, such as offsite clinics, rural settings, schools in mid- to high-income communities, and with younger children. Experimenting with telehealth, as well, could provide SBHCs with valuable insights and avenues for cost-saving and therapeutic effectiveness.

SBHCs and the Complementary Role of the School Nurse/School Nurse Practitioner

There is a distinct difference in the services provided by school nurses and the SBHC. The National Association of School Nurses (NASN) issued a position statement in 2015 endorsed by the School Based Health Alliance (SBHA) that SBHCs do not duplicate or replace school nursing services. This position paper further details the work of the school nurse as (Cornell & Selekman, 2013):

- Management of chronic disease and life-threatening health conditions
- Individual and population-based disease surveillance
- Health promotion
- Assistance in securing insurance and healthcare providers
- Preparation for and response to medical emergencies
- Care for students dependent on medical technology
- Mental health services
- Screenings and referrals
- Immunization compliance
- Medication management
- Healthcare planning and education
- Follow-up care
- Care coordination

In a complementary role, the SBHC, provides a variety of health care services which may include (Barnett & Allison, 2012):

- Primary care
- Comprehensive health assessments
- Treatment of acute illness
- Prescriptions for medication

Additionally SBHCs improve access to care by removing barriers that may include (Guo, Wade, Pan, & Keller, 2010; Keeton, Soleimanpou, & Brindis, 2012):

- Financial (lack of insurance or low income)
- Providers who will accept the student's insurance
- Lack of transportation to appointments
- Scheduling conflicts
- Parent/guardians work schedules

This position statement remains current, but will automatically expire in 2020, if not reaffirmed. The reader is confronted with the overlap between the work of the school nurse and the SBHC, which usually employs nurse practitioners. This position statement deserves immediate revisiting.

An additional area which requires study is the responsibilities and relevance of the school nurse practitioner (SNP). This is a higher education role which was designed to be inserted into school practice, complementing or expanding the scope of practice of the school nurse, by assuming many of the primary care duties which have since been included in the SBHC. The nurse practitioner role has morphed into full acceptance by the public for many specialized populations and many health care sites. But it seems there is less talk of the SNP. Advanced practice nurses, family-pediatric-reproductive-adult nurse practitioners, will become the mainstay of SBHCs, but where will the certified school nurse and the SNP fit in the equation. Will school services be segmented into traditional school services and the SBHC, or would they be better off coming together as one? It should be noted that the SNP certification awarded by the American Nurses Credentialing Center (ANCC) has been closed to new applicants, and can only be accessed for renewals of the credential (ANCC, 2019).

Originally the SNP was the embodiment of the NP prepared to deliver primary care to the school age population, and additionally to teach and serve as the liaison between the school and the community. She/he would serve on the Child Study Team and counsel administration on health related public policy. The SNP should be easily certifiable as a School Nurse, and would elevate the Certified School Nurse role to the minimum of master's preparation. Has certification of SNPs been blocked because preparation for the role has been abandoned? The intersection of these roles should be carefully studied.

Meanwhile, it is the position of the NASN that licensed professional registered nurses (RNs) who work in the specialty of school nursing require advanced skills to address the complex health needs of students within a school community setting. These skills are attained through a *minimum* of a baccalaureate degree in nursing and validated by voluntary specialized certification in school nursing through the National Board for Certification of School Nurses (NASN, 2019). It should be noted that there may be additional state-specific requirements for practice as a school nurse. This role is regulated by states' rights and the Board of Nursing or Department of Education of the particular state in question should be consulted. No nurse is allowed to practice within the school without conforming to state requirements. There has never been any attempt at preemptive legislation to create a national standard which would supersede the state standard. The National Council of State Boards of Nursing (NCSBN) moved from seeking national consensus on licensure to multi-state compacts which aim for the same outcome, but preserve each state's autonomy (NCSBN, 2019).

Conclusion

SBHCs may promote social mobility and improve health equity by meeting the needs of disadvantaged populations and removing barriers to health care services (Knopf et al., 2016). The SBHC financial and physical benefits are well documented, if not statistically proven, but more research is needed on their impact on mental health and educational outcomes. The reader should also be aware of the proliferation of charter, religiously affiliated and private schools. The SBHC has only been tested in public schools, though similar health programs may be forthcoming in private schools. They should be included in the Alliances' database. They often have freer reign to be creative, being excluded from some governmental regulations. Their inventiveness could provide interesting innovations to consider.

It is appropriate to close this chapter with a few comments on start-up. The process of start-up must build within the context of community, its population, and its health care resources, rather than where the experts say you should go. The experts should be used as consultants, not decision-makers. The most important constituency is the families of the students you wish to serve, and be aware that students have opinions too. In fact, opinion should be invited from anyone who lives in the community and/or pays taxes. Each citizen will be an invaluable asset as you develop your initial program, and then as service-recipients if you decide to expand. The SBHC is a collaborative venture between the community, and the school district. The community must feel ownership, and the school is part of the community in that broader sense. The community brings all of its resources including strengths and weaknesses to the table. A careful assessment should be completed on the community, including its health problems, health profile, and demographics. The stages of this assessment, who to include, when to include them, and the identity of a leadership team to pull everything together, should be thought out carefully and strategically. Opinions of community leaders should be sought; and focus groups are a good vehicle. And remember that private, religiously affiliated, or charter schools will each have a different constituency.

References

American Nurses Credentialing Center. (2019). *School nurse practitioner certification (SNP-BC)*. Retrieved from https://www.nursingworld.org/our-certifications/school-nurse-practitioner-renewal/

American Public Health Association. (2018). *Preventing gun violence*. Retrieved from https://www.apha.org/~/media/files/pdf/factsheets/160317_gunviolencefs.ashx

Atkins, M. S., Cappella, E., et al. (2017). Schooling and children's mental health: Realigning resources to reduce disparities and advance public health. *Annual Review of Clinical Psychology, 13*, 123–147.

Barnett, S. E., & Allison, M. A.; Council on School Health. (2012). School-based health centers and pediatric practice. *Pediatrics, 129,* 387–393. doi:10.1542/peds.2011-3443

Basch, C. E. (2011, October). Healthier students are better learners: A missing link in school reforms to close the achievement gap. *Journal of School Health, 81*(10), 593–598. doi:10.1111/j.1746-1561.2011.00632.x

Bersamin, M., Coulter, R. W., et al. (2019). School-based health centers and school connectedness. *Journal of School Health, 89*(1), 11–19. doi:10.1111/josh.12707

Brodeurk, P. (1986). *School-based health clinics.* Retrieved from Rwjf.org

Brom, H. M., Salsberry, P. J., & Graham, M. C. (2018). Leveraging health care reform to accelerate nurse practitioner full practice authority. *Journal of the American Association of Nurse Practitioners, 30*(3), 120–130. doi:10.1097/JXX.0000000000000023

Bureau of Primary Health Care. (2016). *Uniform data system.* Rockville, MD: Health Resources and Services Administration.

Centers for Disease Control and Prevention. (2009). *School connectedness: Strategies for increasing protective factors among youth.* Atlanta, GA: U.S. Department of Health and Human Services. Retrieved from https://www.cdc.gov/healthyyouth/protective/pdf/connectedness.pdf

Cornell, M., & Selekman, J. (2013). Collaboration with the community. In J. Selekman (Ed.), *School nursing: A comprehensive text* (2nd ed., pp. 176–179). Philadelphia, PA: F. A. Davis Company.

Department of Education. (2019). *Improving basic programs operated by local educational agencies (Title I, Part A).* Washington, DC: Author. Retrieved from https://www2.ed.gov/programs/titleiparta/index.html

Gunderson, G. W. (2019). *National school lunch program: Early programs by state.* Washington, DC: U.S. Department of Agriculture. Retrieved from https://portal.ct.gov/SDE/Nutrition/School-Nutrition-Programs

Guo, J. J., Wade, T. J., Pan, W., & Keller, K. N. (2015). School-based health centers: Cost-benefit analysis and impact on health care disparities. *American Journal of Public Health, 100*(9), 1617–1623.

Health Resources and Services Administration. (2019, February). *HRSA awards $11 million to increase access to critical services at school-based health centers.* Retrieved from hrsa.gov/about/news/press-release/hrsa-awards-11-million-school-based-health-centers

Kanaan, S. B. (2007). *Making the grade: State and local partnerships to establish school-based health centers.* Princeton, NJ: Robert Wood Johnson Foundation. Retrieved from https://www.rwjf.org/en/library/research/2007/02/making-the-grade.html

Keeton, V., Soleimanpour, S., & Brindis, C. D. (2012). School-based health centers in an era of health care reform: Building on history. National Institutes of Health Public Access, Author Manuscript, pp. 1–31.

Kerns, S. E., Pullman, M. D., Walker, S. C., Lyon, A. R., Cosgrove, T. J., & Bruns, E. J. (2012). School-based health center use and high school dropout rates. *Archives of Pediatrics & Adolescent Medicine, 166*(7), 675–677. doi:10.1001/archpediatrics.2012.550

Knopf, J. A., Finnie, R. K., Peng, Y., Hahn, R. A., Truman, B. I., Vernon-Smiley, M., … Fullilove M. T.; Community Preventive Services Task Force. (2016, July). School-based health centers to advance health equity: A community guide systematic review. *American Journal of Preventive Medicine, 51*(1), 114–126. doi:10.1016/j.amepre.2016.01.009

Larson, S., Chapman, S., Spetz, J., & Brindis, C. D. (2017). Chronic childhood trauma, mental health, academic achievement, and school-based health center mental health services. *Journal of School Health, 87*(9), 675–686. doi:10.1111/josh.12541

Lear, J. G. (1996). School-based services and adolescent health: Past, present and future. *Adolescent Medicine, 7*, 163–180. Retrieved from https://europepmc.org/article/med/10359965#impact

Leroy, Z. C., Wallin, R., & Lee, S. (2017). The role of school health services in addressing the needs of students with chronic health conditions. *Journal of School Nursing, 33*(1), 64–72. doi:10.1177/1059840516678909

Love, H. E., Schlitt, J., Soleimanpour, S, Panchal, N., & Behr, C. (2017, May). Twenty years of school-based health care growth and expansion. *Health Affairs, 38*(5), 755–764. doi:10.1377/hlthaff.2018.05472

National Association of School Nurses. (2015). *The complementary roles of the school nurse and school based health centers (Position Statement).* Silver Spring, MD: Author.

National Association of School Nurses. (2019). *Education, licensure, and licensure of school nurses.* Retrieved from nasn.org

National Council of State Boards of Nursing. (2019). *APRN Consensus model.* Retrieved from ncsbn.org/aprn-consensus.htm

National Research Council, Institute of Medicine. (2009). *Adolescent health services: Missing opportunities.* Washington, DC: National Academies Press.

Porter, P. J., Avery, E. H., & Fellows, J. A. (1974). Model for the reorganization of child health services within an urban community. *American Journal of Public Health, 64*(6), 618–619. doi:10.2105/ajph.64.6.618

Ramos, M. M., Sebastian, R. A., Stumbo, S. P., McGrath, J., & Fairbrother, G. (2017). Measuring unmet needs for anticipatory guidance among adolescents at school-based health centers. *Journal of Adolescent Health, 60*, 720–726. doi:10.1016/j.jadohealth.2016.12.021

Runton, N. G., & Hudak, R. P. (2016, May–June). The influence of school-based health centers on adolescents' youth risk behaviors. *Journal of Pediatric Health Care, 30*(3), 1–9. doi:10.1016/j.pedhc.2015.07.005

School-Based Health Alliance. (2016). *National school-based health care census.* Retrieved from https://www.sbh4all.org/school-health-care/national-census-of-school-based-health-centers/

School Based Health Alliance. (2017). *2013-14 Census of school-based health centers: Methodology, key report data details, and acknowledgements.* Retrieved from http://www.sbh4all.org/wp-content/uploads/2015/02/2013-14-Census-Data-and-Methods.pdf

U.S. Department of Health and Human Services. (2014). *Federal Tort Claims Act. Health center policy manual.* Retrieved from HHS-FTCA-Claims@hhs.gov

Vessey, J. A., & McGowan, K. A. (2006, May–June). A successful public health experiment: School nursing. *Pediatric Nursing, 32*(3), 255–256, 213.

Young, T. L., & Ireson, C. (2003). Effectiveness of school-based telehealth care in urban and rural elementary schools. *Pediatrics, 112*(5), 1088–1094. doi:10.1542/peds.112.5.1088

SPECIAL EDUCATION
JOHN M. DEWITT

LEARNING OBJECTIVES

- Define the following terms: Special Education, Classification, Child Study Team, Free and Appropriate Public Education, Individualized Education Program, Mainstreaming/Inclusion.
- Compare the Individuals with Disabilities Education Act (IDEA) and Section 504 of the Rehabilitation Act.
- Recognize the factors in the special education referral process.
- Identify the spectrum of services that are available, and how qualification for these services occurs.
- Differentiate the roles of each member of the Child Study Team, including the role of the school nurse.

■ Introduction

When one examines the origins and history of the special education system in America's schools, dramatic changes can be observed over its tenure of the past 100 years. Long gone are the days of segregation and ignorance of the needs of our neediest students, thanks to laws such as the Individuals with Disabilities Education Act (IDEA) and Section 504 of the 1973 Rehabilitation Act. These federal laws helped to pave the way to guard against discrimination of people with disabilities. With the advent of these laws, which have since been refined and cultivated, dramatic changes have occurred which help to provide appropriate opportunities for students with special needs to not only learn but to thrive to meet their individual potential.

In today's school system, special education programs are designed to meet the ever-changing needs of the spectrum of disabilities. Special education laws require school districts to follow federal and state mandated rules which not only govern their actions, but monitor timelines, programs, curricula, placements, and various other areas. School systems have entire teams dedicated to ensuring that the specific laws are followed and the needs of the special education students are met.

Although the origins of the American education system's handling of our neediest students is not something we can be proud of, dramatic changes to our understanding of the differences among children and the understanding of disabilities as a whole has led to significant pedagogical changes for our education system.

An Initial Guide Into the World of Special Education

To the outside observer, whether it be a parent, regular education teacher, school nurse, or administrator, the world of special education can be a confusing place due to its many laws, guidelines, timelines, and terms. In an effort to speed through these aspects, special education teachers and school specialists (defined herein as Child Study Team members) often discuss aspects of their field through the use of acronyms and initialisms.

A conversation between these staff members may sound something like this:

Staff member 1: "Hi, I am just wondering about the new case that was referred to the CST?"

Staff member 2: "Do we have any I&RS records that we can review?"

Staff member 1: "I seem to recall that the student was in an EIP before, possibly due to issues with PT, OT, and speech, and may have even been in a PSWD program early on. Are we sure the child didn't qualify for SERS in the past?"

Staff member 2: "I'm not sure, but we need to review the evaluations before we have the IPM. That way we can determine which areas the student may have an issue in, so we can evaluate the right areas."

Staff member 1: "I'm thinking that they may have an SLD based on the recent state testing, but who knows, it could be OHI based on ADD or even MD if they are both impacting learning."

Staff member 2: "Maybe this case will end up with a 504 if the child doesn't meet the NJAC code requirements. Well, you know we'll figure it out by the time we have the EC and then provide an IEP if the child is eligible."

Staff member 1: "Well, it may be a matter of mainstreaming or inclusion—and we do have Resource classrooms to address the needs."

Confused yet? Don't be. Although this may sound like a conversation that has more to do with the alphabet and less to do with special education, understand that the terms are often shortened but have significant meaning behind them. The key terms are limited, and with a little bit of background information, one can decipher this often strange and confusing conversation. The federal guidelines of the IDEA are a mandate for each state level department of education, but slight variations are often adopted at the individual state level. This may reveal slight variations in terms, as some state's adherence to the federal guidelines has resulted in the adoption of more stringent laws and regulations. The terms from the preceding conversation are an example of a conversation that may have been held in a school in a town in New Jersey, but the conversation and terms will be similar in other states. With so many abbreviations, the federal government has even provided a guide for parents on the IDEA website (IDEA, n.d.).

Now, read through the following terms:

CST = Child Study Team: A group of specialized staff members, who are either licensed or certified in their individual state to work in a school system. Members may include: School Psychologist, School Social Worker, Learning Disabilities Teacher Consultant, and Speech-Language Pathologist. Additional ancillary members may include: Physical Therapist, Occupational Therapist, and Behaviorists.

I&RS = Intervention and Referral Services: An in-school support team composed of staff members to support teachers by brainstorming pre-referral interventions. This group of individuals may go under a different name, but they provide systematic direction and feedback before a child is referred for an evaluation.

EIP = Early Intervention Program: A program in which a student would qualify for additional support in specific areas, such as Speech/Language Therapy, Occupational Therapy, Educational Interventions, and so forth. These services are available to students who qualify based on specific, objective criteria, from birth to age 3.

PT = Physical Therapist: A professional who evaluates and provides therapy to help a student's weaknesses in the area of gross motor skills.

OT = Occupational Therapist: A professional who evaluates and provides therapy to help a student's weaknesses in the area of fine motor skills.

PSWD = Preschool Child With a Disability: A child who has been classified as eligible to receive special education services from the ages of 3 to 5.

SERS = Special Education and Related Services: A designation of qualifying for and receiving a specific set of services to address a student's individual, documented needs.

IPM = Initial Planning Meeting: A meeting with specific members of the school and parents, to determine the need for evaluations and a plan/timeline to complete the evaluations.

SLD = Specific Learning Disability: A significant discrepancy between a child's intellectual ability (their intellect or intelligence quotient which they were born with—think brain capacity) and their academic achievement (the baseline of what they have learned in school). These scores are measured through individually administered, standardized evaluations.

OHI = Other Health Impairment: A classification that may cover a specific health impairment, such as attention deficit disorder, or other specific medical conditions which are determined to adversely affect a student's educational performance. For this, a medical assessment is required to document the health problem.

ADD = Attention Deficit Disorder: A developmental disorder, diagnosed by a medical professional, which is marked by a specific set of symptoms.

Inattentive symptoms may include but are not limited to issues with organization, distractibility, and forgetfulness.

Hyperactive symptoms may include but are not limited to restlessness, fidgeting, and an observed inability to maintain typical classroom rules (sitting still, standing in line, etc.).

MD = Multiple Disabilities: A classification that covers a student who has two or more disabling conditions, necessitating a composite program designed to meet their specific needs.

504 = Section 504: A plan developed to help "level" the playing field, not specific to schools (Civil Rights Law).

NJAC = New Jersey Administrative Code: A specific set of guidelines, including definitions, regulations, and timelines, established by the New Jersey Department of Education (New Jersey Administrative Code, n.d.) to align with the federal law (IDEA).

EC = Eligibility Conference: A meeting with specific members of the school and parents, to discuss the results of the evaluations which have been completed, and determine a student's eligibility to receive services through an IEP.

IEP = Individualized Education Plan: A legally binding document developed to provide a student with specific services to meet their unique needs.

Mainstreaming or **Inclusion:** When a special education student is placed into a regular education classroom with typically developing peers.

Here are a few additional key terms to know, as they will provide a deeper understanding of special education as we move through the chapter:

IDEA = Individuals with Disabilities Education Act: A federal law that guarantees a Free Appropriate Public Education to all students ages 3 to 21

FAPE = Free Appropriate Public Education: The legal rights provided to students under the federal laws (U.S. Department of Education, 1999).

Free: An education provided by the government at no cost to families.

Appropriate: A program designed to meet each child's unique needs.

Public: Supervised by the public school system.

Education: A plan to educate the student and meet their school-based needs, including related services (Speech/Language Therapy, Occupational Therapy, Physical Therapy, etc.).

LRE = Least Restrictive Environment: A measure under IDEA which requires children who are eligible for special education to receive as much opportunity to learn with peers who do not receive special education services

PLAAFP = Present Levels of Academic Achievement and Functional Performance: The narrative portion of an IEP, designed to help understand who, what, when, where, and why about the student. This includes a history of the student's evaluations, summaries of evaluations, parental feedback, and narratives from the child's teachers.

G&O = Goals and Objectives: The specific, objective, measurable areas which are targeted in each of the child's areas of weakness, developed to create a baseline of their weaknesses or needs and measure growth in these areas over a specific length of time (generally, on a quarterly basis).

Now that you have read through and have a basic understanding of some terms, let's review the conversation:

Staff member 1: "Hi, I am just wondering about the new case that was referred to the Child Study Team?"

The staff member wants to review the case to have a deeper understanding of what is happening before meeting with the parents and staff.

Staff member 2: "Do we have any Intervention and Referral Services records that we can review?"

The staff member wants to review any pre-referral interventions that the teachers may have implemented in class. This will help the team members determine what intervention may have helped a student, rule out or pinpoint any specific trends and issues that may be occurring in the classroom, and ensure that areas of need are being assessed.

Staff member 1: "I seem to recall that the student was in an Early Intervention Program before, possibly due to issues with Physical Therapy, Occupational Therapy, and speech, and may have even been in a PreSchool Child With Disability program early on. Are we sure they didn't qualify for Special Education and Related Services in the past?"

The staff member wants to determine if the student required a program before entering the public school system, or during their time within the public school system, which would be due to a specific area(s) of weakness. Prior evaluations are invaluable as they may pinpoint areas of delay, need, and growth—or lack of.

Staff member 2: "I'm not sure, but we need to review before we have the Initial Planning Meeting. That way we can determine which areas the student may have an issue in, so we can evaluate the right areas."

The staff member wants to review records to pinpoint areas of need, so that they are informed of the educational history prior to meeting with a parent to discuss the decision of electing to evaluate the student.

Staff member 1: "I'm thinking that the child may have a Specific Learning Disability based on the recent state testing, but who knows, it could be Other Health Impairment based on Attention Deficit Disorder or even Multiple Disabilities if they are both impacting learning."

Based on a review of available records, the staff member will attempt to hone in on areas of potential weakness. These are the areas that the team will request to evaluate through individually administered, standardized evaluations. The team will generally make an effort to focus only on the areas of suspected disability to avoid overburdening a student with unnecessary evaluations. Understanding the time and effort that these evaluations impose on a student, it is prudent to limit them to areas that are recognized as potential weaknesses.

Staff member 2: "Maybe this case will end up with a 504 if the child doesn't meet the New Jersey Administrative Code requirements. Well, you know we'll figure it out by the time we have the Eligibility Conference and then provide an Individual Education Program if the child is eligible."

Each team is required to determine if the results of the specific evaluation meet the state-mandated criteria for eligibility. A student's specific weaknesses must impact their ability to receive an appropriate education. The results of the evaluations are reviewed at a conference with parents and staff members. Generally, the results will provide eligibility for special education, and a specific plan will be created to meet the child's specific individual needs. In the case that a child is determined to not be eligible for special education they may meet the criteria for a 504 plan.

Staff member 1: "Well, it may be a matter of mainstreaming or inclusion—and we do have resource classrooms to address the needs."

The team members are beginning to brainstorm about possible placements, based on the initial information that they have been provided. Of course, an entire evaluation would be necessary to determine the specific strengths and needs, and to determine an appropriate placement with the Individual Education Program team members (including the parents).

▉ The First Steps—Pre-referral Interventions

So how does a student get from their reported struggles in the classroom to a possible referral and evaluation? The next steps are a careful process to determine the current functioning level and possible struggles that may be impacting their ability to function in the class and/or school. This may include academic, social, emotional, behavioral, communication, or other specific needs.

The first steps, generally, are pre-referral interventions. Each state has a screening process for regular education students to be screened to determine which types of support they may require. This can be the first, and possibly only, stop on their journey, if the interventions prove to solve the problem.

As noted earlier, the screening process may have a name such as Intervention and Referral Services (I&RS), Pupil Assistance Committee (PAC) or some other fancy title. In essence, the purpose of this group is to provide support for the teacher to assist the student in the area where the student is struggling. The group will generally include other educators, such as an administrator, guidance counselor, regular and special education teachers, Child Study Team member, and school nurse. The parent(s) or guardian(s) can be a key member providing feedback and the history of the child's education.

The group meets to review all available data on the student and determine whatever additional support the teacher may need.

EXAMPLE 1: Johnny is in fifth grade and struggling in math. The teacher noted that his grades on tests are good, but homework is inconsistent. Additionally, he doesn't always respond when the teacher asks him a question.

EXAMPLE 2: Sarah is in the third grade. She is new to the school district and seems to be struggling on assignments posted on the board. In class, her teachers note that she is polite and respectful but does not seem to be interacting with any of the students. Additionally, she asks for frequent bathroom breaks.

So what is the process to help intervene in these situations? The first step is for the general education teacher to implement all of the proverbial "tools" in their toolbox. The teacher may make suggestions, modifications, and interventions. Once the teacher has exhausted all of their own tips and tricks, they would turn to the group for assistance.

A meeting is scheduled with the key players (as listed previously). At the meeting, the members will review all available data, which may include:

- Academic examples from class, such as writing/math samples
- Tests, quizzes, measurable data
- Emails to and from parents
- A list of all attempts at help that the teachers or staff members have made, the results of those interventions, and the length of time that they have been in place
- Report cards
- Statelocal testing (available standardized measures)
- Vision/hearing screening results
- Available health records

Each member of the team provides a unique perspective and can help to frame the potential issues that may be occurring, and offer insight that may help:

EXAMPLE 1: Johnny is in fifth grade and struggling in math. The teacher noted that his grades on tests are good, but homework is inconsistent. Additionally, he doesn't always respond when the teacher asks him a question.

Potential Role in the Discussion

Regular Education Teacher: Review attempted interventions and present the student's areas of struggle.

Special Education Teacher—Examine any trends in weaknesses on work samples.

Child Study Team Member—Review standardized test to see if any weaknesses are present.

School Administrator—Review parental correspondence and previous report cards.

School Nurse—Review attendance to see if any patterns of days of absenteeism may be occurring. Additionally, review hearing/vision screening results.

EXAMPLE 2: Sarah is in the third grade. She is new to the school district and seems to be struggling on assignments posted on the board. In class, her teachers note that she is polite and respectful but does not seem to be interacting with any of the students. Additionally, she asks for frequent bathroom breaks.

Potential Role in the Discussion

Regular Education Teacher—Review observations of the student in structured (classroom) and unstructured (lunch, playground, etc.) areas.

Special Education Teacher—Examine any trends or weaknesses on work samples.

Child Study Team Member—Review standardized test to see if any weaknesses are present.

School Administrator—Review available records from the previous district.

School Nurse—Review health history forms.

Teachers, both general and special education, come to the classroom with a wealth of experience. Many teachers have taught multiple grades or subjects, have spent countless hours in classrooms, and have completed student teaching experiences. Even with the vast knowledge that they may have, the group discussion allows them to hear perspectives from other professionals and find solutions beyond those in their educational "tool box."

The main goal of the group is to brainstorm about what may be occurring, document new interventions and set a timeline for review. The group will decide on an appropriate time to meet again—generally anywhere from 4 to 8 weeks—to review. That meeting may involve the same members or add new members, if required. If the interventions have made an impact and growth is noted, the team may simply keep them in place and monitor student progress going forward. If interventions have not made a significant impact, the next step may be a referral to the Child Study Team.

■ What Is the Child Study Team?

As noted earlier in this chapter, the Child Study Team (CST) comprises specialized staff members whose role is to analyze a student's current functioning levels and, if necessary, perform evaluations to determine the child's functioning level in suspected areas of disability. Although each state has members assigned based on their laws, the core members generally include a School Psychologist, Learning Disabilities Teacher Consultant, and School Social Worker. In specific cases, ancillary members such as a Speech-Language Pathologist may join the team. Additional evaluations may be sought from Physical Therapists, Occupational Therapists, Behaviorists, and specialized medical professionals (as deemed necessary). The case manager, who is generally the School Psychologist, Learning Disabilities Teacher Consultant, or School Social Worker, will coordinate meetings, gather required documents, and act as the liaison for all parties.

Child Study Team Members (Core)

School Psychologist: Utilizes standardized evaluative tools to assess a student's intellectual, social, and emotional needs. Their role may eventually include providing counseling services (group, individual, consultation) along with the creation of specific IEP driven Goals and Objectives under their area of expertise.

Learning Disabilities Teacher Consultant: Utilizes standardized evaluative tools to assess a student's academic strengths and weaknesses (only a few states continue to have this role—for those states that do not, the School Psychologist is trained to administer evaluations in this area). Their role may eventually include providing consultation services to teachers, including classroom guidance along with the creation of Specific IEP-driven Goals and Objectives under their area of expertise.

School Social Worker: Gathers and documents a student's case history, including all pertinent information about their home life, developmental history, and so forth. Their role may eventually include providing counseling services (group, individual, consultation) along with the creation of specific IEP-driven Goals and Objectives under their area of expertise.

Child Study Team Members (Ancillary)

Speech-Language Pathologist: Utilizes standardized evaluative tools to assess a student's overall communication abilities, including their expressive and receptive language abilities. Their role may eventually include therapy along with the creation of specific IEP-driven Goals and Objectives under their area of expertise.

Other Staff Members Who May Be Part of the Evaluative Team

Physical and Occupational Therapists: Utilizes evaluative tools to assess a student's overall gross and fine motor skills. Their role may eventually include therapy along with the creation of specific IEP-driven Goals and Objectives under their area of expertise.

Behaviorists: Utilizes evaluative tools to measure objective behaviors which may be impeding a student in school. Based on the data, may create a specific plan (Behavior Intervention Plan) to address those needs. Their role may eventually include consultation with staff, parents, or students.

School Nurse: Provides results of hearing and vision screenings, which are required, prior to evaluations. They will also help to provide medical history, student needs, and other health information which are vital to the evaluation process

■ The Next Step—Referral to the Child Study Team

A student can be referred to the CST by someone who has knowledge of the child's struggles that are impacting them in school. This can include a parent or staff member who formally requests a meeting to review their concerns. The CST will hold an Initial Planning Meeting to review all available data, including pre-referral interventions, such as those completed through the I&RS process, or similar meeting. The goals for the CST are to narrow down the area(s) of concern and determine the appropriate evaluations that should be performed based on the data they have reviewed. In all cases, a parent will provide input and consent to move forward with the evaluations. In many cases, a school nurse's input is vital and essential. The CST will need to understand any medical issues which may be impacting the student, their previous medical history, and their most recent vision and hearing screening. Due to the need to schedule meetings within a timely fashion and in accordance with state laws, not all staff may be available to attend the meeting. In this case, it is imperative for them to provide their feedback as it may impact the status of the evaluations—or, more specifically, which evaluations may be agreed upon.

A main concern is the time that it will take to complete the necessary evaluations, once a parent has formally agreed to move forward with the case. Each state has specific timelines and regulations which must be followed. This also includes state imposed requirements and rationale (State of New Jersey–Department of Education, 2020).

The names of the stages may change based on each state, but a basic outline for the process is:

- Referral to the Child Study Team
- Initial Planning Meeting
- Evaluations (once parents have formally agreed to move forward)
    - May include, but not limited to: Psychological Evaluation, Educational Evaluation, Speech/Language Evaluation, Social Case History, Func-

tional Behavior Analysis, Occupational Therapy Evaluation, Physical Therapy Evaluation, Neurological Evaluation, Psychiatric Evaluation.

■   In all cases, updated **Hearing/Vision screenings** must be completed to ensure that the student's hearing and vision are within normal limits and are not the base cause of their struggles.

■   Eligibility Conference (to discuss the results and the next steps).

Upon completion, copies of all evaluations are provided to the parents so they can review them prior to meeting. The CST will invite the parent back to review the results and let the parents know if they qualify for Special Education and Related Services. As each state has specific criteria, the team will determine if the current issues are impacting the student's ability to receive an appropriate education. Upon qualification, the CST will discuss their recommendations with the parents and other meeting members.

Two distinct paths:

If the child qualifies … (a quick guide)

1. An Individualized Education Plan is created to meet the student's specific, unique needs.

2. Feedback from the teachers and reports are included in this document to paint a picture of the student.

3. Goals and Objectives are created for each of the child's special education classes and/or related services. These specific, measurable criteria will provide the basis for the child's program and allow an objective measurement tool over time (generally feedback on these areas is provided to the parents three to four times a year).

4. Accommodations and Modifications are provided for regular/special education settings, standardized testing, and so forth.

5. Classroom placement is determined by the data that are available from the evaluations completed and reviewed at the Eligibility Conference. Each student's IEP must define the placement and the amount of special education and related services a student will receive (minutes/hours) per school day/week/month.

Here are a few common placements:

Mainstream/Inclusion: A student may have additional accommodations and modifications which can be addressed in the mainstream classroom. This classroom model in a public school places the student with their general education peers, where they may have access to the general education materials (which may be modified to meet their specific needs).

Resource Program: A student may require remediation on a specific skill or skills. This classroom model in a public school removes the student from the general education classroom for a specific subject or subjects (e.g., Mathematics).

The student will have specific Goals and Objectives which will drive instruction in the classroom and focus on the student's weaknesses.

Self-Contained Program: A student may require a more intensive, structured classroom to address multiple needs and skills. This classroom model in a public school removes the student from the general education classroom for all academic subjects (i.e., Mathematics, Language Arts, Science, Social Studies). The student will have specific Goals and Objectives which will drive instruction in the classroom and focus on the student's weaknesses. In this case, students may be mainstreamed for non-academics as deemed appropriate, including Physical Education, Art, Lunch, Recess, and so on.

Out of District Programs: A student may require intensive services to meet their specific skill deficits, which cannot be addressed in the public school setting. This intensive model is one of the most restrictive as it removes the student from interactions with their mainstream peers. The student will have specific Goals and Objectives which will drive their intensive program.

If the child does not qualify … (a quick guide)

In the event that a child does not meet the specific criteria for special education services through an IEP, the team will often provide recommendations to the teachers and other staff members.

The child remains a regular education student, and the teacher may continue to receive guidance from the I&RS committee or they may be referred to the 504 committee to determine their need for a plan to assist them.

Some tips to keep in mind when thinking about special education and related services:

- FAPE requires that students with a disability qualify in one of the specific categories detailed in the law.
- IDEA requires that the Child Study Team develop an IEP based on the student's demonstrated/measured need. It also requires parental notice and consent for evaluations and implementation of the IEP. The law provides parents with the right to consent or decline evaluations and services.
- Although a student may not meet the stringent requirements under the special education laws, they may meet the requirements for a "504 plan." Section 504 is a part of the Rehabilitation Act of 1973 (U.S. Department of Labor, n.d.), which requires schools to provide appropriate, reasonable adaptations and accommodations to eligible students with a disability. In short, it is a civil rights law to prevent discrimination by institutions who receive public funds.
- Section 504 requires schools to inform parents about how they intend to accommodate students with a disability. In short, it requires the school district to level the playing field for those students (and staff members) with a disability. This may be as simple as additional time for a student

with documented issues with attention, or use of an elevator for a student in a wheelchair.

■   When comparing IDEA and Section 504, the evaluations for the former tend to be more comprehensive because those students' needs tend to be more complex. Generally speaking, a 504 plan is the most appropriate when a student has a documented disability that does not directly interfere with their ability to learn.

See Table 20.1 for a comparison of 504 Plans and IEP.

TABLE 20.1 504 PLAN AND IEP COMPARISON

504	IEP
Broad Civil Rights Law which protects the rights of the handicapped in programs that receive financial assistance. Identifies children with a physical or mental impairment which substantially limits a major life activity. The student must be permitted "equal access," not individualization. There is no requirement to re-evaluate though it is always in the student's best interest to do so. Requires notice only before a significant change in placement.	Federally funded statute, the purpose of which is to provide financial aid to states. Identifies all school-aged children who fall within one or more specific categories of qualifying conditions. The IEP is a plan developed for the individual student specific to the child's needs. Parents must be given written notice prior to any change in placement.
Discrimination is not permitted because of any disability.	Students are protected with behavioral issues by requiring schools to perform a functional behavior assessment and develop a positive behavioral support plan to teach appropriate behavior.
The issue is handled in a similar fashion.	Discipline is dealt with on an individual basis. It must be determined if the behavior is related to the disability.
No required re-evaluation but should be evaluated annually and goals reassessed and changed as needed.	Re-evaluation is conducted every 3 years and sooner when requested by parent/teacher request.
Parents are free to file a complaint with the Office of Civil Rights. The school then appoints a neutral party to intervene.	Parents are entitled to dispute the placement or evaluation of the student and may have a hearing. This is to be a neutral state-appointed officer.
Prior notice is not required.	Parents must receive 10 days notice before any changes in educational placement can be made.

504, section 504; IEP, Individualized Education Plan.
SOURCE: Data from MetroKids. (n.d.). IEP vs. 504: What's the difference? Retrieved from http://www
.metrokids.com/MetroKids/November-2012/IEP-vs-504-Whats-the-difference/

The School Nurse's Role

As a key team member, the school nurse provides an array of information about the health of the student, their daily habits and medical issues, their family support system, and a broader understanding of the school system/school building. As each school building has an internal, systemic climate, the school nurse's knowledge and insight can be an essential key in the effectiveness of any plan.

Some key thoughts:

- The school nurse's knowledge of the student's medical history (including but not limited to Vision and Hearing screenings) is key to understanding the student's personal history and potential issues—whether I&RS, CST, or Section 504 Committee planning.

- The school nurse has a strong working knowledge of the day-to-day building and classroom routines, which can be helpful when developing effective interventions.

- The school nurse's observational skills and knowledge of child development provide a wealth of information needed for decisions throughout the process.

- The school nurse's willingness to serve as a liaison to support families can greatly reduce anxiety and stress.

- The school nurse can help to create a climate of acceptance of the special education students within the school building and among other students.

- Although not a member of the Child Study Team, the school nurse's insight, knowledge, and contributions as part of each process is invaluable.

References

IDEA. (n.d.). *IDEA-related acronyms, abbreviations, and terms.* Retrieved from https://sites.ed.gov/idea/acronyms/#A

MetroKids. (n.d.). *IEP vs. 504: What's the difference?* Retrieved from http://www.metrokids.com/MetroKids/November-2012/IEP-vs-504-Whats-the-difference/

New Jersey Administrative Code. (n.d.). *N.J.A.C. 6A:14, special education.* Retrieved from https://www.state.nj.us/education/code/current/title6a/chap14.pdf

State of New Jersey–Department of Education. (2020). *List of state-imposed special education rules, regulations, or policies in accordance with 20 U.S.C. §1407(a).* Retrieved from https://www.nj.gov/education/specialed/rules.pdf

U.S. Department of Education. (1999). *Free appropriate public education for students with disabilities: Requirements under Section 504 of the Rehabilitation Act of 1973.* Retrieved from https://www2.ed.gov/about/offices/list/ocr/docs/edlite-FAPE504.html

U.S. Department of Labor. (n.d.). *Section 504, Rehabilitation Act of 1973.* Retrieved from https://www.dol.gov/agencies/oasam/civil-rights-center/statutes/section-504-rehabilitation-act-of-1973

VIOLENCE TOWARD SELF AND OTHERS

DAPHNE JOSLIN

LEARNING OBJECTIVES

- Identify the major types of violence affecting children and adolescents at home, in schools, in institutions, and communities.
- Recognize risk factors associated with children being a victim of and/or committing violent acts.
- Identify physical and mental health effects, academic and behavioral consequences of violence victimization.
- Apply a public health framework to consider primary, secondary, and tertiary prevention efforts.
- Propose initiatives to prevent/reduce violence affecting children and adolescents in schools and communities.

■ Introduction

Interpersonal violence toward and by children and adolescents occurs at home, in school, and in public spaces—playgrounds, streets, concerts. Disproportionately, the assailant is a relative, close friend, or date. Physical, sexual, and emotional abuse of children is committed most often by a family member, but also by caregivers, coaches, physicians, even clergy. Current or former students, not strangers, are the typical assailants in school shootings. Community violence often results from gang retaliation that targets individuals but also kills or injures children in playgrounds or even in their homes. Hate crimes traumatize vulnerable children and teens targeted because of religion, ethnicity, color, sexual orientation, immigrant status. Violent interactions between police and communities of color result not only in deaths and injuries but also trauma, especially among African American boys and their families. The increasing number of suicidal attempts and deaths among children and teens is alarming. Violence-related posttraumatic stress disorder (PTSD) affects not only physical and mental health but also academic progress and behavior. In this chapter, school nurses will recognize how they are pivotal in promoting initiatives to prevent child violence toward themselves and others, creating interventions for healing, and in helping school staff to recognize the impact of PTSD and on learning and behavior.

A 9-year-old girl commits suicide because of racist bullying. An 8-year-old boy sees his baby sister killed as bullets fly through an open window, a result of a gang shooting. A transgender teen takes their life after family and church rejection. A 13-year-old girl intentionally cuts herself out of loneliness and self-hatred. An 11-year old boy comes to school without proper clothes for cold weather, with bruises on his face that he refuses to identify.

Scope of Violent Behavior

Stories of physical, emotional and sexual violence toward children and adolescents shock us with graphic details of deaths, injuries, physical and emotional pain, trauma, and loss. In the wake of school shootings, schools themselves have become places of danger. In examining factors that contribute to being a victim or assailant and identifying victimization symptoms and consequences, this chapter offers school nurses the opportunity to move beyond a sense of horror and helplessness that many feel in the wake of such violence.

In the World Report on Violence and Health, the World Health Organization (WHO) defines violence as "the intentional use of physical force or power, threatened or actual, against oneself, another person, or against a group or community, that either results in or has a high likelihood of resulting in injury, death, psychological harm, maldevelopment or deprivation" (WHO as cited by Krug, Dahlberg, & Mercy, 2002, p. 5). This definition distinguishes injuries, deaths, and trauma that result from unintended events such as accidents and natural disasters from those resulting from an individual or group's threatened or actual use of force or power. Whether an act is seen as violent is variable, depending upon cultural norms and legal definitions that may legitimize intentional acts such as police use of lethal force (Alvarez & Bachman, 2017), disciplining children, or forced sexual relations upon wives by their husbands. School nurses identifying violence-based injuries and psychological trauma may encounter parents, community members, and even school staff who differ in their views of what constitutes violence.

Underlying causes of aggression and violent acts are studied with the hope of uncovering the causes of intentional harm to another human being. This wealth of research has examined factors such as serotonin and testosterone levels, brain injuries, personality disorders, stress related to economic deprivation, social learning, societal alienation and dislocation, and the effects of media and social media (see Alvarez & Bachman, 2017). Because the research is inconclusive regarding one explanatory factor, practitioners who develop programs to prevent violence draw upon multidimensional frameworks.

Rather than a criminal justice approach to violence, as a multidisciplinary field committed to program and policy initiatives to reduce the risk of being either a victim or perpetrator of interpersonal violence, public health offers conceptual frameworks and successful evidence-based models that school nurses might adopt or propose to school colleagues, administrators, and community partners. Two frameworks are discussed here with a third offered later in the chapter.

Public Health Frameworks and Evidence

Public health considers three levels of prevention: Primary, secondary, and tertiary. Primary prevention strategies seek to prevent exposure to risk factors that contribute to disease, injuries, and death. Storing unloaded guns at home in a locked cabinet so that children and teens cannot use them is an example of primary prevention of accidental and intentional gun-related injuries and deaths. Educating teens about the dangers of drug and alcohol consumption as they relate to being a victim or perpetrator of sexual assault/rape is another. Advocating reduction or elimination of graphic acts of violence in the media is a primary prevention policy approach.

Secondary prevention strategies address the risk of an individual engaging in or being a victim of violent behavior because of predisposing factors. For example, parents who were abused as children have a greater likelihood of abusing their own children. Effective programs screen new parents and provide comprehensive services to reduce the likelihood of them hurting their children. Secondary prevention also includes efforts to screen potential victims of violence so that the risk of violence is interrupted and emotional trauma addressed. A secondary prevention program implemented at Children's Hospital of Philadelphia screens young emergency department violence victims to reduce reinjury and retaliation (Children's Hospital of Philadelphia, n.d.).

Tertiary prevention seeks to minimize the effects of disease, injury, and trauma so that the quality of an individual's life can be maximized. Assisting survivors of domestic violence to have financial self-sufficiency and avoid potentially violence relationships is an example. Batterer intervention programs attempt to resocialize men who are violent toward their domestic partners by giving them skills, values, and norms that build nonviolent relationships (Alvarez & Bachman, 2017).

The Social Ecological Model (Figure 21.1) also uses systematically gathered data to design public health interventions that recognize the dynamic interplay of contributing factors. The model encourages practitioners to understand how these sets of factors impact one another and to develop interventions that address the interplay (Centers for Disease Control and Prevention [CDC], 2020). The CDC's website describes four levels of intervention: individual, relationship, community, and societal. An expanded ecological approach used by the American College Health Association (2018) refines the social ecological model by including an institution or organization level. Consistent with the CDC model, the levels include: *Intrapersonal or individual* which includes biological or personal history factors including attitudes, beliefs, knowledge, behavior, age, education, history of abuse; *relationship or interpersonal* focuses on family members, peers and other informal social networks; *institutions or organizations* such as schools, neighborhood organizations, religious institutions, military, workplaces; *community* includes characteristics in a geographical area such

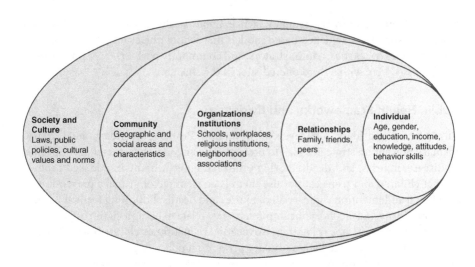

FIGURE 21.1 Social ecological model.

as unemployment levels, public green spaces, local drug trade, population density, lack of community organizations; *societal and public policy* focuses on laws and policies as well as broad cultural norms governing behavior.

Using these two models, public health practitioners are guided in designing and evaluating programs and interventions by data collected by a variety of organizations, including the CDC the National Incident-Based Reporting System, the Federal Bureau of Investigation, the National Intimate Partner and Sexual Violence Survey, the U.S. Bureau of Justice, the National Justice Center, the U.S. Bureau of Labor Statistics, local and state agencies, and research centers, such as the University of California at Davis Violence Prevention Research program and the University of Chicago Center for Youth Violence Prevention. These resources are listed at the end of the chapter.

Child Abuse

Child abuse includes four types of harm:

■ **Physical abuse:** The "intentional use of physical force that can result in physical deaths and injuries. Examples include hitting, kicking, shaking, burning, shoving, or other shows of force against a child" (CDC, 2018a). Resulting harm includes death or physical injuries, including broken bones, cuts, bruises, burns, scalds.

■ **Sexual abuse:** "… pressuring or forcing a child to engage in sexual acts. It includes behaviors such as fondling, penetration, and exposing a child to other sexual activities" (CDC, 2018a). This includes sexual exploitation and sex trafficking.

■ **Neglect:** "… failure to meet a child's basic physical and emotional needs," including housing, food, clothing, education, and access to medical care (CDC, 2018a).

■ **Emotional Abuse:** Physically invisible, emotional abuse refers to "behaviors that harm a child's self-worth or emotional well-being. Examples include name calling, shaming, rejection, withholding love, and threatening" (CDC, 2018a).

Children may suffer from one or more types of abuse.

The statistics presented here are based on data collected by child protective services agencies and reported to the National Child Abuse and Neglect Data System (NCANDS). Child abuse is underreported because of children's fear, inability to verbalize, or even the normalization of abuse within families. Significantly, the highest percentage of reported referrals to Child Protective Services were from educational professionals (19%) followed by law enforcement (18%), social services (12%), medical professionals (10%), mental health providers (6%), day care providers (<1%, with nonprofessionals—relatives, neighbors and friends making 17% of referrals (U.S. Department of Health and Human Services [DHHS], 2019).

The very young are the most vulnerable, with children under 1 year having the highest percentage of reported referrals for abuse. Girls have a slightly higher rate of victimization. Children with developmental delays, behavioral and emotional issues, and medical conditions face higher risk of abuse. Also vulnerable are children whose parents abuse alcohol and/or drugs, and/or are themselves in abusive relationships, or have financial difficulties. Neglect including medical neglect (63%) and physical abuse (11%) are the most prevalent types of reported single abuse, followed by sexual abuse (7%) and psychological or emotional abuse (2%). The most prevalent combination is neglect and physical abuse, both being more easily identified and thus reported (DHHS, 2019).

Parents are most likely to be the reported abusers (78%), followed by other relatives (6%), foster care (4%), legal guardians (4%), unmarried partner of parent (2%), and friends/neighbors (1%). Mothers are as likely to be physically abusive as fathers (CDC, 2019).

Domestic violence toward a parent but not the child increases the risk of children's physical abuse and neglect and also impaired psychological development. A comprehensive review of the literature by Holt, Buckley, and Whelan (2008) suggests multiple affected areas, including behavioral, aggression toward others, depression, anxiety, and being a victim of bullying. Notably, children may also display somatic symptoms.

Schools are prime locations for teachers and other personnel to identify the impact of child abuse. Attention, memory, and cognitive deficits may occur, along with PTSD symptoms, impaired social-emotional skills, behavioral problems, depression, and anxiety (DHHS, 2019). The National Association of School Nurses (NASN) underscores the vital role of school nurses. "School nurses can be involved in prevention, early identification, reporting, and treatment related to child maltreatment because of their opportunity to interact with children daily. School nurses are professionally and ethically accountable to do the following:

- Know local laws, regulations, policies, and procedures for reporting child maltreatment.
- Know the signs and potential indicators of child maltreatment including sexual exploitation.
- Provide clear nursing documentation that includes questions asked and answers given and use a body diagram when appropriate for suspected child maltreatment and sexual exploitation.
- Provide students with personal body safety education and advocate for school health education policies that include personal body safety.
- Educate and support staff regarding the signs and symptoms of child maltreatment.
- Identify students with frequent somatic complaints which may be indicators of maltreatment.
- Provide support to victims of child maltreatment.
- Facilitate the linkage of victims and families to community resources, including a medical home.
- Collaborate with community organizations to raise awareness and reduce the incidence of child abuse and neglect." (NASN, 2018a)

Rape and Sexual Violence

Shocking revelations of child rape and sexual abuse by Roman Catholic priests and by trusted coaches shattered the myth of stranger-perpetrated sexual assault of minors. The latter occur, but the majority of sexual assault and rape cases are perpetrated by family members, trusted friends, neighbors, and other adults. According to the Administration for Children and Families, 674,000 children were victims of abuse or neglect nationwide during 2017, with 8.6% being raped or sexually abused (DHHS, 2019).

The government report titled Child Maltreatment 2012 estimates the overall prevalence of sexual abuse to be about 9.3% (DHHS, 2012). Of the approximately 63,000 victims of sexual abuse reported in the United States in 2012, 2.6% were ages 2 and younger, 14% were 3 to 5 years old, and 17.2% were 6 to 8 years old. Sexual abuse was most prevalent among older children and adolescents: 18.4% were 9 to 11 years old, 26.3% were 12 to 14 years old, and 20.9% were 15 to 17 years old. Because of the shame, stigma, and denial among victims and their families, experts believe that most child sexual abuse is unreported and that the actual number of sexually abused children is not known.

To estimate the prevalence of sexual abuse and sexual assault by the age of 17, Finkelhor, Turner, Shattuck, and Hamby (2015) used three national U.S. telephone surveys (pooled sample of 2,293 15- to17-year-olds). The lifetime experience of sexual abuse and sexual assault was 26.6% for girls and 5.1% for boys, with 11.2% of females and 1.9% for males being abused/assaulted only by adults. The National Center for Victims of Crimes (2018) states that one in 20 boys and one in five girls are victims of sexual abuse, with children between the ages of 7 and 13 being the most vulnerable.

Being female, living in rural areas, and/or those with high poverty and unemployment, foster care, and with a parent's live-in partner are particular risk factors (Briere & Elliot, 2003).

A review of the research by Collin-Vézina, Daigneault, and Hébert (2013) found that children who had been sexually abused had more mental health symptoms and behavioral issues than those who had experienced other types of trauma. These include anxiety, depression, suicide ideation and attempts, alcohol and drug abuse, high risk sexual behavior, PTSD, eating and dissociative disorders, and pregnancy.

School nurses can educate teachers about potential indicators of sexual abuse that teachers may observe in the classroom. These include not only touching genital areas, complaining of genital irritation, and trouble sitting, but also age inappropriate sexual knowledge, interest, and sexually acting out (Briere & Elliott 2003; Collin-Vézina et al., 2013).

Sex Trafficking

According to the U.S. Department of Justice and the National Center for Missing and Exploited Children, it is estimated that 100,000 to 300,000 children are forced to provide sex to others each year in the United States (U.S. Department of Homeland Security, n.d.). Child neglect, maltreatment, and abuse increase the risk of sexual exploitation or trafficking (Clayton, Krugman, & Simon, 2013) as do developmental delays and learning disabilities. Because of feelings of rejection and alienation, lesbian, gay, bisexual, transgender, or questioning (LGBTQ) youths are more likely than heterosexual youths to be victims of trafficking. Family members and peers may promote sexual exploitation.

Frequent truancy or absences, signs of physical abuse and neglect, nervousness, excessive amounts of cash, inconsistent explanation of events can be sign of a child's sexual exploitation (Children's Hospital of Philadelphia, n.d.). The National Center for Safe Supportive Learning Environments also reports "hunger, malnourishment, or inappropriate dress for the weather, signs of drug addiction, coached or rehearsed responses to questions, a sudden change in attire, behavior, relationships, or material possessions (e.g., expensive items), a 'boyfriend' or 'girlfriend' who is noticeably older and/or controlling, an attempt to conceal scars, tattoos, or bruises" (National Center for Safe Supportive Learning Environments, n.d.).

Dating Violence

Abusive behaviors occur in millions of adolescent dating relationships. These behaviors include physical violence (hitting, kicking, punching, or threats of violence), forced or attempted forced sexual acts, "sexting" (posting sexual pictures online), and stalking (a pattern of unwanted attention and contact that causes fear) and psychological abuse that harms or exerts control; CDC, 2019b).

Among teens who dated or went out with someone in the prior year, 8% reported being a victim of physical violence and nearly 7% a victim of sexual dating violence.

Physical abuse included being pushed, hit, bitten, scratched, choked, or injured with an object or weapon, with varying degrees of seriousness (Foshee, Bauman, Fletcher, Rice, & Wilcher, 2007). Being socially humiliated, berated, cursed at, threatened with physical violence, threatened as responsible for the person's suicide are forms of psychological violence (Draucker & Martsolf, 2010).

Females were significantly more likely to be victims of physical abuse (9%) than were males (7%). While there were no significant differences in the percentage of Hispanic and White students who experienced dating violence, African American students (10%) were more likely to be victims than White (7%) or Hispanic students (7.6%; CDC, 2018c).

Among the identified risk factors for teen dating violence are traditional beliefs about gender roles, physical child abuse (Foshee, Benefield, Ennett, Bauman, & Suchindran, 2004), and witnessing parental violence (Foshee et al., 2004, 2007). Having friends in violent dating relationships also increases the risk of abuse (Arriaga & Foshee, 2004).

In addition to injuries, unwanted pregnancy, and STIs, dating violence is also associated with using tobacco, alcohol and drugs, unsafe sex, suicide attempts, depression, and anxiety. Dating violence during adolescence can also be a precursor to intimate partner violence during adulthood (Wolfe, Crooks, Jaffee et al., 2009).

Adolescents do not always recognize that some behaviors, like name calling or controlling forms of jealousy can be patterns of abusive and potentially violent behavior. Teens may also be afraid to tell friends, family, or teachers (CDC, 2019b).

Educational programs can help to support teens in developing nonviolent, healthy relationships. The CDC program *Dating Matters: Strategies to Promote Healthy Teen Relationships* offers skill-based curricula for students, peers, families, schools, and neighborhoods to foster healthy relationships for preteens 11 to 14 years old (CDC, 2018b).

Hate Crimes

The Office of Justice Programs Bureau of Justice Statistics cites The Hate Crime Statistics Act (28 U.S.C. § 534) that defines a hate crime as "crimes that manifest evidence of prejudice based on race, gender or gender identity, religion, disability, sexual orientation, or ethnicity" (Office of Justice Programs, n.d.). According to the Bureau of Justice, about 54% of hate crimes were not reported to police during 2011 to 2015 (Masucci & Langton, 2017). With under-reporting, analysis of the 7,106 single-bias (only one type of bias) incidents reported in 2017, 58.1% were motivated by a race /ethnicity/ancestry bias, 22.0% by religious bias, 15.9% by sexual-orientation bias, 1.7% by gender-identity bias, 1.6% disability bias, and 0.6% by gender bias. Of the 5,803 victims in 2017 whose age was reported 12% ($n = 678$) were juveniles (U.S. Department of Justice: FBI, 2018b). Youth are also perpetrators of hate crimes. According to the FBI, U.S. Department of Justice, 2017 Hate Crime Statistics, 17% of perpetrators were 18 years old or younger whose victim(s) may be children, adolescents or adults.

Hate crimes directed toward children or school personnel occur in elementary, middle, and high schools. Of the 340 hate crimes at elementary, middle, or high schools reported to the FBI in 2017, 61% were biased against the victim's race or ethnicity, 20% religion, 12% sexual orientation, 7% gender identity, 2% disability, 7% multiple bias, and less that 1% against gender (U.S. Department of Justice: FBI, 2018a). Although victims or perpetrators may not always be juveniles, hate crimes that occur in playgrounds and parks reflect attitudes and norms in the larger community that contribute to hate crimes by and against children and teens and out of school.

Prejudiced-motivated harassment does not, in itself, constitute a hate crime. However, bias incidents of verbal, written slurs, symbols, or graffiti may reflect or can foster the cultural climate of a school or community where hate crimes occur. In a Southern Poverty Law Center survey of elementary, middle, and high schools, two thirds of the 2,776 K–12 teacher educators who responded to the questionnaire witnessed a hate or bias incident in their school during the fall of 2018, a total of 3,265 hate incidents. In the vast majority of cases there was no discipline of the offender. Reaffirming inclusive values, providing professional staff development, communicating with families, issuing public statements condemning the acts, and supporting marginalized students and staff were actions taken to repair the harm (Costello & Dillard, 2019).

School Violence

Violent acts in schools, on school grounds, or in transit to and from school are directed at students, teachers, and staff. While it is often suggested that the media have sensationalized school violence, school administrators and teachers perceive that violence in schools has increased significantly in the past two decades (Wynne & Joo, 2011). School safety data are published annually in *Indicators of School Crime and Safety* (National Center for Education Statistics, 2019*)*. In 2017, about 16% of students in grades 9 to 12 reported that they had carried a weapon such as a gun, knife, or club anywhere at least 1 day during the previous 30 days, and 4% reported carrying a weapon on school property at least 1 day during the previous 30 days (Musu, Zhang, Wang, Zhang, & Oudekerk, 2019). According to the U.S. Department of Education in 2013, 7% of students in grades 9 to 12 in 2011 reported a threat or injury with a weapon, such as a gun, knife, or club, on school property (King, 2014).

The most recent data on school-associated deaths released by the CDC School-Associated Violent Death Surveillance System (SAVD-SS) report a total of 38 students, staff, and other nonstudent school-associated violent deaths (30 homicides, 7 suicides, and 1 legal intervention) between July 1, 2015 and June 30, 2016. Analysis of single and multiple victim homicides occurring on school grounds or in transit found that multiple victim homicide rates "increased significantly from July 2009 to June 2018" while single victim rates were stable during that time period (CDC, 2019a).

School-based violence also includes simple assault and serious violence crimes of rape, sexual assault, robbery, and aggravated assault/assault with a weapon (Musu et al., 2019). In the Youth Risk Behavior Survey (YRBS), students in grades 9 to 12 were asked about their involvement in physical fights, in general and on school property. The percentage of students in grades 9 to 12 who reported having been in a physical fight anywhere decreased from 33% to 24% between 2001 and 2017 and those who reported having been in a physical fight on school property also decreased from 13% to 9%. A higher percentage of male students (30%) than female students (17%) in grades 9 to 12 reported having been in a physical fight anywhere during the previous 12 months. Twelve percent of male students, compared with percent of female students reported having been in a physical fight on school property (Musu et al., 2019). Strawhacker (2002) reported on Jackson and Foshee's (1998) research that found that as parents' lack of concern, monitoring, and responsiveness to children declined, there was a greater risk of 9th and 10th graders engaging in physical fights, carrying a weapon, or threatening another student with a weapon.

Teachers are subject to threats and physical attacks by students. According to a national survey, during the 2015–2016 school year, 10% of public school teachers reported being threatened with injury; 6% reported having been physically attacked by a student from their school. A greater percentage of elementary school teachers than of secondary school teachers reported being threatened (11% vs. 9%) or being physically attacked (9% vs. 2%). A higher percentage of female public school teachers were physically attacked than were males (6% vs. 4%) although there were no gender differences in threats of injury (10%). Twelve percent of Black public school teachers reported being threatened, compared with 10% of White and 8% of Hispanic teachers (Musu et al., 2019).

Tragically, school staff vocabulary now includes "active shooter," a term used to identify the threat of "an individual actively engaged in killing or attempting to kill people in a confined and populated area" (U.S. Department of Homeland Security, 2017). According National Center for Education Statistics, "From 2000 to 2017, there were 37 active shooter incidents at elementary and secondary schools and 15 active shooter incidents at postsecondary institutions" (U.S. Department of Education, 2018). "Mass shootings" defines a mass casualty event where more than three or four individuals are killed (U.S. Department of Justice: Office of Victims of Crime, n.d.).

Analyzing conditions that contributed to averted school shootings, Daniels found that most school attacks were averted because students report concerns regarding another student's threat, behavior, or plot (Daniels, 2019). Plotter's parents or parents of other students were also key in alerting authorities. These findings are relevant to the role of school nurses in creating a culture of alert response by students, faculty, families, and the community. Daniels calls for a school culture where students are treated with respect by school staff and learn to treat one another in the same manner to reduce bullying and isolation and to encourage communication.

Langman cautions against a stereotypical view of school shooters that casts them as having been bullied and being socially isolated. As an expert who is called upon by local police and the FBI, Langman identifies a range of personality factors of school shooters and recommends threat assessment teams include mental health experts and psychologists (Martin, 2017). Peterson and Densley, who have studied every mass school shooting since 1966, argue that a precipitating personal crisis and suicidal ideation are common among school shooters, as are childhood trauma and exposure to violence early in life that contribute to thought disorders, suicidality, depression, and anxiety (Peterson & Densley, 2019).

Proactive violence prevention starts with schools, colleges, faith-based communities, and employers initiating conversations about mental health and establishing systems for identifying individuals in crisis, reporting concerns and reaching out, not with punitive measures but with accessible, affordable social services, mental health resources and long-term intervention for those with trauma-related histories of abuse, depression, and anxiety. Wellness programs in schools and the workplace that teach resilience and social-emotional skills as well as policies and practices that decrease the stigma around mental illness are needed (Petersen & Densley, 2019).

The unique position of school nurses enables them to prevent and respond to school-based violence by virtue of their ability to identify subtle symptoms of trauma that often underlie violent reactions. King (2014) proposes that because of "their nondisciplinary and nonacademic role" they may learn of weapons brought to school, situations of escalating violence, and planned or intentional violent behaviors in reaction to peer, academic or family-related issues. Nurses have the potential to "develop a therapeutic relationship" (King, 2014, p. 4) to prevent violent episodes through assessment and appropriate referrals. In addition, the NASN proposes that the school nurse's office can be a safe space where conflicts can be prevented from escalating and where school nurses can assist students in developing skills such as anger management and problem-solving as strategies to prevent violent situations. School nurses can participate in crisis management teams and help to support the development of curricula and evidenced-based programs that are effective in preventing and reducing violence in children and adolescents (NASN, 2012). King also proposed that school nurses work to create a culture of nonviolence, nonbullying, and gun safety through school-community partnerships and activities (King, 2014). As health educators, they may also be able to approach the issue of gun safety from the perspective of harm reduction without threatening the charged issue of gun rights. School nurses are able to support the efforts of administration to provide and maintain security; to offer programs to parents that support building skills in the areas of communication, problem-solving, and monitoring of their children; and assist in the development of district and school discipline policy or code of conduct documents. School nurses are able to serve on school safety and curriculum committees, identifying, advocating and implementing prevention programs within the school community (NASN, 2012).

Selekman and Melvin (2017) recommend that the school nurse be a part of the safety or crisis team whose mandate should be to develop a safety plan, update it, and initiate practice drills. In addition, school nurses can help teachers and other staff to recognize the need for an evaluation if a student is being bullied, abused, or is a loner, as well as a student's fascination with guns and violent images. Both FERPA (Family Educational Rights and Privacy Act) HIPAA (Health Insurance Portability and Accountability Act) have exceptions—an actual, impending, or imminent emergency—that allow disclosures if someone—student or staff—presents a danger themselves where there is a written or audible threat. Information can be shared with law enforcement without parental consent.

Community Violence

Many children and teens living in communities with a high volume of street crime and gang violence have witnessed homicides and violent assaults in their neighborhoods; many have had family members or friends killed by random bullets or gang retaliation in playgrounds or at home. Witnessing or being aware of violence in their communities robs them of a sense of safety and protection that other children and their families take for granted. Elementary and middle school students in two urban communities that had a high volume of homicides, rapes, assault, robbery, and gang violence were very fearful about being bullied, assaulted, robbed, attacked by dogs, sexually harassed or assaulted, or kidnapped as they traveled to and from school (Meyer & Astor, 2002). These findings are consistent with other studies of children who have witnessed violence in their communities or have had family members, friends, or neighbors who have been victims.

Researchers studying the effects of exposure to "prolonged and intense neighborhood violence" in a northeastern city state that "... violence and level of danger does not stop at the school door but is carried into the building.... Childhood exposure to violence increases reactivity and worsens impulse control, both of which contribute to the perpetuation of aggression, violence and retaliatory behavior" (Lane, Rubenstein, Bergen-Cico, Jennings-Bet, & Fish, 2017). Children, their families and even school staff experience traumatic stress and PTSD. Emotional numbing in response to trauma may also increase the risk of aggressive behavior.

Homicide is the leading cause of death for African Americans ages 15 to 24 and 25 to 43 and the second leading cause of death among 1 to 4 year olds and 10 to 14 year olds, making traumatic loss a mental health issue in urban communities of color. Parental incarceration and negative interactions with police compound the traumatic-based grief experienced by Black and Latinx children and teens, grief that is unhealed, often displaced and misunderstood when it manifests in behavior and academic problems (Dutil, 2019). Dutil urges school-based therapeutic services, given the absence of sufficient services in the community. While these would typically be the domain of social workers and counselors, school nurses can provide culturally sensitive and supportive trauma-informed professional attention for students and improve awareness by teaching and other staff.

Gangs

Although gang presence in schools has been decreasing since the 1990s, with 12% of students reporting gangs in their schools in 2013, down from an estimate of 28% in 1995, gangs continue to threaten safety and disrupt learning and healthy peer interaction (Carson & Esbensen, 2017; Zhang, Musu-Gillette, & Oudekerk, 2016); increase substance use and drug sales (Decker & Van Winkle, 1996); increase fear of school-based crime (Bachman, Randolph, & Brown, 2011); increase physical, verbal, and cyber bullying and fighting and violent victimization (Kupchik & Farina, 2016). They also foster a culture of "retaliatory violence" that other students who are not gang members may imitate as a way of solving conflicts (King reports on Melde & Esbensen, 2013). In a 2010 study, periods of active gang membership were associated with a 10% to 21% increase in the odds of involvement in violent incidents (King, 2014).

School nurses can reach out to gang violence prevention programs, like Cure Violence also known as Ceasefire in Chicago or Safe Streets in Baltimore and New York City that aim to reduce retaliatory violence in communities, using former gang members as outreach workers. The Gang Resistance Education and Training (GREAT) Program is a school-based, gang violence prevention curriculum for middle school students that teaches social and self-management skills.

Violence Toward Oneself

Intentional acts of violence toward oneself include nonfatal self-injury and suicide. Dramatic increases in both, notably among preteens as well as teens, underscore the need for school-based and community interventions.

Nonsuicidal Self-Harm

Self-harm includes burning, cutting, poisoning, and other injuries. While it is not usually fatal, those who self-harm are at higher risk of suicide (American Academy of Pediatrics, 2018). Olfson et al. (2018) report that self-harm rates among "females ages 10 to 24 nearly doubled from 2009 to 2015 while for males rates increased at a slower pace" (p. 1). Fifteen percent of students self-harm, with a higher prevalence among girls (20%) than boys (9%; Monto, McRee, & Deryck, 2018).

Laye-Gindu and Schonert-Reichl (2005) found that the intent to injure oneself but not end one's life was motivated by self-hatred and anger, a need to manage one's emotions (e.g., anxiety, depression, or stress), self-punishment, cope with feelings of alienation and loneliness, and as a distraction. Boys also self-harm out of boredom, and in the company of others as a game or "test of will." Girls are more likely to self-harm out of despair and in isolation.

In recommending that professionals screen for self-harm and suicidal intent, Petersen, Freedenthal, Sheldon, and Andersen (2008) urge a "therapeutic alliance" without judgment of the behavior as "attention grabbing," and offering positive coping skills and problem-solving (Laye-Gindu & Schonert-Reichl, 2005). Given the rising prevalence of self-injury and the overlap between it and suicide (25% of those who self-harm reported a prior suicide attempt), regular screening for self-injury is needed as is suicide risk and unhealthy behaviors (e.g., alcohol and drug use) among those who self-harm (Laye-Gindu & Schonert-Reichl, 2005).

Suicide

Suicide was the second leading cause of death among 10 to 14 year olds and 15 to 24 years olds in 2017. According to the CDC, "the suicide rate among 11 to 14 [year olds] has doubled since its decade low in 2007, from 1.6 to 3.2 deaths per 100,000 population" (CDC, 2019d).

Especially disturbing is the increase of children ages 5 to 12 who consider or attempt suicide (Burstein, Agostino, & Greenfield, 2019). According to the CDC Youth Trends Report (CDC, 2017), suicide risk indicators increased from 2007 to 2017. The proportion of high school students who reported persistent feelings of sadness and hopelessness increased from 28% to 32%. Those who seriously considered suicide rose to 17% in 2017, from 14% in 2007. According to CDC's Youth Risk Behavior Survey

2015 (YRBSS2015), 17% of high school students reported seriously considering suicide in 2017 (females 22%, males 11%), nearly 15% made a plan, and 7% attempted suicide.

Risk Factors

Due to homophobic attitudes and rejection in schools, family, and religion, bullying, threats or acts of violence, and internalized homophobia, LGBTQ youth are at significant risk. According to the 2015 YRBSS, among youth identifying as LGBTQ, 43% seriously considered suicide, 29% attempted suicide one or more times, and 9% made a serious attempt requiring medical intervention (reported in Aranmolate, Bogan, Hoard, & Mawson, 2017).

The increase in suicides among 10 to 14 year olds calls for attention to the risk of preteens and young teens being vulnerable to "all or nothing" solutions to problems because they lack certain emotional and cognitive skills (Stoep, McCauley, Flynn, & Stone, 2009). A convergence of puberty's physical and hormonal changes, parent–child conflict, poor communication, peer relationship issues, bullying victimization and perpetration, school problems, accompanied by alcohol and drug use, a history of self-harm and mental health issues leaves pre- and young teens at risk (Stoep et al., 2009). Feelings of "unimportance, thwarted belongingness, and perceived burdensomeness as a family member" were common in the "premeditative thoughts about suicide" among adolescents who took their lives (Stoep et al., 2009).

The dramatic, persistent increase in suicides by African American youth led the Congressional Black Caucus to convene an Emergency Task Force on Black Youth Suicide and Mental Health, citing the Bridge, Horowitz, Fontanella, and Sheftall (2018) study of racial disparity in youth suicide that reported that suicide rates among Black children aged 5 to 11 years increased between 1993 and 1997 and 2008 and 2012 while they decreased among White children of the same age, and that the rate for Black children ages 5 to 12 is twice as high as that of White children. Yet African American children and teens are consistently less likely than their White peers to be treated for depression. Harsh disciplinary practices toward African American boys compound the risk as acting out and anger being misinterpreted rather than being seen as signs of depression. At the same time, children who are withdrawn are overlooked or neglected, because they are not disruptive (Lindsay, Brown, & Cunningham, 2017).

School nurses can initiate programs to de-stigmatize mental health help-seeking and treatment; to educate teachers, parents and the community about depression, PTSD, anxiety and suicide; and to encourage referrals of students/children/teens for assessment. Because parents can be resistant to facing mental health issues, fearing that it reflects bad parenting or assuming that behavior is the fault of a defiant or lazy child (Lindsay et al., 2017), school nurses can help families, community members, and organizations to understand children's and teens' emotional needs, development, and behavior. Efforts can also be directed to help to enhance parenting skills so that discipline and conflict with children do not contribute to suicidal ideation (Holland, Vivolo-Kantor, Logan, & Leemis, 2017). Stroep et al. recommend suicidal risk screening at developmental moments of high risk, such as school transitions, family loss or disruption, or when communities experience tragedies.

Students can learn to identify suicide risks and warning signs in themselves, friends, and peers and encourage help-seeking. The Signs of Suicide (SOS) program has demonstrated effectiveness among high school students in reducing suicide attempts among teens at risk, increasing knowledge of depression and suicide, and fostering positive attitudes about intervening with friends seeking help for themselves (Schilling, Asselstine, & James, 2016).

School Nurses and Public Health Approaches to Violence Reduction and Prevention

The Position Statement *School Violence, Role of the School Nurse in Prevention* of the NASN states:

> *It is the position of the NASN that registered professional school nurses (hereinafter referred to as school nurses) advance and encourage safe school environments by promoting the prevention and reduction of school violence. School nurses serve on the front line and are readily able to identify potential violence and intervene to diminish the effects of violence on both school children as individuals and populations in schools and the community (King, 2014). School nurses collaborate with school personnel, healthcare providers, parents, and community members to identify and implement evidence-based programs promoting violence prevention. These evidence-based programs promote violence prevention through early intervention, communication, positive behavior management and conflict resolution. As identified in the* Framework for the 21st Century School Nurse Practice™ *(NASN, 2015), the school nurse supports evidence-based practices and care coordination to provide an environment where students can be healthy, safe, and ready to learn." (NASN, 2018b)*

Public health's conceptual frameworks and evidence-based programs are needed to address the intrapersonal and interpersonal violence discussed in this chapter. School nurses are familiar with the model of primary, secondary, and tertiary prevention that can be applied to the attitudes, values, knowledge, and behaviors that contribute to being a perpetrator or victim of violence, and to healing associated trauma. The social-ecological model provides a dynamic context for understanding the interplay of factors that need to be addressed in order to prevent/reduce violent behavior. These two frameworks are complementary and can be programmatically integrated.

The spectrum of prevention framework (Rattray, Brunner, & Freestone, 2002) has been used by used by the Prevention Institute in violence prevention initiatives. Developed to "conceptualize, implement and coordinate ... public health programs" (Rattray et al., 2002, p. 1), the framework uses strategies at six complementary and synergistic levels: influencing policy and legislation, mobilizing communities and neighborhoods, fostering coalitions and networks, changing organizational practices, educating providers, promoting community education, and strengthening individual knowledge and skills. Multi-level interventions with collaboration and coordination across agencies and institutions are necessary to address complex public health problems, like violence. As an example, we can apply the spectrum of prevention to the problem of suicide among African American children to consider strategies at each level.

Influencing policy and legislation: Advocating for new and changed policies and laws could include changing the harsh disciplinary practices against children of color, lobbying local, state and national elected officials to increase funding of community- and school-based mental health/counseling services.

Mobilizing communities and neighborhoods: Outreach to and collaboration with parents, other community residents, and with local organizations are necessary to ensure that initiatives have their support and participation in community forums, speak outs, and other neighborhood-based initiatives on depression, suicide, and seeking mental health services, and to build and support more culturally sensitive police patrols, reducing the fear and hopelessness that African American men and youth feel in relationship to law enforcement.

Fostering coalitions and networks: Building upon community/neighborhood mobilization, partnerships can be created with health departments, social and recreational organizations, local businesses such as hair salons and barbershops, and faith-based institutions to create a network of services and education about mental health and suicide. Community-specific resources and strategies are shared to build advocacy for changed policies and to develop and implement effective programs.

Changing organizational practices: Developing and implementing depression and suicide screening tools for elementary, middle, and high school students and within pediatric practices as well as implementing nonpunitive disciplinary practices for students could help to reduce suicidal ideation and identify at-risk children and teen.

Educating providers: The respect and authority accorded nurses offers the opportunity to educate teachers, administrators, coaches, and other school staff about suicide and depression.

Promoting community education: Similarly, school nurses, working collaboratively with community partners, can develop community events, focus groups, and media campaigns to educate children, teens, parents, family members, and clergy in order to counter denial, lack of information and stigma regarding depression, suicide, mental health services and help-seeking. Peer-lead education is vital.

Strengthening individual knowledge and skills: School nurses can improve teachers' and other school staff's capacity to identify and refer students who are depressed and at suicidal risk, rather than defining them as disciplinary problems. They can also develop programs that teach positive coping and nonviolent conflict resolution skills among students, families, and community members.

Ensuring access to quality care: In collaboration with community partners, professional associations of nurses, social workers, teachers, and school counselors, school nurses can advocate for expansion of mental health services for children and their families.

Conclusion

School nurses have the experience, perspective, and authority to be leaders in initiatives to reduce and prevent violence that affects children and adolescents in school and in their families and communities. They can serve as resources for teachers, administrators, and school staff as well as community members and families who are seeking ways to prevent and respond to violence. Finally, they can offer an informed, compassionate presence in a school where children and teens can find safety, concern, and professional guidance.

■ References

Alvarez, A., & Bachman, A. (2017). *Violence: The enduring problem* (3rd ed.). Los Angeles, CA: SAGE.

American College Health Association. (2018). *Ecological model.* Retrieved from https://www.acha.org/HealthyCampus/HealthyCampus/Ecological_Model.aspx

Aranmolate, R., Bogan, D. R., Howard, T., & Mawson, A. R. (2017). Suicide risk factors among LGBTQ youth: Review. *JSM Schizophrenia, 2*(2), 1011. Retrieved from https://www.jscimedcentral.com/Schizophrenia/schizophrenia-2-1011.pdf

Arriaga, X. B., & Foshee, V. A. (2004). Adolescent dating violence: Do adolescents follow their friends' or their parents' footsteps? *Journal of Interpersonal Violence, 19*(No. 2), 162–184. doi:10.1177/0886260503260247

Bachman, R., Randolph, A., & Brown, B. L. (2011). Predicting perceptions of fear at school and going to and from school for African American and White students: The effects of school security measures. *Youth and Society, 43*(2), 705–711.

Bridge, J. A., Horowitz, L. M., Fontanella, C. A., Sheftall, A. H., Greenhouse, J. Kelleher, K. J., & Campo, J. V. (2018). Age-related racial disparity in suicide rates among U.S. youths from 2001 through 2015. *JAMA Pediatrics, 172*(7), 697–699. doi:10.1001/jamapediatrics.2018.0399

Briere, J., & Elliot, D. M. (2003). Prevalence and psychological sequelae of self-reported childhood physical and sexual abuse in a general population sample of men and women. *Child Abuse and Neglect, 27*(10), 1205–1222. doi:10.1016/j.chiabu.2003.09.008

Burstein, B., Agostino, H., & Greenfield, B. (2019). Suicidal attempts and ideation among children and adolescents in U.S. emergency departments, 2007-2015. *JAMA Pediatrics, 173*(6), 598–600. doi:10.1001/jamapediatrics.2019.0464

Carson, D. C., & Esbensen, F. (2017). Gangs in school: Exploring the experiences of gang-involved youth. *Youth Violence and Juvenile Justice, 17*(1), 3–23. doi:10.1177/1541204017739678

Centers for Disease Control. (2020). *The social-ecological model: A framework for prevention.* Retrieved from https://www.cdc.gov/violenceprevention/publichealthissue /social-ecologicalmodel.html#:~:text=CDC%20uses%20a%20four%2Dlevel,%2C%20 community%2C%20and%20societal%20factors

Centers for Disease Control and Prevention. (2017). *Youth risk behavior survey 2007–2017.* Retrieved from https://www.cdc.gov/healthyyouth/data/yrbs/pdf/trendsreport.pdf

Centers for Disease Control and Prevention. (2018a). *Child abuse and neglect: Risk and protective factors.* Retrieved from https://www.cdc.gov/violenceprevention/ childabuseandneglect/riskprotectivefactors.html

Centers for Disease Control and Prevention. (2018b). *Dating matters®: Strategies to promote healthy teen relationships.* Retrieved from www.cdc.gov/violenceprevention/ datingmatters

Centers for Disease Control and Prevention. (2018c). *National youth risk behavior survey data summary and trends report, 2007-2017.* Retrieved from https://npin.cdc.gov/ publication/youth-risk-behavior-survey-data-summary-trends-report-2007-2017

Centers for Disease Control and Prevention. (2018d). *Web-based injury statistics query reporting system (WISQARS)* [online]. Retrieved from https://www.cdc.gov/injur/wisqars/index.html

Centers for Disease Control and Prevention. (2019a, October 24). *School-associated violent death study.* Retrieved from https://www.cdc.gov/violenceprevention/youthviolence/schoolviolence/SAVD.html

Centers for Disease Control and Prevention. (2019b). *What is teen dating violence?* Retrieved from https://www.cdc.gov/violenceprevention/intimatepartnerviolence/teendatingviolence/fastfact.html

Children's Hospital of Philadelphia. (2019). *Child sex trafficking.* Retrieved from https://injury.research.chop.edu/violence-prevention-initiative/types-violence-involving-youth/child-sex-trafficking#.XWFvBy2ZNmA

Chiodo, D., Wolfe, D. A., Crooks, C., Hughes, R., & Jaffe, P. (2009). Impact of sexual harassment victimization by peers on subsequent adolescent victimization and adjustment: A longitudinal study. *Journal of Adolescent Health, 45*(3), 245–252. doi:10.1016/j.jadohealth.2009.01.006

Clayton, E. W., Krugman R. D., & Simon, P. (2013), Confronting commercial and sexual exploitation and sex trafficking of minors in the United States. Washington, DC: National Academies Press.

Collin-Vézina D., Daigneault, I., & Hébert, M. (2013). Lessons learned from child sexual abuse research: Prevalence, outcomes, and preventive strategies. *Child and Adolescent Psychiatry and Mental Health, 7*, 22. doi:10.1186/1753-2000-7-22

Costello, M., & Dillard, C. (2019). *Special report: Hate at school.* Montgomery AL: Southern Poverty Law Center.

Daniels, J. (2019). *A preliminary report on the police foundation's averted school violence database (police foundation).* Retrieved from https://schoolshooters.info/sites/default/files/Averted-School-Violence.pdf

Decker, SH & Van Winkle, B. (1996) Life in the Gang: Family, Friends and Violence. New York: Cambridge University Press.

Deckler, S., Deckler, S. H., & Van Winkle, B. (1996). Life in the gang: family, friends and violence. New York: Cambridge University Press.

Draucker, C. B., & Martolf, D. (2010). The role of electronic communication technology in adolescent dating violence. *Journal of Child and Adolescent Psychiatric Nursing, 23*(13), 33–42.

Dutil, S. (2019). Adolescent traumatic and disenfranchised grief: Adapting an evidence-based intervention for Black and Latinx youths in schools. *Children & Schools, 41*(3), 179–187. doi:10.1093/cs/cdz009

Finkelhor, D., Turner, H. A., Shattuck, A., & Hamby, S. L. (2015). Prevalence of childhood exposure to violence, crime, and abuse: Results from the National Survey of Children's Exposure to Violence. *JAMA Pediatrics, 169*(8), 746–754. doi:10.1001/jamapediatrics.2015.0676

Foshee, V. A., Bauman, K. E., Fletcher, L., Rice, J., & Wilcher, R. (2007). Typologies of adolescent dating violence: Identifying typologies of adolescent dating violence perpetration. *Journal of Interpersonal Violence, 22*(5), 498–519. doi:10.1177/0886260506298829

Foshee, V. A., Benefield, T. S., Ennett, S. T., Bauman, K. E., & Suchindran, C. (2004). Longitudinal predictors of serious physical and sexual dating violence victimization during adolescence. *Preventive Medicine, 39* (5), 1007–1016. doi:10.1016/j.ypmed.2004.04.014

Holland, K. M., Vivolo-Kantor, A. M., Logan, J. E., & Leemis, R. W. (2017). Antecedents of suicide among youth aged 11–15: A multistate mixed methods analysis. *Journal of Youth and Adolescence, 46*(7), 1598–1610. doi:10.1007/s10964-016-0610-3

Holt, S., Buckley, D., & Whelan, G. (2008). The impact of exposure to domestic violence on children and young people: A review of the literature. *Child Abuse and Neglect, 32*(8), 797–810. doi:10.1016/j.chiiabu.2008.02.004

Jackson, C., & Vangie, A. F. (1998). Violence-related behaviors of adolescents: Relations with responsive and demanding parenting. *Journal of Adolescent Research, 13*(3), 343–359. doi:10.1177/0743554898133006

King, K. K. (2014). Violence in the school setting: A school nurse perspective. *Online Journal of Issues in Nursing, 19*(1), 4. doi:10.3912/OJIN.Vol19No01Man04

Krug, E., Dahlberg, L., & Mercy, J. (2002). *World report on violence and health*. Geneva, Switzerland: World Health Organization.

Kupchik, A., & Farina, K. A. (2016). Imitating authority: Students perceptions of school punishment and security, and bullying victimization. *Youth Violence and Juvenile Justice, 4*, 34–54.

Lane, S. D., Rubinstein, R. A., Bergen-Cico, D., Jennings-Bey, T., & Fish, L. S. (2017). Neighborhood trauma due to violence: A multilevel analysis. *Journal of Health Care for the Poor and Underserved, 28*(1), 446–462. doi:10.1353/hpu.2017.0033

Laye-Gindhu, A., & Schonert-Reichl, K. A. (2005). Nonsuicidal self-harm among community adolescents: Understanding the "whats" and "whys" of self-harm. *Journal of Youth and Adolescence, 34*(5), 447–457. doi:10.1007/s10964-005-7262-z

Lindsay, M., Brown, A., & Cunningham, D. R. (2017). Boys do(n't) cry: Addressing the unmet mental health needs of African American boys. *American Journal of Orthopsychiatry, 87*(4), 377–383. doi:10.1037/ort0000198

Martin, S. (2017). 5 questions for Peter Langman. *American Psychological Association, 48*(10), 33. Retrieved from https://www.apa.org/monitor/2017/11/conversation-langman

Masucci, M., & Langton, L. (2017). *Hate crime victimization, 2004-2015* (NCJ 250653). Washington, DC: U.S. Department of Justice: Office of Justice Programs Bureau of Justice Statistics. Retrieved from https://www.bjs.gov/content/pub/pdf

Melde, C. & Esbensen, F.-A. (2013). Gangs and violence: Disentangling the impact of gang membership on the level and nature of offending. *Journal of Quantitative Criminology, 29*(2), 143–166.

Meyer, H. A., & Astor, R. A. (2002). Child and parent perspectives on routes to and from school in high crime neighborhoods. *Journal of School Violence, 1*(4), 101–128. doi:10.1300/J202v01n04_07

Monto, M. A., McRee, N., & Deryck, F. S. (2018). Nonsuicidal self-injury among a representative sample of U.S. adolescents, 2015. *American Journal of Public Health, 108*(8), 1042–1048. doi:10.2105/AJPH.2018.304470

Musu, L., Zhang, A., Wang, K., Zhang, J., & Oudekerk, B. A. (2019). *Indicators of school crime and safety: 2018* (NCES 2019-047/NCJ 252571). Washington, DC: National Center for Education Statistics, U.S. Department of Education, and Bureau of Justice Statistics, Office of Justice Programs, U.S. Department of Justice. Retrieved from https://nces.ed.gov/programs/crimeindicators/

National Association of School Nurses. (2012). *School violence, role of the school nurse in prevention issue brief*. Retrieved from https://files.eric.ed.gov/fulltext/ED539208.pdf

National Association of School Nurses. (2018a). *Prevention and treatment of child maltreatment—The role of the school nurse* (Position Statement). Retrieved from https://www.nasn.org/advocacy/professional-practice-documents/position-statements/ps-child-maltreatment

National Association of School Nurses. (2018b). *School violence—The role of the school nurse* (Position Statement). Silver Spring, MD: Author. Retrieved from https://www .nasn.org/advocacy/professional-practice-documents/position-statements/ps-violence

National Center for Educational Statistics. (2019). Indicators of school crime and safety: 2018. Washington, DC: US Department of Education, US Department of Justice

National Center for Victims of Crime. (2018). Retrieved from https://members .victimsofcrime.org/media/reporting-on-child-sexual-abuse-statistics

Offenhauer, P. & Buchalter, A. (2011). Teen dating violence: A review and annotated bibliography. Washington, DC: U. S. Department of Justice.

Olfson, M., Wall, M., Wang, S., Crystal, S., Bridge, J. A. Lui S., & Blanco, C. (2018). Suicide after deliberate self-harm in adolescents and young adults. *Pediatrics, 141*(4), e20173517. doi:10.1542/peds.2017-3517

Peterson, J., & Densley, J. (2019). Op-Ed: We have studied every mass shooting since 1966. Here's what we've learned about the shooters. *Los Angeles Times.* Retrieved from https:// www.latimes.com/opinion/story/2019-08-04/el-paso-dayton-gilroy-mass-shooters -data

Petersen, J., Freedenthal, S., Sheldon, C., & Andersen, R. (2008). Nonsuicidal self-injury in adolescents. *Psychiatry, 5*(11), 20–26. Retrieved from https://www.ncbi.nlm.nih.gov/ pubmed/19724714

Polanin, M., & Cooper, R. (2019). *Self-injury is increasing in teenage girls: What can parents do?* Washington, DC: National Center for Health Research. Retrieved from http://www .center4research.org/self-injury-increasing-teenage-girls-can-parents/

Rattray, T., Brunner, W., & Freestone, J. (2002). *The new spectrum of prevention: A model for public health practice.* Martinez, CA: Contra Costa Health Services. Retrieved from https://www.preventioninstitute.org/tools/spectrum-prevention-0

Schilling, E. A., Aseltine, R. H., & James, A. (2016). The SOS suicide prevention program: Further evidence of efficacy and effectiveness. *Prevention Science, 17*(2), 157–166. doi:10.1007/s11121-015-0594-3

Selekman, J., & Melvin, J. (2017). Planning for a violent intruder event: The school nurse's role. *NASN School Nurse, 32*(3), 186–191. doi:10.1177/1942602X16686140

Stoep, A. V., McCauley, E., Flynn, C., & Stone, A. (2009). Thoughts of death and suicide in early adolescence. *Suicide & Life-Threatening Behavior, 39*(6), 599–613. doi:10.1521/ suli.2009.39.6.599

Strawhacker, M. (2002). School violence: An overview. *The Journal of School Nursing, 18*(2), 68–72. doi:10.1177/10598405020180020201

U.S. Department of Education. Institute for Education Sciences. National Center for Education Statistics. (2018). *Indicators of school crime and safety.* Retrieved from https:// nces.ed.gov/programs/crimeindicators/

U.S. Department of Health and Human Services, Administration for Children and Families, Child Welfare Information Gateway. (2012). *Child maltreatment 2012: Summary of key findings.* Washington, DC: Children's Bureau. Retrieved from https://www.acf.hhs.gov/ sites/default/files/cb/cm2012.pdf

U.S. Department of Health and Human Services, Administration for Children and Families, Child Welfare Information Gateway. (2019). *Child maltreatment 2017: Summary of key findings.* Washington, DC: Children's Bureau. Retrieved from https://www.childwelfare .gov/pubs/factsheets/canstats/

U.S. Department of Homeland Security. (2017). *Active Shooter.* Washington, DC. Retrieved from www.dhs.gov/xlibrary/assets/active_shooter

US Department of Homeland Security. (n.d.). *From the FBI: Active shooter Incidents of 2016 and 2016*. Washington, DC. Retrieved from https://www.hsdl.org/c/from-the-fbi -active-shooter-incidents-of-2016-and-2017

U.S. Department of Homeland Security. (n.d.). *Human trafficking 101 for school administrators and staff*. Washington, DC: Blue Campaign. Retrieved from https://www .dhs.govsites/default/files/publications/DHS%20Blue%20Campaign.pdf

U.S. Department of Justice: Federal Bureau of Investigation. (2018a). *Hate crime statistics, 2017: Offenders*. Retrieved from https://ucr.fbi.gov/hate-crime/2017/topic-pages/offenders

U.S. Department of Justice: Federal Bureau of Investigation. (2018b). *Hate crime statistics, 2017: Victims*. Retrieved from https://ucr.fbi.gov/hate-crime/2017/topic-pages/victims

U.S. Department of Justice: Office of Victims of Crime. (n.d.). *Mass casualty shootings*. Retrieved from https://ovc.ncjrs.gov/ncvrw2018/info_flyers/fact_sheets/2018NCVRW _MassCasualty_508_QC.pdf

Wolfe, D. A., Crooks, C., & Jaffee, P. (2009). A school-based program to prevent adolescent dating violence: A cluster randomized trial. *Archives Pediatric Adolescent Medicine, 163*(8), 1692–1699. doi:10.1001/archpediatrics.2009.69

Wynne, S., & Joo, H. (2011). Predictors of school victimization: Individual, familial and school factors. *Crime & Delinquency, 57*(3), 458–488. doi:10.1177/0011128710389586

Zhang, A., Musu-Gillette, L., & Oudekerk, B. A. (2016). *Indicators of school crime and safety: 2015* (NCES 2016-079/NCJ 249758). Washington, DC: National Center for Education Statistics, U.S. Department of Education, and Bureau of Justice Statistics, Office of Justice Programs, U.S. Department of Justice.

Online Resources

Centers for Disease Control and Prevention. *Self-directed violence and other forms of self-injury*: https://cdc.gov/ncbddd/disabilityand safety/self-injury.html

Cruise, T. K., & Canter, A. S. (2004). Sexual abuse of children and adolescents. In A. S. Canter, L. Z. Paige, M. Roth, I. Romero, & S. Carroll (Eds.), *Helping children at home and school II: Handouts for families and educators* (pp. S5-95–S5-98). Bethesda, MD: National Association of School Psychologists.

Cure Violence: https://cvg.org

National Center for Safe Supportive Learning Environments: https://safesupportivelearning .ed.gov/human-trafficking-americas-schools/risk-factors-and-indicators

National Gang Center of Bureau of Justice: https://www.nationalgangcenter.gov/#about

National Sexual Violence Resource Center: http://www.nsvrc.org/projects/child-sexual -assault-prevention/preventing-child-sexual-abuse-resources

Polaris Project: http://www.polarisproject.org

University of California-Davis Health Violence Prevention Research Program Home: https://health.ucdavis.edu/vprp/

University of Chicago. Chicago Center for Youth Violence Prevention: https://voices .uchicago.edu/ccyvp/about/

U.S. Department of Homeland Security. (n.d.). *Human trafficking 101 for school administrators and staff*. Washington, DC: Blue campaign. Retrieved from https://www .dhs.gov/sites/default/files/publications/DHS%20Blue%20Campaign.pdf

U.S. Department of Homeland Security Iowa. *The school shooter: A quick reference guide*. https://www.homelandsecurity.iowa.gov/documents/misc/FBI_School_Shooter _Guide.pdf

SCHOOL-BASED CRISIS MANAGEMENT

CARLEA D. M. DRIES

LEARNING OBJECTIVES

- Identify the characteristics of a crisis event.
- List the elements related to promoting physical and psychological safety.
- Identify the variables used when conducting psychological triage.

▮ Introduction

All schools have the legal and moral responsibility to safeguard the well-being of students and staff in the event of a crisis. Recent and continuing crises have made the need for schools to develop and rehearse comprehensive plans encompassing prevention, planning, response, and recovery an imperative. Schools need to have the capacity to respond to a range of crises, from an accidental injury (e.g., an arm broken on campus) to more significant events such as a staff or student death, school shooting, natural disaster, or health epidemic.

Children spend a considerable portion of their formative years on school grounds. Thus, schools are the context within which they typically experience psychosocial and accidental situational crises, and where they learn how to resolve and cope with these negative situations. The Sandy Hook Advisory Commission (2015) recognized that schools might offer the most realistic possibility for children to access supports. Schools are responsible for creating positive school climates, preventing negative behaviors such as bullying and harassment, and being prepared to respond to potential threats such as weather emergencies, fires, and acts of violence. Effective crisis protocols are essential for schools to meet this responsibility (Cowan, Vaillancourt, Rossen, & Pollitt, 2013). Responding to a school-based crisis is unique and requires specialized training and knowledge of schools, the learning process, physical health, mental health, and children's crisis reactions. Appropriate crisis planning and response can help build students' resilience and expedite a return to learning.

▮ The Benefits of Early Crisis Intervention

It has been understood that long-term or permanent damage can develop if an individual experiencing crisis remains untreated. Early recognition of potential crises encourages timely, proactive responses that may prevent or minimize impact. Crisis training may help to increase knowledge, skills, and confidence levels and maximize opportunities for efficient intervention. According to landmark research conducted by Johnson, Casey, Ertl, Everly, and Mitchell (1999), crises that are ignored or ineffectively resolved can create posttraumatic stress responses that compromise the achievement of the goals of education in the following ways: (a) creating negative reactions that impact learning; (b) reducing the ability to focus on instruction; (c) interfering with attention; (d) disrupting social exchanges; (e) decreasing memory retention and retrieval skills; (f) becoming obsessed or engrossed with the traumatic experience; (g) reverting to prior coping levels; and (h) increasing physiological arousal and startle responses. The study implies that school personnel can misinterpret many of these problems and associated crisis-related behaviors as discipline issues, and thus students are frequently punished as opposed to being provided with appropriate intervention services. It would follow that students who are experiencing crisis reactions that are not recognized or validated will have a more difficult time restoring equilibrium and assimilating the experience. Presently there is a class action lawsuit against the Compton Unified School District wherein the plaintiffs allege the typical response was to punish students who were traumatized by continual community-based violence rather than offer help. The case cites research suggesting that children who experience community violence are at an increased risk for depression, suicidal ideation, and lowered academic achievement. In 2015, a class action suit was brought against the Compton Unified School District, maintaining that trauma is a disability and therefore schools are required to make modifications and/or accommodations for traumatized students, rather than enforce penalties such as suspension or expulsion. The plaintiffs want the school district to provide teacher training, mental health support for students, supports for staff who are experiencing secondary trauma, and the use of conflict-mediation prior to punishment. This case highlights the continued importance of providing educators with specialized crisis response skills.

Children represent a particularly vulnerable population whose reactions or symptomatology are typically different than those of adults. Trauma exposure in early years can undermine child and adolescent development in a variety of areas that influence academic, personal, and interpersonal success: communication skills, an intact sense of self, peer and adult relationships, attention and focus, executive functioning skills, morale, and personality development, as well as influence coping skills (e.g., De Bellis, Woolley, & Hooper, 2013). Adverse experiences also place children at risk for negative academic, social, emotional, and professional outcomes (Rossen & Hull, 2013). The strong association between measures of school safety and average student achievement suggests that students are unable to concentrate on academics when they fear for their physical well-being. This again speaks to the importance of being able to intervene with children in crisis situations. Because most children spend much of their time within the school setting, school-based health providers are in a powerful position to be able to address their unique needs and issues. Further, outside providers might not know or understand the individual culture or climate of the specific school and therefore would be challenged to deliver sufficient support. This provides a rationale not only for appropriately training and utilizing the skills of school-based health professionals, but also to encourage schools to have their own crisis teams.

■ Definition of Terms

Coping is the process of using various, healthy or unhealthy, cognitive and/or behavioral strategies to adapt to stressors.

Crisis can be used to cover a broad range of anticipated and unanticipated events. Examples of crises that fit this definition include severe illness and injury, unexpected death, threatened death or injury, acts of war, natural disasters, and man-made disasters. This term may be used synonymously with *critical incident*.

Crisis intervention or *crisis response* involves the immediate provision of assistance to individuals experiencing a crisis. It is a short-term, goal-directed helping process focused on resolution of an immediate problem and stabilization of the resulting emotional conflicts. Prompt intervention should be geared toward re-establishing emotional and behavioral stability, providing support, and facilitating the needs of those most closely impacted by the crisis. Crisis intervention is also referred to as *secondary care* (Caplan, 1964).

Crisis resolution is the goal of crisis intervention. Resolution involves the restoration of equilibrium, cognitive mastery of the situation, and the development of new coping strategies. However, in cases of perpetual crisis stressors (e.g., chronic community-based violence), the resolution is less about recovery and becomes more focused on survival and increasing effective coping skills.

Disequilibrium is the disruption of an individual's homeostatic balance as a result of a crisis event. It is associated with the inability to maintain emotional control and characterized by confusing emotions, increased vulnerability, somatic complaints, and erratic behavior.

Postvention involves the provision of services (including counseling and debriefing activities) designed to reduce the long-term effects experienced by those directly and indirectly impacted by crises. The recovery process includes learning new ways of coping with stress through positive crisis resolution. Postvention is also referred to as *tertiary care* (Caplan, 1964).

Prevention, for the purpose of this chapter, is the provision of education, training, consultation, and crisis intervention designed to reduce the occurrence of mental distress, reduce the incidence of crises, and promote growth, development, and crisis resistance in individuals and the community. Prevention is also referred to as *primary care* (Caplan, 1964).

Psychological triage is the manner in which each individual's unique risk factors are assessed in order to determine the appropriate level of intervention and postvention services. Included in this evaluation are the individual's proximity to the critical incident, vulnerability (e.g., coping skills, support network), and reactions to the event.

School crisis is an incident occurring either at school or in the community that negatively impacts students, staff, and/or other members of the school community. Any situation that creates, or has the potential to create, a disruption of the educational process or normal school operations can be considered a school crisis.

Trauma is an emotional response to adversity, stress, or a crisis (American Psychiatric Association [APA], 2015). Immediately following a critical incident, shock and denial are expected. Longer-term responses include emotional lability, flashbacks, and disrupted relationships, as well as somatic complaints.

Definitions of Crisis

Crisis situations inevitably occur throughout the routine course of life and may be prompted by either a single catastrophic event (such as the school shooting at Sandy Hook Elementary School, Superstorm Sandy, Hurricane Katrina, or the terrorist attacks of September 11, 2001), or the cumulative effect of successive stressors (such as repeated physical abuse or chronic community violence). It is important to note that the term *crisis* covers a wide array of incidents, and does not automatically mean a single traumatic event, such as a school shooting. Common situations could include fire or structural damage, an earthquake or tornado, or hazardous material exposure. Despite their seemingly omnipresent status on news outlets, situations of violence are statistically rare, as cited by the National Center for Educational Statistics (2019). According to the School-Associated Violent Deaths (SAVD) Surveillance Study, from the time period of July 1, 2015 through June 2016 (the most recent information available), there were a total of 38 school-associated violent deaths in elementary and secondary schools in the United States. Of those incidents, 30 were homicides, 7 were suicides, and 1 was a legal intervention (i.e., involving a law enforcement officer). Additional information gathered from media reports can provide a glimpse of specific SAVD cases. For example, the Sandy Hook Elementary School shooting incident (Newtown, Connecticut) on December 14, 2012, resulted in 20 child homicides, 6 adult homicides, and 1 adult suicide. On its website, the Everytown for Gun Safety organization has been chronicling school shootings since the Newtown tragedy (Everytown, n.d.). In the first 2 years since the incident at Sandy Hook Elementary School, there were 92 reported school shootings. It is important to note that the SAVD and Everytown use different measures to categorize their data. The former only reports an incident when a fatality occurs on the school grounds of elementary and secondary schools, whereas the latter records any situation in which a firearm is discharged on a campus from elementary school to college. When the Everytown chart is reviewed using the SAVD criterion, the number of school shootings since December 15, 2012 through December 15, 2014 declines to 35.

Reactions to Crisis

Although once considered pathological, crisis reactions are now recognized as typical responses to atypical situations. Of course, there does remain the possibility that what begins as a common response can lead to pathology, but this is less often the case; recovery is expected. According to the seminal work by Caplan (1964), crises challenge coping resources, jeopardize an individual's sense of emotional balance and stability, create psychological distress, and cause individuals to feel trapped (i.e., unable to escape or effectively deal with the problem at hand).

Leading training programs, such as the PREPaRE curriculum (Brock et al., 2016) developed by workgroups sponsored by the National Association of School Psychologists, denote specific characteristics for assessing the significance of a crisis. The situation must be perceived as extremely negative, thusly leading to physical or emotional pain. It needs to generate feelings of helplessness, powerlessness, and/or entrapment. The incident may occur suddenly, unexpectedly, and without warning. There is also a hierarchy of crisis classifications in terms of traumatic impact. The highest impact events have a greater sense of assaultive violence and typically have a higher fatality rate, such as acts of war and/or terrorism. The lower impact events are generally less intentional, such as natural disasters or severe (nonfatal) illness or injury. Four features influence the resultant devastation from a crisis: predictability, consequences, duration, and intensity. Each of these characteristics can mitigate the level of response needed, as well as the length of the trauma impact. It is important to recognize that duration and intensity can be affected by media exposure.

The crisis state creates significant upset, feelings of anxiety, and/or disequilibrium, all of which are associated with an inability to cope with or adapt to the situation. In other words, the circumstances are outside the individual's typical coping skills and the resulting confusion leaves the person feeling unsettled. The emotional experience of a crisis may range from intense pain to numbness, but usually includes confusion, vulnerability, disorganization, helplessness, and disequilibrium. An individual in crisis often exhibits changes in attention span (usually decreased), reflection, emotional responses (typically becoming more overt and less restrained), impulsivity, and help-seeking behaviors. Within schools, responders must consider the individual's unique perception to the whole of the critical incident and only provide services to an individual who is demonstrating, in overt or covert ways, a need.

Crisis Drills

In response to incidences of school-based violence in recent decades, there has been a surge in the number of materials to support school personnel in intervening with school crises. Likewise, legal requirements have been created requiring schools to take crises into consideration. In addition to federal legislation (e.g., Every Student Succeeds Act, 2015; Obama, 2011), many states now require schools to have protocols for harassment, intimidation and bullying; suicide intervention; and disaster preparedness. As of 2010, the New Jersey Department of Education requires that districts must have one fire drill and one security drill per month. Security drills include active shooter, evacuation (non-fire), bomb threat, lockdown, shelter-in-place, and reverse evacuation. Further guidance is provided for the maintenance of a district-wide emergency management manual, which should contain contact information for all school personnel, building schematics, and specific instructions of how to respond to a host of potential crises (e.g., chemical spill, missing person).

It is not essential for districts to take the same actions when trying to resolve a critical incident, therefore this text will not dictate a specific protocol. However, as will be discussed, comprehensive school safety planning and engagement in crisis drills is of utmost importance for appropriate crisis response.

Given the relative novelty of the field, recommended practices may not have been thoroughly vetted. However, although there is a lack of research on crisis prevention and intervention in schools, there is consistency across best-practices recommendations. Specific crisis preparation and preparedness strategies typically recommend developing a comprehensive crisis management plan, forming a multidisciplinary crisis response team, and conducting emergency exercises. Although developing crisis response plans and forming multidisciplinary crisis teams have face validity and are supported by the military model, empirical data can be considered lacking. Crisis drills, often referred to as emergency or security drills, particularly those that provide children with active practice, an explanation for the rehearsal, and opportunities to discuss how each protocol would help in an emergency situation, have been found to lead to better skill performance and reduced fears about fires. Rehearsing procedures has been found to increase the prospect of members of the school community adhering to the protocols in the event of a real crisis. Lockdown drills practiced according to such models have been suggested to increase knowledge and skills of how to respond appropriately without increasing anxiety or perceived safety risk.

Utilizing a multilevel approach for practicing security drills can be beneficial. After orienting the school community to the protocols for each emergency drill, it is recommended to practice the same. Such rehearsals can occur in a typical format, such as a fire drill. The next level of training would be a tabletop exercise wherein a scenario of a critical incident is created and members of the multidisciplinary crisis team evaluate their hypothesized response. These are often conducted in real time to allow for the participants to truly understand how long each step might take (e.g., after calling 911, it might take 10 minutes for the first responder to arrive on the scene). The next level is called a functional exercise, which is a stressful simulation of what happens during a crisis event without deploying all school and local resources to respond. For example, a functional exercise of a fire may involve the use of a smoke machine in the building or artificially heating an exit door. Both of these simulate realities of a fire emergency and force staff and students to practice evacuation under convincing conditions.

The last level of training is a full-scale drill. This typically takes about 3 to 6 months of advance planning and may last several hours or a full school day to conduct. The full-scale drill involves the school and all local emergency response agencies that would be relevant to the simulated crisis event. Schools would practice a foreseeable critical incident (e.g., a fire caused by an explosion in the chemistry lab) by going through the steps of the crisis response protocol. This could include assessing the need for medical attention, family reunification steps, mental health support, and so on.

Most schools do not conduct a functional exercise or full-scale drill each school year. However, schools should not conduct either of these more advanced trainings without first preparing the entire school community with orientations, emergency drills, and tabletop exercises. In all cases, training must be developmentally appropriate, minimize traumatic exposure and impact, avoid the use of unnecessary and potentially frightening props (such as rubber bullets), and provide support in the aftermath for those individuals who were frightened. It is essential for school personnel to work with law enforcement in order to conduct these exercises in a manner that does not compromise physical or psychological safety. Parent and staff consent also need to be considered.

In the event that a district would like to conduct full-scale drills, the Federal Emergency Management Agency (2003) provides four key recommendations: (a) The focus should be on preparing and learning, while being sensitive to the needs of students and staff who may be vulnerable to the realism associated with a full-scale drill; (b) support must be available to address the needs of the school community in the event of emotional responses during or after an exercise; (c) trauma histories must be considered prior to the selection of volunteers to participate in the drill as victim or perpetrator; and (d) notification must be made to the public so as to not lead people to believe the rehearsal is an actual critical incident.

Training staff in recognizing risk factors and having structures in place to systematically assess these risks are critical to prevention. Additionally, students and staff need to be informed of what to do if they detect a risk. As discussed elsewhere in this text, schools should be equipped to conduct risk assessments for suicide, homicide, and other threats. Mitigation of threats can be invaluable in preventing loss. Everyone inside the school and in the community needs to work together to achieve the goal of having a safe learning environment. Collaboration with local emergency agencies, neighborhood resources, the school community, and national assistance teams is essential in promoting physical and psychological safety. As indicated earlier, legislation requires interagency cooperation in creating school safety plans (U.S. Department of Education Readiness and Emergency Management for Schools, 2008; U.S. Department of Education, Office of Elementary and Secondary Education, Office of Safe and Healthy Students, 2013).

Preventive Measures

In an op-ed article, Cornell (2016), a forensic clinical psychologist and professor of education who is Director of the University of Virginia Youth Violence Project wrote, "Prevention does not require prediction.... Violence prevention cannot wait until there is a gunman at the door, but must start long before problems escalate into violence." Schools can incorporate preventive strategies in an effort to reduce instances of school-based violence. Some facilities have opted to implement zero tolerance policies, which may use metal detectors or security checks to deny entry to anyone carrying a weapon, in attempts to prevent incidents of violence. A significant body of research reviewed by the American Psychological Association Zero Tolerance Task Force suggests that these policies are ineffective as the means to increase positive student outcomes. Such policies have limited empirical support as well as a propensity to create unintended negative consequences, such as student resentment and escalation of behavior.

Instead, the research suggests that social supports, resilience, and hope are critical to help children successfully cope in the aftermath of a traumatic experience (Hines, 2015). These prevention programs use instructional methods to teach the student body about violence and character education. Educational approaches implemented within the framework of a comprehensive and integrated mental and behavioral health program may be more effective. Interventions such as character education, wellness programming, positive behavioral intervention supports (PBIS), peer mediation, and social-emotional learning programs have been shown to support student growth. For decades it has been documented that a positive school climate can be the foundation for effective instruction, learning, and student success (e.g., Thapa, Cohen, Guffey, & Higgins-D'Allesandro, 2014). Further, it promotes a physically and psychologically safe learning environment to support academic and social-emotional learning, as well as increasing school attendance, decreasing dropout rates, and closing the achievement gap. The final report of the Sandy Hook Advisory Commission (2015) reiterated several key tenets of prevention components, including crime prevention through environmental design (CPTED), utilizing multidisciplinary school committees to address school climate and responses to critical incidents, and the importance of access to effective treatment for those affected by trauma.

Physical Safety

It is important to consider crime prevention through both physical safety and psychological safety. The former emphasizes three concepts: natural access control, natural surveillance, and territoriality. Natural access control and surveillance design help to promote students' taking ownership of their school and increase a potential offender's perception of risk because they know the school community will not tolerate negative behaviors. More detailed descriptions of these components of CPTED follow.

Access control is a concept aimed at decreasing the opportunity for a crime to occur. Such things as guards, locks, closed doors/windows, double entryway doors, limiting entry to one centralized location with clearly enforced visitor procedures, established procedures for deliveries, fences, gates, or other physical design elements can discourage access by unintended users. It is important to note zero tolerance is not the same as access control, although zero tolerance sites may use the same features.

Natural surveillance allows people to observe events that occur both inside and outside the building. As such, it can be one of the first steps in creating a safer school environment. A clear line of sight to the outside of the building, use of cameras, proper lighting (including in the parking areas), clearly marked parking spaces for visitors, landscaping, as well as increased supervision within the building (e.g., monitoring the hallways during passing periods) can all contribute to surveillance.

The final component of physical safety is territoriality, which is essentially the delineation between the school campus and community property. In addition to the boundaries created, it also represents school pride. Helping to keep the school clean, displaying student work, and demonstrating school spirit can all increase territoriality.

Psychological Safety

A primary concept in promoting psychological safety is establishing a school-wide PBIS (or comparable social/emotional and character development) program. Nearly 18,000 schools across the United States have shifted to using the universal system as an effective, evidence-based approach to reduce problem behaviors and increase positive behaviors (Fallon, McCarthy, & Sanetti, 2014). Supportive approaches to discipline are more effective than those that rely on punitive consequences given that such programs have the capability to generate various options when dealing with problem behaviors or preventing behaviors from occurring. Attention is focused on creating and sustaining universal (school-wide), targeted (classroom or group), and intensive (individual) systems of support. Positive behavior intervention support helps in reducing problem behaviors, increasing academic success and improving the quality of life. Schools that are unfamiliar with the PBIS system often respond to problem behaviors with office discipline referrals, suspensions, or other zero tolerance policies.

In addition to PBIS, school officials may consider incorporating social–emotional learning. Students lacking social–emotional skills experience challenges in following directions, managing their emotions, and getting along with the other children and the adults that share their classroom. Such programs can be a fundamental part of the curriculum from preschool through high school as ways to help children explore and identify feelings that may contribute to concerning behaviors. Likewise, social–emotional curriculum can directly teach children how to utilize social problem-solving skills in challenging situations. It has been found that social-emotional learning initiatives promoted academic success, health, and well-being in urban, suburban, and rural schools and after-school programs across K–12 grade levels while simultaneously preventing a variety of problems such as substance abuse, violence, truancy, and bullying. Bettencourt, Gross, and Ho (2016) conducted a longitudinal study using the Personal and Social Development domain of the Maryland Model for School Readiness (MMSR) to examine the relationship between kindergartners' social–emotional readiness and important educational outcomes in more than 9,000 elementary school students enrolled in Baltimore City Public Schools. The investigators tracked the same students through fourth grade and found that students who entered kindergarten behind in social–emotional skills were up to 80% more likely to have been retained; up to 80% more likely to require special education services; and up to seven times more likely to be suspended or expelled at least once. Additionally, socia–emotional readiness in kindergarten was a significant predictor of grade retention even after controlling for student scores on the other readiness domains of the MMSR, such as language and literacy development, cognition and general knowledge, and physical development and health.

Another aspect of psychological safety is school connectedness, which was defined by the Centers for Disease Control and Prevention (2009) as "the belief by students that adults and peers care about their learning *as well as* about them as individuals" (p. 5) [emphasis added]. School connectedness is related to the natural surveillance discussed earlier, specifically in the increased presence of school staff members in the hallways, lunchroom, and so on. It reduces the prevalence of deviant behaviors regardless of the socio-economics of the community and for students with and without disabilities. As with territoriality, school connectedness can lead to higher academic motivation, greater school competence, and more positive perceptions of the overall school climate. It results in higher grade point averages and the development of supportive relationships with teachers and peers. Kraft, Marinell, and Yee (2016), in collaboration with the Research Alliance for New York City Schools, recently completed a multiyear exploration of the relationship between school organizational contexts, teacher turnover, and student achievement in New York City middle schools. The researchers analyzed multiple data sources to evaluate their impact on overall school climate. These were distilled into four main categories: school safety and order, leadership and professional development, high academic expectations, and teacher relationships and collaboration. The study tracked those indicators over a period of 4 years (2008–2012) and compared them with student test scores and school data on teacher retention. Increases in school safety and academic expectations for students correspond with increases in student achievement. Safety had the strongest relationship with student gains across both English language arts and mathematics. Increases in measures of school safety and high academic expectations alone boosted math scores enough to account for an extra month and a half of instruction.

■ Safety Teams, Crisis Teams, and Planning

Due to the significance of school climate in crisis prevention and preparation, it is of paramount importance for campuses to have comprehensive safety teams and plans in addition to the physical and psychological safety precautions. Many schools already have crisis teams set up to address crisis planning, without a focus on overall school safety and climate. Attention to both overall safety and prevention programming, in addition to crisis planning, is recommended. Safety teams focus on prevention, whereas crisis teams focus on response. In an ideal situation, the two teams would have overlapping personnel so that the response teams are able to contribute to the development of the plans. Unfortunately, some of the professional groups most often left out of the safety team model, and resulting safety planning, are school-based mental and overall health professionals. Such personnel can introduce safe school initiatives and quality prevention programs, help establish effective safety and crisis plans, provide guidance and support to administrators regarding system-level issues for consideration in plan development, advise school leaders on physical and psychological responses in the event of a crisis and provide direct interventions, conduct program evaluation regarding the effectiveness of the safety and crisis plans, facilitate plan modifications, and, perhaps most importantly, help students and staff return to pre-crisis levels of functioning in the event of a critical incident. When they are unable to contribute to safety planning, school-based health providers miss out on the opportunity to build self-efficacy through performance attainments, or to build vicarious self-efficacy through observation of others' response practices.

When considering members of these teams, it would be wise to look at the specific skills held by school personnel. Often, the first people thought of are the administration, but other employees may have attributes that would serve the team; it is important to have representation from different disciplines, such as academic (e.g., lead teacher), social–emotional (e.g., school psychologists), medical (e.g., school nurses), safety (e.g., school resource officer), and technology. Additional participants from the community may be helpful too, such as your local emergency responders and private practitioners. Team members should have positive leadership and personality characteristics, such as being open-minded, well-respected, an ability to remain calm in tenuous situations, strong decision-making skills, and reliability to name a few. It is important to note that members should not be assigned to the safety team; rather, it should be a voluntary position suggesting that the person is confident in their ability to respond to critical incidents. As indicated throughout this chapter, school-based health personnel can be integral to effective planning and response teams. Figure 22.1 depicts a sample of a team hierarchy. It is encouraged to have three levels of redundancy for each position.

A comprehensive district safety plan specifically addresses district needs, provides direction for safety and academic programming for all schools, and directs guidance, leadership, and training. Similarly, the comprehensive school safety plan focuses on meeting school-level needs and following the guidelines set forth by the district. The goal of the safety plan is, through data-based decisions, to ensure a common understanding of crisis response plans that address the physical and psychological safety of the school community as mandated through legal requirements.

In developing response plans, it may be helpful to consider the items deemed essential for different "go-kits" or "grab bags." Among other things, school-based medical providers likely would ensure their ready bags include a listing of all medications required by school community members (and administration times), the medications themselves, bandages, latex-free gloves, gauze, sunscreen, and ice packs (Table 22.1). Some providers are including items such as portable privacy commodes as well as activity books and materials.

■ Assessing Psychological Trauma: Conducting Psychological Triage

Regrettably, even the most comprehensive prevention plan cannot guarantee a critical incident will not occur. Therefore, significant attention should be paid to appropriate crisis response. Once physical and psychological health and safety are reinstated, personnel can begin to assess psychological trauma. Note that treatment cannot begin until physical needs have been addressed, as one cannot begin to heal from trauma when still in harm's way; the medical health and mental health go-kits are useful tools to facilitate comfort. The goal would be to identify those who are considered at risk for becoming psychological trauma victims and to help make initial decisions for treatment. It must be highlighted that multiple tools are used for this evaluation and the resultant psychological intervention are continuing. As presented during PREPaRE

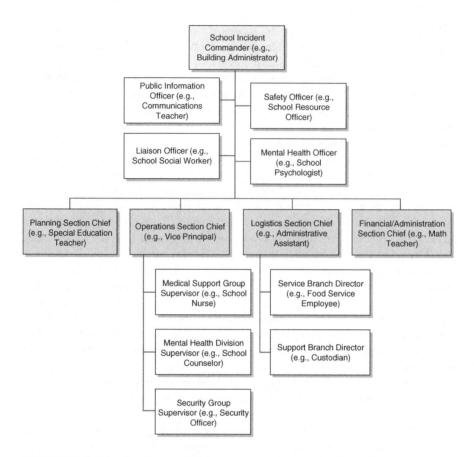

FIGURE 22.1 School safety team hierarchy sample organizational chart.

The figure represents a typical hierarchy for school safety teams. It is important to consider specific skills held by school personnel. Often, the first people thought of are the administration, but other employees may have attributes that would serve the team; it is important to have representation from different disciplines, such as academic (e.g., lead teacher), social-emotional (e.g., school psychologists), medical (e.g., school nurses), safety (e.g., school resource officer), and technology. Additional participants from the community may be helpful too, such as your local emergency responders and private practitioners. Three levels of redundancy are recommended for each position.

training, "triage is a process, not an event" (Brock, personal communication, July 20, 2015). It is ongoing and changeable based upon the presentation of the individuals in crisis. It is important to note again that recovery is typical and expected. Not everyone who experienced the crisis may be so affected that intervention would be warranted; therefore, the providers would respond only to those demonstrating need. Delivering support to those who have *not* indicated necessity may cause undue harm

TABLE 22.1 SCHOOL NURSE'S GO-KIT COMPONENTS

DOCUMENTS	
Crisis management plan	School blueprints
Emergency cards	Individualized and emergency plans
Teacher and student class lists	Absentee list for the day
Alert list	Standing orders
Medication list for students and staff	Emergency evacuation plans
Class pictures or yearbook	Important phone numbers
SUPPLIES	
Emergency medications	Daily medications
Students' personal medications	Spill kit
Gloves, gowns	Bandages, splints, ice packs
Biohazard bags and masks	Flashlight
Communication devices	Blood pressure machine, stethoscope
Master keys for building	Hand sanitizer
Pens, paper, markers	Name tags, triage tags

SOURCE: Reproduced from Loschiavo, J. (2020). *Fast facts for the school nurse* (3rd ed.). New York, NY: Springer Publishing Company.

to the individual because of a continued exposure to the crisis, as well as reducing the student's perception of independent problem-solving abilities and safety However, individuals with pre-existing psychopathology would be the exception. School-based health providers often have the benefit of knowing their student population so they would be aware of such personal sensitivities. This provides further support for having school-based health professionals serve as members of safety and crisis teams.

In assessing psychological trauma, the providers should evaluate the individual's unique experience of the critical incident. Particular attention would be paid to the student's proximity, both physical (i.e., where they were when the event took place) and emotional (i.e., who they knew who might have been involved in the event). In both situations, the further removed the student was, the less likely becomes the need for intervention. As previously mentioned, media coverage can affect perceptions, so care providers should be mindful of individuals' exposure to the news, Internet, and social media. Further, a key consideration is the individual's perception of the situation as a threat. The subjective interpretations can be more important to the overall crisis perception than the exposure. It should be noted that children will often mirror the level of response given by the adult.

The second variables to consider during the evaluation process are the personal vulnerability risk factors (i.e., who the person was when the incident took place). Again, school-based personnel would likely have knowledge about the students' pre-crisis stability and coping strategies. If an individual had sufficient coping skills, no pre-existing psychiatric challenges or trauma history, strong social support resources, and an ability to regulate their own emotions, crisis intervention is typically not required. However, if the student has an avoidant coping style, a poor ability to self-regulate, a psychiatric or trauma history, and is generally alone, the necessity of intervention is increased.

In looking at these vulnerability risk factors, care providers must also consider cultural and developmental variations. Culture (e.g., socioeconomic status, religion, community location) influences the types of events that appear to be threatening and affects how individuals assign meaning to a threat. It also impacts how individuals or communities express traumatic reactions, and how the affected individuals or communities are viewed or judged. The care provider must be aware of the cultural differences and seek the assistance of community cultural leaders for guidance. While crisis interveners should be mindful of the variability in cultures, they should also be aware that their own frame of reference might differ from those affected by the critical incident. Similarly, the individual's view of the responder is to be considered. In some cases, a female crisis responder might not be able to provide support to a male in crisis based on cultural parameters.

As mentioned earlier, the responses of preschoolers and early elementary students often relate more to the reactions of their parents. These individuals are also more vulnerable to psychological trauma, due in part to less sophisticated coping skills and reasoning abilities. These students may demonstrate more regression in achieved milestones (e.g., self-toileting), reduced ability to separate from a caregiver, and increased acting out behaviors (e.g., tantrums, fighting with peers). Trauma-related play is often present, appearing as frightening themes (e.g., monsters) for preschoolers and more direct re-enactments of the critical incident for school-aged children. Older students have more developed abstract reasoning skills. As a result, their crisis reactions are more adult-like. They too might demonstrate more resistant and aggressive behaviors, though this is generally as a means to reassert control. Self-injurious or risky behavioral choices or thoughts can increase, as can revenge fantasies. Such maladaptive coping behaviors may decrease the individual's ability to concentrate or regulate emotions, and may ultimately impact academic progress. Although these behaviors are typically temporary, intervention should be considered.

Once the variables are fully assessed, students' levels of risk are documented to ensure the appropriate level of intervention. For instance, an individual who had limited proximity (physical, emotional), no personal vulnerabilities, a typical response to the situation, and a healthy perception of the threat, as well as adaptive coping skills would be considered a low risk. Conversely, if a student was directly involved in the incident, has pre-existing trauma history, no network of outside support, and is demonstrating continued maladaptive coping strategies, the student would be considered a high risk and therefore a high priority for intervention.

■ Supports and Interventions

After these initial steps of triage have been documented, the crisis responders would begin to provide psychoeducational supports or psychological interventions. Again, these measures are only taken for those who demonstrate substantial need. Psychoeducation is the direct instruction and/or dissemination of information with the goal of having crisis survivors and their caregivers being able to understand, prepare for, and respond to the critical incident, as well as acknowledging the challenges and common responses typically associated with trauma. These sessions can take place through informational bulletins, caregiver trainings, classroom meetings, and student psychoeducational groups. Providing informational handouts to parents and teachers has been debated because of the lack of empirical support. However, opportunities for parents/guardians to participate in caregiver training sessions result in improved coping and reduced psychopathology.

Psychological interventions differ from psychoeducational supports primarily because they allow for the impacted individual to share their own trauma stories, thoughts, perceptions, feelings, and reactions. As a result, these are more active and direct attempts to foster adaptive coping and respond to symptoms of trauma-related stress. Psychological interventions are provided to those individuals who were assessed to be at higher risk. The goal is to re-establish immediate functional coping and not the resolution of the crisis. The interventions are designed to help students cope with problems stemming from the trauma and facilitate referrals to more intensive therapeutic treatments if necessary. Crisis responders should know when, where, and how to refer for outside supportive services.

Role of School-Based Health Providers

As highly trained school-based health specialists, school nurses are in the unique position to support student progress in a variety of areas. Their expertise extends beyond administering daily medications, doling out ice packs, and placing bandages. Concurrently, there is increased awareness of the need for effective crisis prevention and intervention in schools. Less than 30 years ago, responsibility for school crisis intervention was not clearly defined, with community resources often implementing care. However, many school districts are now increasingly relying on professionals within school systems for crisis intervention services.

Although there is heightened emphasis on crisis response in the schools, the field of school crisis intervention is still relatively young. Education and training have not kept pace with the mounting need for the application of crisis intervention skills in the schools. A national survey conducted by Berman (1983) revealed that few professional schools, specifically programs for health and other human service professionals, included formal coursework on crisis theory and practice (Hoff & Hoff, 2012). More recently, Allen et al. (2002) conducted a study of Nationally Certified School Psychologists regarding different aspects of crisis intervention, including university preparation, continuing education, and involvement with school crisis plans and crisis teams. The majority of those who received university training believed they were minimally or not at all prepared to respond to a school crisis; only 2% indicated feeling well-prepared or very well-prepared. As a result, many school psychologists feel they have inadequate training for the crisis intervener role, or that they prefer an administrator take the lead in intervention. Research assessing future school administrators' perceptions of the role of school-based mental health services provider indicated that responding to crisis and working with teachers in crisis situations were of primary importance (Fitch, Newby, Ballestero, & Marshall, 2001). Graduate educators can use this information in preparing school health care providers to better fulfill the expectations of their positions. Because school administrators often view crisis management as an essential task, specific training in that area should be available.

The competent handling of a crisis can forge a strong relationship within the school community. The unifying experience of a critical incident creates an opportunity for connection. However, trivializing or ignoring the effects of crisis implies that the situation was not meaningful enough for the school to acknowledge, or suggests that the crisis was so tremendous that school staff were not able to deal with it directly.

References

Allen, M., Jerome, A., White, A., Marston, S., Lamb, S., Pope, D., & Rawlins, C. (2002). The preparation of school psychologists for crisis intervention. *Psychology in the Schools, 39,* 427–439. doi:10.1002/pits.10044

American Psychiatric Association. (2015). *Trauma.* Retrieved from http://www.apa.org/topics/trauma/

Berman, L. (1983). *Survey of professional schools: Committee report to AAS board of directors.* Denver, CO: American Association of Suicidology.

Bettencourt, A., Gross, D., & Ho, G. (2016). *The costly consequences of not being socially and behaviorally ready by kindergarten: Associations with grade retention, receipt of academic support services, and suspensions/expulsions.* Retrieved from http://baltimore-berc.org/wp-content/uploads/2016/03/SocialBehavioralReadinessMarch2016.pdf

Brock, S. E., Nickerson, A. B., Louvar Reeves, M. A., Connolly, C. N., Jimerson, S. R., Pesce, R. C., & Lazzaro, B. R. (2016). *School crisis prevention and intervention: The PREPaRE model* (2nd ed.). Bethesda, MD: National Association of School Psychologists.

Caplan, G. (1964). *Principles of preventive psychiatry.* New York, NY: Basic Books.

Centers for Disease Control and Prevention. (2009). *School connectedness: Strategies for increasing protective factors among youth.* Atlanta, GA: U.S. Department of Health and Human Services. Retrieved from http://www.cdc.gov/healthyyouth/protective/pdf/connectedness.pdf

Cornell, D. (2016). Be proactive to cut school violence. *Atlanta Journal-Constitution.* Retrieved from http://www.ajc.com/news/news/local-education/be-proactive-to-cut-school-violence/nqjH6/

Cowan, K. C., Vaillancourt, K., Rossen, E., & Pollitt, K. (2013). *A framework for safe and successful schools* [Brief]. Bethesda, MD: National Association of School Psychologists. Retrieved from www.nasponline.org/schoolsafetyframework

De Bellis, M. D., Woolley, D. P., & Hooper, S. R. (2013). Neuropsychological findings in pediatric maltreatment: Relationship of PTSD, dissociative symptoms, and abuse/neglect indices to neurocognitive outcomes. *Child Maltreatment, 18,* 171–183. doi:10.1177/1077559513497420

Every Student Succeeds Act. (2015, December 10). *Public Law No: 114-95. S. 1177.* Retrieved from https://www.gpo.gov/fdsys/pkg/BILLS-114s1177enr/pdf/BILLS-114s1177enr.pdf

Everytown.org. (n.d.). *Everytown for Gun Safety.* Retrieved from http://everytown.org/

Fallon, L. M., McCarthy, S. R., & Sanetti, L. M. (2014). School-wide positive behavior support (SWPBS) in the classroom: Assessing perceived challenges to consistent implementation in Connecticut schools. *Education & Treatment of Children, 37*(1), 1.

Federal Emergency Management Agency. (2003). *Talking about disaster: Providing safety information to the public.* Washington, DC.: National Disaster Education Coalition.

Fitch, T., Newby, E., Ballestero, V., & Marshall, J. L. (2001). Future school administrators' perceptions of the school counselor's role. *Counselor Education and Supervision, 41*(2), 89–99. doi:10.1002/j.1556-6978.2001.tb01273.x

Hines, L. (2015). Children's coping with family violence: Policy and service recommendations. *Child and Adolescent Social Work Journal, 32,* 109–119. doi:10.1007/s10560-014-0333-9

Hoff, M. R., & Hoff, L. (2012). *Crisis education and service program designs: A guide for administrators, educators, and clinical trainers.* New York, NY: Routledge/Taylor and Francis Group.

Johnson, K., Casey, D., Ertl, B., Everly, G. S., Jr., & Mitchell, J. T. (1999). *School crisis response: A CISM perspective.* Ellicott City, MD: The International Critical Incident Stress Foundation.

Kraft, M. A., Marinell, W. H., & Yee, D. (2016). *School conditions matter for student achievement, new research confirms.* Retrieved from http://ny.chalkbeat.org/2016/03/24/school-conditions-matter-for-student-achievement-new-research-confirms/#.VvlG5uIrLcs

Obama, B. (2011). Presidential policy directive: National preparedness. *Council on Foreign Relations.* Retrieved from http://www.cfr.org/world/presidential-policy-directive-national-preparedness/p24731

Rossen, E., & Hull, R. (Eds.). (2013). *Supporting and educating traumatized students: A guide for school-based professionals.* New York, NY: Oxford University Press.

Sandy Hook Advisory Commission. (2015, March 6). *Final report of the Sandy Hook Advisory Commission.* Retrieved from http://www.shac.ct.gov/SHAC_Final_Report_3-6-2015.pdf

Thapa, A., Cohen, J., Guffey, S., & Higgins-D'Allessandro, A. (2013). A review of school climate research. *Review of Educational Research, 83,* 357–385. doi:10.3102/0034654313483907

U.S. Department of Education, National Center for Educational Statistics. (2019). *Digest of Education Statistics.* Washington, DC: Author.

U.S. Department of Education, Office of Elementary and Secondary Education, Office of Safe and Healthy Students. (2013, June). *Guide for developing high-quality school emergency operations plans.* Washington, DC: Author. Retrieved from http://rems.ed.gov/docs/rems_k-12_guide_508.pdf

U.S. Department of Education, Readiness and Emergency Management for Schools (REMS) Technical Assistance Center. (2008). *REMS express: Collaboration: Key to a successful partnership, 4,* 1–9. Retrieved from http://rems.ed.gov/docs/REMSX_Vol4Issue1.pdf

ETHICAL ISSUES IN THE SCHOOL SETTING

WAYNE A. YANKUS | DAVID NASH

LEARNING OBJECTIVES

- Identify at least five ethical issues faced in the school setting.
- List three reasons why ethical conflict is inevitable in some instances.
- Discuss how school nurses are empowered to act always in the best interest of the child.

▪ Introduction

Throughout the school day the nurse is confronted with many different, challenging situations.

School-physician directed Standing Orders guide the routine care and Individualized Healthcare Plans deal with the special needs of many students.

However, there are situations that arise which do not have a right or wrong answer. Local school policies, state mandates, or personal ethics may be in conflict. Families differ and administrators have varying expectations from the professional school nurse.

School nurses are probably at higher risk for liability than many of their colleagues. This is due to the wide range of responsibilities, professional isolation, and the inevitable conflicts between educational and healthcare policies.

This chapter introduces the ethical dilemma of a number of *Emerging Health Issues* and discusses the legal implications. It is *not* intended as a legal reference but more as an opportunity to raise awareness of potential problems and, if possible, avoid these issues entirely.

It is important to recognize that state laws (and for international students, U.S. law as compared to other countries) vary considerably on the topics addressed in this chapter. Readers are encouraged to consult legal and medical experts and review relevant legal requirements in their jurisdiction.

▪ Vaccine Refusal

School nurses are in the forefront of medical decision-making for the health and safety of their students. Their decisions often have major health and legal implications, and may at times be misunderstood or unpopular with parents, students and/ or staff. Such is the case when enforcing the state rules on immunization. State rules are enforced by audit from the Department of Health in most states. The requirement for student immunizations may be the single most important public health achievement of the 20th century. School is where the children are and where the diseases often foment. Having an immunized student body above 97% usually ensures the suppression of outbreaks of communicable illnesses such as measles, mumps, rubella, pertussis, and a host of diseases suffered by the young and the older student.

However, in recent years usually among the educated, there has been a movement to refuse immunization—some or all—for the child. This is in direct opposition to state and school health code and statute.

In all states, medical exemptions exist for those students who are undergoing treatments preventing immunization. They are protected by the immunized "herd" of students receiving timely immunization in their class cohort. Medical exemptions to immunization generally have a beginning and an ending and can be reviewed episodically by the school and the child's primary physician.

Religious exemptions to immunization exist in some states. A parent must declare that their religion forbids or is incompatible with immunization. In some states such as New Jersey, simply mentioning the word "religious" in a request is sufficient to exempt a child from protective immunization. In other states, the requirements are more rigorous.

There are a few remaining states where philosophical exemptions to immunization continue to exist. They are rapidly disappearing as state health departments have become more aggressive in fighting preventable contagious diseases by legislative action. Some states have realized the human and financial costs of fighting epidemic illness.

Under federal law (McKinney-Vento Act), homeless children must be allowed to enroll and begin attending classes even if they have not received immunizations. However school districts are also required to assign a homeless liaison to work with such children and their families to assist children in receiving the required immunizations.

In addition, where students are entering the United States from another country, state rules vary relative to student enrollment without evidence of immunizations. As a best practice, school officials should work closely with such families, as they would with homeless students, to assist them in identifying available resources for students to receive immunizations. In the case of unaccompanied minors, federal agencies will ensure that such students receive their initial round of immunizations as needed.

Gatekeeping is the task of the school nurse with the support of the administration. When a family has not cooperated with immunization regulations, it is up to the nurse to notify administration so that academic code and health laws are applied, which may mean that the student is unable to attend school until the needed immunizations are obtained. The nurse may also give families options of where to receive immunizations, from public health authorities or health care providers who have been advised of the rules and regulations existing for their state.

Avoiding adversarial situations is difficult when a family refuses to immunize. Provisional admission with the plan to complete each first vaccine of each series will be sufficient to permit the student to attend school; however, noncompliance often brings an unpleasant exchange between the parent and nurse. In such cases, it is critical for the school nurse and school administration to be on the same page.

Principals and superintendents of school systems have a legal obligation to promote and adhere to state immunization regulations and may personally face disciplinary action, as well as exposing their school district to legal liability where immunization requirements are not followed. However, school principals also face competing demands to do everything possible to ensure that all students are being educated and are being properly supervised, as opposed to being home, often in an unsupervised setting.

One strategy for reducing potential conflict is for the school nurse to proactively educate the administrative team on the health risks associated with failure to immunize, and the growing number of examples of outbreaks of diseases that had been thought to have been virtually eradicated in the United States.

School administrators may not have the same level of understanding regarding the potential health risks associated with a student attending classes for even a short period of time without proper immunizations. Educating administrators, parents, and students on critical health issues is an important part of the role of the school nurse and school physician. By working together, the school nurse and school physician are often able to overcome hesitancy about vaccines.

Too often parents trust the Internet far more than a health professional. In today's society, it is our job to have good and useful information to assist educators, administrators, and families to understand why these public health rules exist. Herd immunity is critical to each vulnerable child in school.

The ethics of reversing this trend is that the public health overrides private wishes. Schools are public places and is where most children spend their day. As medical staff and educators we are obligated to provide a safe learning space which includes the elimination of contagious disease. We also assume that nurses understand the science and wisdom of healthy schools by maintaining state-required vaccine laws. A key role is to work with families who are hesitant to vaccinate and provide information and interpretation to allow for sound decision-making.

While we are the child's advocate and respect the rights of parents, our obligation is to serve the child's best interest. School nurses are respected and play key roles in building trust within their schools, and providing for a safe school which includes a greater than 94% immunization rate to guarantee herd immunity. Catch up or provisional immunization status is a start for some parents and the Advisory Committee on Immunization Practices (ACIP) and the American Academy of Pediatrics (AAP) publish yearly catch-up charts to assist schools with this task as well as information on what is not a viable bloc to immunization.

It is not improper to ask yearly if vaccine status has changed for those who have previously refused. Sometimes a family illness requires those who are around or care for the parent or relative to be up to date on immunizations. Regardless, it is up to the school nurse to promote, record, educate, and advise on the safety of immunizations for the health of the school. Close conferencing with the school physician can be a reliable partnership.

▉ Medical Marijuana in the School Setting

Medical marijuana is an issue that has come to bear on school medical services. Some states have passed laws that allow for students while at school or at board of education sanctioned activities to receive an oil, pill, or liquid containing THC or tetrahydrocannabinol, the active ingredient in recreational pot or marijuana. Common use diagnoses are seizures, multiple sclerosis, HIV, wasting diseases, and intractable pain. However, in some states more diagnoses have been added to the list.

Due to restrictions on the research of its medical use by the federal government, medical marijuana remains a Schedule I drug available only to a few researchers. Therefore, what is available to students with one exception (Epidiol) is not certified USP pure. Most of the product is from a stash at home and not the pharmacy.

While some states who have licensed recreational marijuana use have dispensaries to obtain the drug, it is still not uniform for each pill, each time, each batch, and each use. Vaping and smoking is not allowed at this time in any school, but we are aware it is happening.

The school nurse is often the one chosen to administer medical marijuana to a student in the absence of parents which usually creates a violation of the Nurse Practice Act in some states. Is what is being administered to this student viable, reliable, and trustworthy? The answer is usually "no," and the adage "do no harm" applies.

In New Jersey and Colorado the law requires that a student have the substance administered by a licensed prescriber or by a parent or guardian and that only non-inhalable products be used. Successful use of the drug has been mostly on students with intractable seizures for whom all other modes of therapy have failed. Often parents will come to the school to administer the dose when the nurse can't, shouldn't, or won't perform the function. This creates another questionable situation in the nurse's office.

We then face the issue of:

- ▉ What is legal in my state?
- ▉ What is the purity of the product?
- ▉ Who is licensed to administer the product, and if unlicensed, are they reliable?
- ▉ How does this affect my license?
- ▉ How do I protect myself?

On the periphery of medical marijuana use in schools is the expanding use in some states. For example, in New Jersey there are specific, permissible reasons to have it prescribed, including multiple sclerosis, migraine, chemotherapy, HIV, PTSD, certain wasting diseases, and terminal pain. However, with more available diagnoses, schools are challenged to respond appropriately to the safety concerns. Typically, if you drove your car to school and had a migraine for which the drug was approved in your state, how do you advise the student about transportation home? They shouldn't drive; that is obvious—another dilemma for the nurse's office to solve.

Or, if taking the medical marijuana did not achieve the intended outcome for the student, did the student take some other form of medication for the same problem (e.g. acetaminophen) and are there interactions?

It is also possible that there may be a period of "trial and error" and a student who is administered medical marijuana may not be able to function appropriately in school. This risk is potentially greater than it would be for other medications given the lack of uniform standards for medical marijuana. Given the potential uncertainties related to the impact of medical marijuana there is also a need to proceed with great caution regarding the participation of such students in athletics, which could potentially place the student who is prescribed medical marijuana and other student athletes at risk of greater harm, and thereby create a risk of greater legal liability as well.

Legislators are working on crafting these laws often without much input from the medical community. What we do know is that more students are taking the drug for various reasons with and without a doctor's prescription. What is the impact on drug testing at school or the existing laws regarding a student's removal? This is ambiguous territory and the school risks the loss of Title I funding. The Justice Department has taken a back seat to observe how states will handle these changes and challenges.

All of this can also apply to faculty. While it is not the nurse's obligation to medicate faculty and staff, they are often pressured into doing so in the name of collegiality. Nurses should be cautioned that this is an area of school health that is unclear and expanding. Dangers include the student who is also abusing other substances. Some states have added laws, codes, and statutes to include emergency recovery drugs such as naloxone in nasal spray form to reverse overdose.

Another ethical issue with medical marijuana relates to the parent who administers the drug on site at school. Careful Board of Education policy, working with the school physician, and administrative support working as a team will be the solution going forward on what is destined to be part of the school nurse's responsibility.

One final issue with medical marijuana relates to staff members and/or parents who may be prescribed the substance. In the absence of clear state guidance permitting use by adults in the school setting, school districts should consult with their legal counsel and be cautious about granting any approval for such use by adults in the school setting. In addition, the school nurse should generally not be involved in any way in administering medical marijuana to such adults in the school setting.

This is new territory for nursing and schools. It is developing state by state with challenges and conflicts between federal and state laws and our practice. Safe school communities remain the stated goal. No student should be denied necessary medications to allow for their presence; however, clear policies protect both the student, family, nurse and administration.

Responding to Suspected Substance Use and Conducting Drug Testing in Schools

While specific protocols will vary depending on your state, ensuring student health must be the overriding priority in responding to incidents of suspected substance use by students. At times, this priority may be in conflict with the desires of other key stakeholders. Law enforcement may wish to focus on the criminal investigation aspect and potentially delay sending a student for a medical examination. Parents may wish to focus on helping their child avoid legal action and/or school disciplinary action, and seek to delay having a student undergo medical examination. School administrators may reach their own conclusions regarding whether or not a student is under the influence, or may request that the school nurse confirm or reject the concerns expressed by other staff, potentially delaying or preventing a student's medical examination. The school nurse has a crucial role to play to ensure that all stakeholders remain focused on student safety and ensure that competing demands do not compromise student safety.

As a school nurse, you need to clearly understand your required protocols related to suspected substance use as defined in state law and/or district policy (which must comply with state law). For example, if a teacher reports that a student may be under the influence, the school nurse should always see the student immediately to determine if the student is in need of immediate medical assistance. In some states, the school nurse will be authorized to make a determination as to whether or not the student must be sent out for a medical examination. In other states, the student will be required to be sent out even if the school nurse does not see any signs that the student is under the influence.

In some states, school systems base their evaluation of students for suspected substance use on the discovery of a student in possession of a dangerous substance or otherwise under suspicion of substance use (in New Jersey see N.J.A.C. 18A:40A-12). Many schools test on site after parents have given blanket permission at the start of the school year. Many do not. In 1995 and again in 2002 the Supreme Court established that school-based testing was legal. Courts have also upheld random testing of students if permitted under state law and local board policy, often for students who participate in athletics or other extracurricular activities, and/or for students who drive to school.

Usually it is up to the nurse as medical officer to evaluate a student and determine what professional follow up or further evaluation is medically needed for safety. The school nurse is put into the position of evaluating the student who has been placed in suspect. It requires the nurse to have a knowledge of the signs and symptoms of substance use. Training for the school nurse and all staff on the signs that a student may be under the influence should occur on an annual basis, at a minimum, and may need to be updated based on emerging trends in substance use and new information regarding the various ways that substance use may manifest in students, as new drugs, delivery methods, and drug purities are introduced. The nurse has a crucial role to play in ensuring that staff are properly trained, since the school nurse cannot be relied upon as the only individual able to identify warning signs. It is important to understand your state's requirements as to the role of the school nurse in training other staff, including how often such training must occur.

When the student is in possession, it also becomes a case for the administration and local authorities (NJAC and NJSA), and may result in disciplinary action and potentially criminal charges under state law. The medical admonition to the school nurse is always: *if there are changes in vital signs and/or cognition, call emergency ser-*

vices and have the student safely transported to the local emergency department of a hospital. Administration or police should not be allowed to alter sound medical decisions where death or harm could happen. This requires a nurse to be professional and clear in concerns for the student. Over the years some schools have required that students be tested for specific substances in order to return. Some schools actually do the testing. This may contradict the statutes and regulations in some states where a medical evaluation is all that is needed to return to class. It is critical that the school nurse understand the definition of "medical examination" in that state, and whether or not drug testing is a uniformly required element, may be a required element under board policy, or cannot be required at all.

The value of on-site testing at the school is, of course, hard copy and proof. However, all substances do not persist in the blood or urine for an indeterminate or uniform amount of time. How do you separate for discipline or counseling the student who smoked marijuana last week but tests positive today? Some substances are readily detected and some are not. While various testing methods exist, some are more invasive and/or more reliable than others. Urine testing is the preferred route for most middle and high schools.

The AAP in the United States has twice published policy statements against in-school testing (2007 and 2014). In 2014 the AAP stated that the "chain of custody" required for accurate testing is rarely available to most local in-school or hospital laboratories. Chain of custody means the student has been observed urinating, the specific gravity and temperature of the urine is taken to prevent fraudulent use of another's urine, and that the containers are sealed and signed at each stop along the way to the laboratory. This is the usual method used by courts and police when sampling urine for drug abuse. It is almost impossible in schools to do the same. When there is a breakdown in this chain of custody, the results of the testing may be challenged, and could potentially result in reversal of disciplinary action. More importantly, having students undergo drug testing at the school site could lead to a delay in a student receiving medical care, or even the student never receiving needed care because the district testing program did not include the specific substance being used by that student. Such delays or failure to receive medical care could endanger student health and safety and result in significant potential legal liability for the school district and for individual decision-makers.

Parents often want to take charge of the situation when they are contacted regarded their child's suspected substance use, which can sometimes be helpful but at other times works against their child's safety. For example, it is in the interest of the school to have an immediate medical examination of the suspected abuser. Families often opt to take the student to their own physician who may not be immediately available. In addition, that physician's office may not be prepared to offer drug testing if the school requires it. Also, some students with ADHD may test positive for amphetamines based on their medical therapy. Families often do not share this information with the school.

School policy must be clear as to school and board of education sponsored events and the suspicion of drug use and what action will be taken. More often than not, these events take place after school, on evenings or weekends such as proms, field trips, and athletic events. The original contact is usually an administrator or faculty member who then refers to the nurse or to the parent for immediate medical evaluation. If given the option, many parents will delay evaluation in order to clear the student which is why school policy must be clear as to what "immediate" really means.

From the evaluator's standpoint, the questions are: Is the student safe to return to the school environment or are counseling and further evaluation necessary? With discovery, can you provide needed services if the student tests positive? And remember that a positive test does not diagnose a substance abuse disorder (Levy et al., 2015). Most cases in school will be resolved without police intervention; however, with the increase in vaping and user devices, nurse services requires full knowledge of abuse behavior and signs and symptoms of use. This requires teamwork involving the medical staff, administration, and guidance and specialized substance abuse counselors if available in your system.

Schools do have a role in combating drug use among the student population which also includes anabolic steroids or other banned performance enhancing drugs (PED) for athletes.

Suspected steroid or PED use is often treated differently than suspected use of alcohol or other substances under state law and district policy. Often, coaches are in the best position to see the signs that a student may be using steroids.

The school nurse needs to ensure that coaches are properly trained to recognize these signs and understand the immediate and long-term health dangers associated with steroid use. This can be a difficult ethical issue, since coaches also face significant pressures to succeed and may therefore be reluctant to report suspected use. Effectively addressing this issue requires a concerted education campaign for coaches, parents, and student athletes in order to change the culture that may encourage looking the other way on suspected steroid or PED use.

In sum, the school nurse needs to understand state law and local policy related to addressing suspected substance use, ensure that student safety always overrides other competing demands and interests, work to educate all stakeholders on the signs and dangers of substance use, ensure informed decision-making related to the dangers of on-site testing, respect the privacy of students and families, and work to build a climate of trust within that community without sacrificing a sober and safe school.

Chronic Absence From School

In schools we promote presence and decry absence. The child is absent from school for various reasons such as illness, family issues, travel, or appointments outside of school. The school nurse will exclude the child from school for vomiting, diarrhea, undiagnosed rash, fever greater than 100.4°F, or conjunctivitis. Students may also be separated for reasons of ongoing medical concerns as described in their medical exclusions such as chemotherapy, bed rest, or infectious disease. Other reasons for chronic absence from school are poverty, food insecurity, caring for a family member, bad grades, bullying, disengagement, development of a school phobia, and illness/injury.

Throughout the United States, addressing chronic absenteeism has become a major priority. For example, nearly three quarters of all states have included chronic absenteeism as a school accountability indicator under the federal Every Student Succeeds Act or ESSA (Attendance Works, n.d.). Under ESSA, chronic absenteeism is defined as missing 10% or more school days within one academic year for any reason. The "for any reason" piece is important, since the larger issue involved is the educational impact of chronic absenteeism, even if the absences are for legitimate reasons.

When a student is out for a prolonged period as determined by board of education policy, the student qualifies for home instruction. In recent years, states have expanded the concept of home instruction beyond the student's home for student and faculty safety. Now, home instruction may involve going to the library to meet a student or students rather than being alone at their home.

Ethical issues arise when absence borders on truancy—which is defined under state law and includes a specific number of unexcused absences which will vary by state.

Nurses may collect the medical notes from providers to prove and define what is needed for a student to return to school. Often, the school nurse will receive a doctor's note that is vague, or may not have been signed, or may otherwise need clarification or authentication. Under the Family Educational Rights and Privacy Act, a school nurse or school physician may contact the doctor's office in such cases and confirm the authenticity of the note and ask relevant clarifying questions. For example, the note may have no anticipated return date. Or the doctor may not have indicated whether the student is capable of attending school for a portion of the school day, rather than not at all. Or the note may have been signed by a staff person in the office without the doctor's knowledge or consent. It is important to note that schools are not permitted to demand a student's medical diagnosis under the Family Educational Rights and Privacy Act (FERPA) or the Health Insurance Portability and Accountability Act of 1996 (HIPAA). However, the school does have the right to know the impact that a student's medical condition may have on a student's ability to function in school, and the school nurse will have the right to specific medical information in some cases, as when the school nurse is required to administer prescribed medications. Generally speaking, schools are governed by FERPA, rather than HIPAA, when it comes to student's medical information. Additional resources are identified for further information on these laws.

When there is a lack of clear or authentic information regarding student absence, and the absence is prolonged, the student risks repeating the grade level or not graduating. This situation is aggravated when the student is chronically absent due to other factors, such as being a caretaker of family members, working late hours, or trying to reach municipal services which are only available during the school day. While school resource officers or attendance officers when present in the school system are helpful, they are not always available and accessible for needy students.

Another complication involves students whose absence may be linked to unexplained or suspicious injuries. In such cases, the school nurse may have specific information that leads to a reasonable suspicion that the student is possibly being abused. For example, the nurse may have treated a student for an injury, where the child's explanation of the injury is not credible, given the nurse's knowledge. While state laws vary, they generally require school officials to immediately report suspected abuse, and then have child welfare agencies conduct the investigation, rather than school officials. In some cases, dual reporting to law enforcement is also required, in part to ensure that immediate action is taken if necessary to address the needs of the student, perhaps even preventing the student from going home that day.

It is up to the administration to discipline those students who are absent because they are "gaming the system" and may need to receive disciplinary action. The nurse becomes a partner when she has knowledge that would aid the individual student to avoid such disciplinary action, perhaps because the student confided in the nurse as to why they were absent. Incarcerated students present a unique set of issues upon release. Such students may have unique medical needs that the school nurse needs to be aware of, including particular physical or mental health issues that could impact that student or others. Again, the nurse's office is the repository of records, information, and screening needed for those students who fail to show up.

So when does it become truancy or a case for the child welfare agencies to step in on behalf of the child? When does chronic absence become a concern?

Much has been written about Munchausens by Proxy or parents willingly keeping students home for various selfish reasons. Often those reasons are for the offending parent to obtain custody, seek notoriety, emotional loneliness in a marriage, and to feel needed and worthwhile. Children are often subjected to various doctor's visits, treatments, hospitalizations, and home care that frustrates the school from providing home instruction. The teacher is often met at the door or in the library when the parent denies access to the student due to fatigue or some concern.

The nurse may have known the student over the years, observed them at school, and been aware of the family's requests for services. Nurses are uniquely positioned to be truth tellers to administrators who are concerned over an absence pattern. An example may be that of a "sick student" according to the parent who has exceeded the absence limit, but shows up at school events, lunch, or riding a bike all over town. When does a nurse feel confident to report such behavior in light of what is on record? When can the nurse consult with the school physician to intervene with colleagues regarding what is observed and what is written?

Working with guidance or social services, the nurse can often resolve these issues. The school physician consultant is also critical in obtaining parent consent to speak on behalf of the school to medical colleagues regarding the ongoing and future care of students who are absent. Again, record keeping is critical should there be a question of the student's need for exemptions or grade achievement.

Parents and children with special needs often require accommodations to guarantee their presence in class. Under Section 504 of the Rehabilitation Act of 1973, schools are required to ensure equal access to an education for students with disabilities. This law requires schools to identify and address the needs of students with a mental health or physical impairment that impacts one or more major life activities (such as learning, concentrating, eating, drinking, etc.), and to provide reasonable accommodations for such students. Similarly, the Individuals with Disabilities Act requires school district's to identify and address the needs of students who have a disability that impacts the ability of that student to receive a free and appropriate public education (FAPE). When a student is eligible under both IDEA and Section 504, the best practice is for the student to have a single individualized educational program (IEP) under IDEA that addresses the student's educational needs and incorporates those elements that would otherwise be included in a 504 plan. As the Office for Civil Rights made clear in guidance released in 2016, a doctor's note is one piece of relevant information in determining whether or not a student is eligible for a 504 plan, but must be considered in concert with other relevant information. In addition, the doctor's input regarding appropriate accommodations is not determinative, and in some cases a doctor may be prescribing accommodations that are inappropriate or less effective than other alternatives. The key is to consider the doctor's information and gather information from other sources, which may include the school nurse, the teacher in the classroom, and other knowledgeable persons about that student's needs and appropriate accommodations. Working with the guidance team and under federal and state statutes and codes, these students benefit from in-class education. However, due to their medical needs and conditions, these students sometimes exceed the normal absences. Usually it is for medical appointments, surgery, or adjustments to the 504 or IEP plans, or transportation issues. Generally, these are excused absences. Sometimes it behooves the school to place a student in out-of-school placement or in a special program to complete their education as standard school is sometimes not a good fit.

Regardless, the nurse should play a role in the committee deliberations on the student's needs at school including the need for an aid or nurse specialist.

Chronic absence may also result from a real school phobia that could develop for a variety of reasons. A student may be struggling with underlying mental health issues. The student may have experienced bullying or a traumatic experience such as the loss of a loved one. There is a growing body of case law in which courts are demanding that school districts work to address the social and emotional needs of students, in addition to academic needs. In some cases, schools may have a child find obligation that is triggered under Section 504 or IDEA when a student is unable to attend school or function in school.

Chronic absence can also be influenced by poverty, recent immigration, work, and religious holidays not on the Board of Education calendar. For all the reasons given for absence, we may excuse medical needs, sometimes excuse absence due to other social service needs, and for religious requirements. But even where such absences are excused, the school nurse and others should continuously explore ways to get the student back into school, even on a partial basis. For example, it may be worthwhile in some cases to arrange transportation for a student to be in school for a portion of the school day. Perhaps a student dealing with school phobia is able to function well in a particular class, and having that positive experience in school could gradually be extended over time in order to facilitate the student's full return. Often the school nurse can help by encouraging such "outside the box" thinking.

Team work by the school nurse with administrators and guidance or social service agents help to keep vulnerable children form forming a pattern of unnecessary absence.

Administrative Support

One of the more ethical concerns for the school nurse points to the working relationship with administrators. Principals and superintendents have a lot to do with a successful school practice. Administrators and school nurses can either work together or can sometimes work at cross purposes. Typically, this occurs where the administrator and nurse do not fully appreciate and/or respect the educational, legal, and/or ethical responsibilities of each party.

An example of working at cross purposes is sometimes seen in the enforcement of vaccine codes, laws, and regulations as they apply to student and public health. School nurses retain the records of student vaccines and their completeness or lack thereof. If a student's family is noncompliant in obtaining the necessary vaccinations for admittance to school or the appropriate grade, they are generally excluded. (Note that there are specific exceptions under federal law that allow for the immediate enrollment of a homeless student even without vaccinations. Additional exceptions may apply depending on your state's requirements.)

Medical exemptions aside, it is expected that the school administration will not grant the student's family extensions or grace periods that are not written into the state's laws. When this happens, it places the nurse in a situation of confrontation or losing all authority. Similarly, it is expected that the school nurse will not prevent a homeless student from enrolling and attending school, even without all vaccinations in place.

Another example is enforcement of district policy on substance use and/or possession at school. It is critical that the school nurse and school administration have a clear understanding of state law when it comes to addressing this issue. In some jurisdictions, it is appropriate for the school nurse to make a medical determination as to whether or not it is reasonable to suspect that a student is under the influence of alcohol or other controlled substances and, therefore, needs to be seen by a doctor. In other states, if any staff member expresses a belief that a student may be under the influence "the train has left the station" and the student must be sent out for a medical examination. The school nurse and school administrator need to know and follow the state's required protocols on this issue. Regardless of state laws, it would always be ill advised for a school principal to disregard or overrule a school nurse who has expressed concerns that a student may be under the influence. As a general rule, school officials should err on the side of student safety and send a student out for medical examination when in doubt.

To provide adequate health services which include the ability to listen to students' and parents' concerns, the school nurse needs the support of the administration of the school. The school nurse has access to sensitive health information on many students. At times, a tension can arise between the school nurse and other school officials who believe they could better serve students if they also had information regarding that student's health status.

Generally speaking, FERPA is the applicable federal law that must be considered in determining what information may be shared by the school nurse with other school staff. The legal standard for sharing information under FERPA is "legitimate educational interest."

For example, a school bus driver may need to know that a student is prone to seizures and the appropriate steps to take if that situation arises.

As another example, the nurse is generally aware of when a new medication is being taken and what the side effects may be, and thus is one step ahead of the classroom teacher who may notice a change in a student's behavior. Here again, teamwork is the critical factor of dual reporting. The classroom teacher may have a legitimate educational interest in receiving some information about the health side effects that a student may experience in class. Physician prescribers and families count on this type of feedback.

Coaches are also a part of that need to know. At the beginning of each sports season, the nurse usually supplies a coach with a list of students who are diabetic, have seizure disorders, are asthmatic, and so forth; these students require attention as well as perhaps have medical devices that need to be on the field for games and practices.

No one is served by the nurse keeping information secret or the administrators pushing coaches and teachers to overlook key medical information. And the reality of pre-participation physical examinations is all about the suitability to participate in sports. Some states have a standard form for admission, continuation in certain grades, and sports; however, when a school system decides to "go it alone" for various reasons, it is mandatory that the nurse be part of the team in deciding on the necessary medical information.

Occasionally a student will suffer a loss, come down with a chronic illness, finish a hospitalization, or be dealing with a newly diagnosed mental status. Confidentiality rules the day. Legally, the question is who has a "legitimate educational interest" in receiving that information. Specific and more restrictive confidentiality rules may apply to particular health issues. For example, the diagnosis of HIV is confidential and does not prevent a student from participation; however, in some states that information is shared only with the superintendent and the nurse.

Team work with administrators, teachers, and coaches when sharing information about student health promotes school student safety. Good record keeping and information sharing with administration is key to not allowing enabling behavior to subvert good healthcare. Often the school nurse is the most informed about the state laws regarding a student's presence in the school building. At no time should a nursing license be jeopardized by administrative behavior and at no time should a school nurse act outside of areas of responsibility. Working closely with the school's physician is critical. It is the physician who, as a non-faculty member, can often apprise the Board of Education, parents, and administration as to current code or statutes regarding immunizations, medical excuses, and return to school situations. The school nurse has many responsibilities, chief among them is ensuring compliance with legal requirements related to student health and safety. By promoting appropriate information sharing among all parties, working to educate key stakeholders on constantly evolving legal requirements, and understanding the responsibilities of school administrators, the potential for conflict is greatly reduced.

Often administrative cooperation is hampered by lack of knowledge of the rules. The responsibility of the head of a school is a daunting task and the number of regulatory agencies and legislative unfunded mandates continues to increase yearly. This makes a principal's or superintendent's job all the more difficult. This often comes into play with immunization regulations, chronic absence, truancy, and exemptions to physical education.

Generally, nurses and counselors at any level can establish a working relationship with administration to enforce the health and safety of all students and ensure legal compliance.

When necessary, nurses have the option of protecting their license by putting the concerns in writing. Good record keeping will always be helpful for school nurses. School nurses should also be aware of other supportive resources, such as the state nursing board, the school nurses association, and the department of education.

Working together to promote good health at a school is the optimum goal. While this takes time, planning, and patience, our children's well-being is worth the effort.

References

Attendance Works. (n.d.). *Policy: ESSA brief for states.* Retrieved from https://www.attendanceworks.org/policy/federal-policy/essa-brief-states/

Levy, S., Schizer, M., & Committee on Substance Abuse. (2015). Adolescent drug testing policies in schools. *Pediatrics, 135*(4), e1107–e1112.

U.S. Department of Education, Office for Civil Rights. (2016, December). *Parent and educator resource guide to Section 504 in public elementary and secondary schools.* Retrieved from https://www2.ed.gov/about/offices/list/ocr/docs/504-resource-guide -201612.pdf

Further Readings

AAP Committee on School Health. (2008). Role of the school nurse in providing health services. *Pediatrics, 121*(5), 1052–1056.

AAP (2014). Testing for Drugs of Abuse in Children and Adolescents. Pediatrics, 133(6), e1798–e1807. doi:10.1542 peds.2014-0865

Allison, M. A., Attisha, E., & Committee on School Health. (2019). The link between school attendance and good health. *Pediatrics, 143*(2).

Ammerman, S., Ryan, S., Adelman, W. P., & and the Committee on Substance Abuse, the Committee on Adolescence. (2015). The impact of marijuana policies on youth: Clinical, research, and legal update. *Pediatrics, 135*(3), e769–e785.

Centers for Disease Control and Prevention. (2012). If you choose not to vaccinate your child, understand the risks and responsibilities. Retrieved from https://www.cdc.gov/ vaccines/hcp/conversations/downloads/not-vacc-risks-color-office.pdf

Committee on Infectious Diseases. (2019). Recommended childhood and adolescent immunization schedule: United States, 2019. *Pediatrics, 143*(3).

Committee on Practice and Ambulatory Medicine and Council on Community Pediatrics. (2010). Increasing immunization coverage. *Pediatrics, 125*(6).

Committee on Substance Abuse and Council on School Health. (2007). Testing for drugs of abuse in children and adolescents: Addendum—Testing in schools and at home. *Pediatrics, 119*(3), 627–630.

Council on School Health and Committee on Substance Abuse. (2007). The role of schools in combating illicit substance abuse. *Pediatrics, 120*(6), 1379–1384.

Flaherty, E. G., MacMillan, H. L., & Committee on Child Abuse and Neglect. (2013). Caregiver-fabricated illness in a child: A manifestation of child maltreatment. *Pediatrics, 132*(3), 590–597.

Green, R., & Reffel, J. (2009). Comparison of administration and school nurse perceptions of the school nurse role. *Journal of School Nurse, 25*(1), 62–71.

Holmes, B. W. (2016, June 20–21). Pediatrician-school nurse partnership vital to child health: AAP policy. *AAP News*.

New Jersey Administrative Code (NJAC).

nurse.org. (2019, June 1). *New law allows school nurses to give medical marijuana-CBD Oil-to Kids in Colorado*. Retrieved from https://nurse.org

State Departments of Health USA for schedule requirements for schools.

Stein, P. (2019, September 19). D.C. approves law to allow licensed students to consume medical marijuana at school. *The Washington Post*. Retrieved from https://www.washingtonpost.com/local/education/d-c-approves-law-to-allow-licensed-students-to-consume-medical-marijuana-at-school/2019/09/18/a0ac3066-da1a-11e9-a688-303693fb4b0b_story.html

21ST CENTURY TECHNOLOGY FOR THE SCHOOL NURSE

JANET HALDER

LEARNING OBJECTIVES

- Identify shifts in technology and electronic documentation and communication in the school nurse setting.
- Describe technology alternatives to handwritten nursing notes and interdepartmental communication.
- Discuss available web-based Student Information Systems.
- Examine the impact of Wearable Technology and Telemedicine.

▌ Introduction

Until the advent of technology, student medical information was handwritten and kept in carefully guarded, locked cabinets in the school nurse's office. Cumbersome amounts of paper documentation followed every student from elementary to middle and then to high school.

Through the years, medical professionals have adapted to an inexhaustible number of new ideas to improve patient care, and technology has undoubtedly been critical to these improvements. Technology has drastically changed the field of clinical nursing and is quickly finding its way into the school health office. School nurses have become increasingly accustomed to digital thermometers and electronic blood pressure cuffs, and many of their offices are now equipped with a computer. Incorporating technology innovations into school health offers boundless possibilities and numerous benefits. School nursing is a unique specialty, challenging the very often lone practitioner to find ways to keep the focus on student care rather than time-consuming and often overwhelming clerical tasks. Advances in technology offer new possibilities for the school nurse and are designed to assist and support critical school nursing goals.

Electronic medical records (EMR) offer easy access to student medical information and facilitate communication with authorized users. Teachers and administrators can share relevant parts of the electronic data, much of which school nurses traditionally had to hand deliver. A well designed, web-based medical information system can track student visits, screenings, medications, athletic physicals, and medical concerns. The enormous amount of stored information is a rich source of well-child data useful for research. In this age of electronics and emerging medical innovations, tiny computerized devices, called wearable medical technology, such as blood glucose sensors, wireless tracking tags, and vagus stimulators, are all part of the exciting future of technology in school nursing.

■ The 21st Century School Health Office

Medical and technological advances have changed healthcare, and therefore nursing, dramatically.

More than a decade ago, the National Education Association co-founded the Partnership for 21st Century Skills (Battelle for Kids, n.d.), encouraging schools to infuse technology into education. That has led to designs for 21st-century classrooms, 21st-century libraries, 21st-century skills for students, and many more "21st-century" ideas for schools and education. Unfortunately, there is no mention of technology for the 21st-century health office in that partnership.

In many school health offices across the country, technology has not kept pace with either medical technology or educational technology. Often, in schools where technology has been well infused, their school information systems leave out components that include the health office. Too often, nurses are given older computers that are hand-me-downs from classrooms or administrative offices, and school nurses are left running both large and small offices without the latest hardware and software to best meet the needs of students. In a time when there is an expanding number of technology-dependent children and limitless technological possibilities for the care of those students, it is of great concern when the health office is under-equipped.

Let's take a peek at the 21st-century school nurse's office: This suburban middle school health office is centrally located, in easy walking distance to the busy gym and adjacent to the administrative offices that also house the Child Study Team. The classroom for special needs students is next door. One of the school's automated external defibrillators (AEDs) is clearly marked just outside the office, and is electronically connected to the local 911 number in an alarmed, steel, unlocked box. The brightly lit, spacious, and clean health office has three areas of activity and a separate, handicapped accessible bathroom. The office desk holds a laptop computer complete with a web-based student information system that includes a health program, a walkie-talkie, and a mini iPad. The iPad is receiving continuous blood glucose data on a sixth-grade boy who is upstairs in math class. There is one more laptop computer at a small standing desk just inside the door. When a student enters and signs in on the entrance computer, the student's name, time stamp, and complaint, which the student chooses from a drop-down menu, shows on the nurse's computer as well. As the school nurse stands up to greet this student and picks up the digital thermometer that is charging in its stand, the nurse already knows the girl's name, what class she is coming from, and what brings her to the health office. The office information systems program is linked to all school services. It can quickly check the past visits of this student, her attendance record, whether the student has any allergies, classroom accommodations, or custody issues. Additionally, the software program has interoperability among community healthcare agencies and providers whom the student has seen in the past. This interoperability makes it possible to see when the child's last visit to her doctor was, a diagnosis if one was determined, and medication dispensed at a pharmacy.

This 21st-century health office could have been the scene for a science fiction movie just 30 years ago. But medical and technological advances have changed healthcare, and therefore nursing, dramatically.

As recently as the 1970s, things were very different; nurses used the second hand on their wristwatch to calculate IV drip rates, and personal diabetes monitors and pumps were in the infant stages of development. In school health offices across the country, mercury thermometers were used to take a student's temperature. Portable AEDs in schools were unheard of, and there were only a few large school computers, often in converted building spaces, usually reserved for advanced math students. There were no computers in any of the administrative offices and certainly not one in the school health office.

School nurses who began their practice in the 1970s or 1980s have lived through the explosion of technology in medicine and education. They have a keen perspective on how that has changed both clinical and school nursing. Technology has improved patient outcomes, and its development and implementation have changed the face of healthcare. Data gathered and stored in computerized school health offices are a huge resource for the analysis of information on school-aged children. It has helped patients modify behaviors, allowed more precise therapies, developed remote patient monitoring, and devised ways to remind patients to take medication or to exercise. Younger nurses who grew up surrounded by technology may take for granted even the small technological advances of electronic IV monitors, electronic sphygmomanometers, state-of-the-art vision screening equipment, and portable defibrillators. The future of school nursing lies in the hands of these tech-savvy registered professional nurses who will help build school health centers that incorporate the time-saving, life-supporting, more comprehensive technology now available.

■ Electronic Medical Records

Nursing documentation has been an essential part of patient care from the earliest days of nursing, but over time documentation responsibility has changed immensely. Years ago, the doctor wrote down what he wanted to be done, and the nurse followed the orders and charted, in narrative form, everything that had been done to carry out the directives. Documentation has progressively become part of a much more significant and wide-ranging complex patient profile; it is expected to cover the steps in the Nursing Process from patient assessment to evaluation. Proper nursing documentation supports the delivery of excellent patient care. With the advancement of technology, electronic documentation has developed as a means of communication among members of the healthcare team, and, in some cases, other off-site medical stakeholders All health documentation, including electronic, describes the health needs of the student, evaluates care delivery effectiveness, and links intervention to outcome. It supports legal requirements and plans for care, and continues to be part of the historical patient care record.

Until recently, all documented patient information was simply a collection of filed paper data that was too unmanageable to deliver information. With electronic capability, large amounts of accumulated electronic data can be analyzed to yield knowledge and improve patient outcomes. Over the last three decades, as medical and nursing technology has advanced, nurses have learned to navigate a long list of technology-related challenges, including electronic charting. Electronic documentation in hospitals, long-term care facilities, home-care settings, and medical offices has become the norm and has now found its way into the school health office. EMRs are here to stay and nurses, including school nurses, must develop proficiency in managing these new dimensions.

◼ School Health Office Technology

Basic computer technology in the health office has streamlined practice and allowed more time to be spent practicing the time-honored skills of our profession: active listening, compassion, patient education, critical observation, and assessment.

When the 21st century dawned on school nursing, many offices were equipped with a computer, Wi-Fi, and an email address, now considered the bare bones of modern medical technology. Armed with those tools, the school nurse had tip-toed into the 21st century. Many school health offices are still operating with only these tools and, with them, nurses have quite successfully organized student health information, and set up systems to communicate with teachers and administrators in their building, as well as parents and the broader healthcare community. The Google search bar alone replaces the *Physicians' Desk Reference* and many other nursing and medical reference books. A computer in the health office puts a world of medical information at the fingertips of a busy school nurse.

Basic computer technology in the health office has streamlined practice and allowed more time to be spent practicing the time-honored skills of our profession: active listening, compassion, patient education, critical observation, and assessment. Even without commercial integrated school and health office informatics systems, the nurse can create spreadsheets for vision, hearing, blood pressure, and scoliosis screening, and data can be entered and stored electronically. From a well-designed spreadsheet, data such as students with distance vision greater than 20/30, hearing deficits, high blood pressure readings, or out of range BMIs can be pulled out of the spreadsheet for analysis. A "home-made" electronic health record database, created in-house, using Microsoft Access or Microsoft Works, makes it possible to keep track of referrals or pull up immunization information that, without electronic records, would take hours to search for.

As professionals in the field of school nursing, we know that healthy children learn better, and children who learn become more productive adults. More than ever before, school nurses are working to minimize the obstacles to learning for students with disabilities or chronic diseases. Medical technology can help support the student and the nurse in delivering 21st-century care. Children with special needs, associated with technology dependencies, who formerly would have been managed at home or in the hospital, are often able to attend school if the school nurse is adequately prepared to support both the child and the family. Children who are oxygen dependent, with tracheostomies with or without ventilators, enteral feeding tubes, or IV infusions, are now able to attend school, and the school health office must have the technology to support them.

The National Association of School Nurses (NASN) describes the professional school nurse as the person who "serves in a pivotal role that bridges health care and education" (NASN, 2019). Equipped with adequate technology, the nurse can better coordinate student health among the medical home, family, and school, and better achieve success in that pivotal role.

The school nurse's role as communicator is enormous. In this age of medically fragile students in school, specialized education, and individual student plans, the nurse is often in the middle of a whirlwind of information. As each day unfolds, a great deal of critical information is gathered and processed in the health office. Parents call about their child's absence which sometimes includes supplemental information ranging from fever or infection to anxiety or a special home situation. Teachers are continually calling with information or questions concerning students with health-related modifications, while administrators may report information about a playground fight that needs nurse follow-up. And, as each student comes into the office, the nurse gathers more pertinent information with health implications. School nurses, with access to a computer in their office, can more easily meet the challenge of gathering, processing, storing, and disseminating essential information.

With a computer and fair proficiency, the school nurse can save time as she meets these and other responsibilities. Documents can be written, sorted, and shared electronically or via email. A Google feature in Google Gmail called Confidential Mode is an easy way to make email even more private. Confidential Mode lets users add an expiration date to a sent document, and once that date is reached the email is no longer viewable. Emails marked as Confidential can't be copied, forwarded, printed or downloaded. Using this confidential feature, teachers who have the "right to know" receive the information, and there is no risk of the message be further shared.

Software designed for online word processing as well as spreadsheet and presentation creation, combined with sharing capability, opens a world of time-saving in a busy health office. The nurse no longer has to leave the office to meet with classroom teachers for the dissemination of simple lists or directives regarding a particular student. Although telephone calls can be used to alert teachers when necessary, an email or shared computer document carries with it a timestamp and verification of notice. Often, and especially when there is only one nurse in a building, it is difficult to leave the activity-teeming office for meetings with faculty. Locking the health office for teacher training or information sharing is likely to result in a long line of children at the door or in the main office when the nurse returns. Two or more people can work on a shared document without having actually to be together. Once a Google document is opened, it can be shared with one or several other people who can view, comment, or edit the document. File sharing makes it simple for different departments in the school to add information to a list of students. For example, the nurse can create and share a list of student athletes with the guidance counselor and assistant principal. The nurse, counselor, and assistant principal can work separately, but at the same time, to fill in pertinent information such as the date of a student's last physical, academic eligibility, and discipline eligibility.

In most districts, school nurses are responsible for staff health education. Some of the required faculty teaching can be done using presentation software such as Microsoft PowerPoint or Google slides. Detailed information with graphs, pictures, and text can be incorporated on slides and sent via email to teachers, and watched at the convenience of individual faculty members. Thus, EpiPen and glucagon delegate training, as one example, could be viewed by teachers online, and then a posttest and hands-on training with the nurse educator could follow. Of course, all sharing and training sent from the health office, whether electronic or not, must comply with Family Educational Rights and Privacy Act (FERPA), and Health Insurance Portability and Accountability Act (HIPAA) regulations.

Creating computer folders that are clearly named and dated is an effective way to store mountains of information. With the computer's editing capabilities, the endless lists of information can be pulled up, often year after year, and added to, or changed, without rewriting entire documents. The concerns list that took hours to compile last year can be electronically stored and easily updated for next September. It can then be sent to the necessary teachers who can print or electronically store it in a folder on their own password-protected computer. The flu shot flyer that took 30 minutes to create last year is quickly retrieved, re-dated, and re-sent to teachers, secretaries, administrators, and custodians. With some good technologic organization, the time-saving possibilities are endless.

▓ Electronic Medical Records and Electronic Health Records

No doubt, a technology system that unites school nurse practice with both educational and out-of-school health systems can improve healthcare and education opportunities for children.

It was in 2004, with the creation of the Office of the National Coordinator of Health Information Technology, that the need to convert paper medical records to EMRs was nationally recognized (Department of Health and Human Services [DHHS], 2018). EMRs replace paper-based medical records and hold everything that would previously have been included in a paper chart. They are considered a secure and useful tool for maintaining patient healthcare data. The electronic record is not just a repository for digitized health information; hospitals, outpatient clinics, pharmacies, insurance providers, diagnostic centers, and patients themselves can share EMRs through an interoperable electronic health records (EHRs) system. Interoperability among stakeholders makes the electronic health record an appropriate tool for all hospitals, medical professionals, insurance companies, imaging centers, and government agencies, and is equally valuable for school nurses (Box 24.1).

While a computer in the health office can save time and facilitate communication within the school district, there are higher goals school nurses must work toward. The school nurse will be standing with both feet firmly planted in the 21st century when the school health office is equipped with the capability to generate EMRs and be part of an EHRs system that interfaces with other members of each student's health systems.

Web-based EHRs with interoperability are in place in some hospitals, private, and out-patient medical offices and are the future for school health offices. When sharing beyond the building and beyond the district becomes possible, the full benefits of the interoperability of EHRs will come to fruition for school health.

A patient's healthcare journey can take them from a doctor's office to a laboratory to a pharmacy.

BOX 24.1

ELECTRONIC MEDICAL RECORDS (EMRs) VERSUS ELECTRONIC HEALTH RECORDS (EHRs)

Electronic Medical Record
A single practice's digital patient cart.

Generated by:

Practitioner	Insurance carrier
Physician	Imaging center
Nurse	Clinic
Specialist	Surgeon
Dentist	

Contains:
Medical history
Diagnoses
Treatments

Electronic Health Record
Designed to reach out *beyond* the single practice that originally compiles the information. A compilation of medical records from all healthcare stakeholders, they are built to share information with other health care providers. Authorized users may instantly access a patients EHRs.

Every stop generates a record of physicians' notes, lab results, and medication, which can all become part of a patient's EHR. Interoperable EHRs allow all coordinating medical professionals to access and transmit patient information instantly, and allows collaboration among providers. Additionally, patients can have access to their own health records; they can see their diagnostic test results, send messages to providers, and make appointments.

The NASN states that "registered professional school nurses should have access to a software platform for student EHRs that includes nursing language/medical terminology and complies with standards of confidentiality, security, and privacy. Interoperability of records with other members of the healthcare and school-based teams facilitates optimal student/population health and academic outcomes." ... "Electronic health records are an essential tool for school nurses to keep students healthy" (NASN, 2019).

No doubt, a technology system that unites school nurse practice with both educational and out-of-school health systems can improve healthcare and education opportunities for children. There were 56.6 million children entering school for the 2019–2020 school year (National Center for Education Statistics, 2019), and many of those children did not have a primary care health provider; a school nurse may be the only medical professional a child sees. School nurses are trained in assessment and documentation, and very often are the first health professional to see an ill or injured student. Information that the school nurse enters into a child's medical record, including assessments, family information, screenings, and immunizations, may be the child's first or only health record. School nurses are an essential part of the total healthcare of students as well as the link between student health and education. Professional school nurses coordinate care for children with chronic conditions or disabilities and afford students access to education. Regardless of a child's health status, school nurses promote student health as a support for learning. The wherewithal to receive and share student EHRs fully incorporates the school nurse in the greater healthcare system. Because the school nurse is a critical provider and central stakeholder for student wellness, the 21st-century school nurse will become a full partner with all community healthcare systems when equipped with a software platform for student EHRs that interface with other clinicians.

Web-Based Student Information and Administrative Software Systems for Schools

In the school environment where the nurse is often practicing alone, it is immensely important to have time-saving tools at one's disposal so care can be devoted to students rather than to time-consuming clerical tasks. The nurse should be aware of the available possibilities designed to streamline health office responsibilities. There is a large selection of commercial pre-kindergarten through grade 12 software systems available for school administrative and student management. Some also have a well-constructed additional module for the school health office (Box 24.2).

BOX 24.2

STUDENT INFORMATION AND ADMINISTRATIVE SOFTWARE SYSTEMS FOR SCHOOLS

1. Cloud-based pre-K–12 Integrated School Management System **without** a health office component, i.e., *Administrator's Plus*.

2. Web-based pre-K–12 Student Information and Administration Software System **with** a health office component, i.e., *Genesis*.

3. Web-based PK–12 software suite that is a **stand-alone health office** system, i.e., *SNAP Health Center*.

---

1. The first category of school software systems manages student, personnel, and financial school records. They generally allow for communication among parents, teachers, administrators, and the community. The products are web- or cloud-based systems that allow vast amounts of information to be stored without taking up space on school computer systems. System features can include attendance tracking, school-wide analytics tracking, district accounting and budgeting, curriculum creation for teachers, assignment management, grade book management, and report card creation. Some advertise access to real-time and longitudinal data to monitor student progress and manage FERPA, HIPAA, and Children's Online Privacy Protection Act (COPPA) compliance. Data about school facilities, bus transportation, and school lunches are often included. One example of this type of system is the Rediker product called **Administrator's Plus**.

2. Another choice for schools is also a web-based Student Information and Administrative Software System that has all of the components noted in item 1 and also includes a comprehensive school health module. An example is **Genesis**, an administrative software system for New Jersey schools. The health program allows the school nurse to check-in a student, chart from a drop-down menu, and add narrative information. It includes many other search and record features such as checking for prior visits, recording and tracking health screenings, recording physicals submitted for students, tracking daily medications, and generating New Jersey-mandated reports for student admission and transfer. Additional health data can be entered and sorted by variables such as grade, age, time, or complaint. The program is compatible with both major operating systems, it has an alert feature for students with special healthcare needs, supports student photo import, facilitates student sign-in on a second computer, and allows the nurse to follow multiple students simultaneously. It is a comprehensive

system that assists the nurse in delivering sophisticated care in a busy, fast-paced school health office.

3. **SNAP Health Center** is a stand-alone health office program, designed by and for nurses and has similar functionality to the Genesis health office module. It has system tracking capability, which could be valuable for tracking student information such as concussions, falls in school, or flu cases. **SNAP** allows access to student's Emergency Action Plans and allows parents to access and update their child's health information. Teachers and administrators can view health information such as student allergies, classroom modifications, and action plans within the confines of FERPA and HIPAA regulations. The program has graphing ability that could be used for medication administration, student vision screening, or BMIs.

New ideas and innovations continually find their way into nursing. New medical technology persistently pushes the limits of our experience as there seems to be an inexhaustible number of new ideas for nursing professionals. While school nurses are encouraged to embrace advances, they must also be aware of potential drawbacks to these new frontiers.

Implementing a new software system is expensive and takes time-intensive training—both precious resources in schools. There are serious legal implications when health records are incomplete or missing; therefore, when a school decides to implement a new technology system, loss of information from previous records, paper or electronic, must be carefully considered. All past information must be completely recoverable. A school health office system is continually communicating with the network and cannot function without reliable network connectivity. Consequently, Wi-Fi systems must function at the highest level. School nurses know that health office information is strictly confidential, and any system implemented in school must guarantee safeguards to unauthorized access to health information.

▪ Selection of a School Health Documentation System

Although EHRs are the gold standard and are inching closer, health information systems still fall short of seamless interoperability.

The selection of a school district's integrated, comprehensive school health documentation system should be made with a great deal of input from the school nurse. Administrators, IT professionals, and school nurses should work together to find a system. The system should be cost-effective and embedded with the necessary security and privacy requirements, including HIPAA and FERPA compliance, individual password capability, overwrite protection, selective limits on sharing information, and a secure back-up system. The system should support data points defined by the NASN, have drop-down and narrative charting capability, and include comprehensive system training at startup and beyond. Additional key elements in the selection of a school health documentation system are found in Box 24.3. Any system purchased should include a legal agreement between the school and the provider regarding the use and maintenance of all student data.

BOX 24.3

ADDITIONAL ELEMENTS TO CONSIDER IN THE SELECTION OF A SCHOOL HEALTH DOCUMENTATION SYSTEM

Multiple students followed simultaneously	504, integrated health plan, individualized education program tracking
Student photo import	
Alert feature for students with health care needs	Medical alert information
Medication tracking	Accident templates and reports
Administration	Screening tracking
Drug reference	Automatic backup
Expiration tracking	Immunization tracking

Many school nurses report access to school electronic documentation systems, such as the ones cited, that do not have the capability of sharing with the greater healthcare system that true EHRs afford. All of these Student Information and Administrative Software Systems with an add-on or stand-alone health module do an excellent job. However, they lack the element of true interoperability with other members of students' healthcare teams.

While the NASA and school nurses may be completely invested in the value of EHRs, we all know that change comes slowly. Although EHRs are the gold standard and are inching closer, health information systems still fall short of seamless interoperability. There are barriers to the goal, and school districts, perhaps more so than private stakeholders, face many challenges of incorporating EHRs with comprehensive interoperability. One would think that full integration and interoperability across systems is doable considering the smartphones we use, the smart cars we drive, and the smart credit cards we carry. Although the NASN and the federal government have set forth initiatives to implement EHRs in all clinical settings, including school health offices, significant obstacles exist and must be resolved before full integration is possible. The reality is that costs are high, there are privacy and security concerns regarding overwrite protection and confidentiality, and there are time-consuming issues with training and system integration. One challenge is the need for a nationally uniform patient identification system. Patient privacy concerns have slowed implementation of electronic systems, and without the ability to identify individuals across all systems, EHR sharing simply doesn't work. Achieving interoperability, that is, connecting EHR systems among providers, regardless of which software program a provider is using, has been another big challenge. Many providers have EHR systems but are unable to share information with other providers because, to date, there is not a single standard interoperability format for sharing data—leaving thousands of EHRs as a disconnected hodge-podge. Another impediment to interoperability is a practice called information blocking by companies or healthcare providers. Providers may not want to share information they have generated for security or privacy reasons, and vendors may charge hefty fees that discourage information sharing.

While schools wait for truly interoperable EHRs, there is some health information sharing that benefits the school nurse. All states have immunization registries that are confidential, population-based, computerized information systems that collect and consolidate vaccination data about children in the state. Nurses who are authorized and registered can search for records of immunizations within a state. States' Departments of Health also collect and disseminate information which can assist the school nurse in surveillance and prevention including data on communicable diseases, animal rabies, and influenza-like illnesses,

An increasing number of Community Health Information Networks (CHINs), which provide the infrastructure of interrelated Health Information Organization's computers on a smaller geographic scale, permit multiple providers to share and communicate healthcare information. For example, Camden, New Jersey, has a Health Information Exchange system that is used by providers in all the area's hospitals and primary care offices, and the city is looking for ways to connect school nurses to that network.

A school nurse who is presently using a well-constructed web-based student information system might question the advantage of EHRs that afford interoperability with a local, state, or national network of providers. School nurses may be reluctant to start over with new, more complete software when it is perfected, affordable, and accessible in the school setting. The question often asked is: Why is the idea of interoperability so important?

The simple answer is data, and the more intricate answer is big data. Whether school nurses like it or not, moving into the 21st century, as critical health practitioners, includes embracing big data.

▇ Big Data

School nurses engage with over 90% of the nation's children. In this data-driven era of analytics, the amount of information school nurses can collect, and its value, is possibly unsurpassed in any other area of healthcare.

A customer buys a pair of sneakers on the Internet and pays with a credit card, gives the company a street address, email address, bank information, shoe size, and even color preference. That's data. When someone goes to the pharmacy to pick up an antibiotic, the pharmacist enters a name, address, birthdate, medical insurance, and drug information into their computer system; that's data. When sports physicals are entered into the school health office program, with the student's age, last physical, sport the child is interested in playing, academic eligibility, injury, and concussion history, that's data. Immunizations that students receive are data, and each student's visit to the nursing office is entered with a complaint, length of stay, temperature, academic subject they are missing, and if they are sent home, that is data. Each student who is absent or tardy is also data.

Large volumes of data are considered Big Data.

School nurses engage with over 90% of the nation's children (U.S. Census Bureau, 2013). In this data-driven era of analytics, the amount of information school nurses can collect and its value are possibly unsurpassed in any other area of healthcare. School nurses stand in a unique and powerful position to shape decisions and policies through data collection and sharing.

Rates of poverty in urban areas are growing, there is increasing acuity of student health problems, and there is a significant disparity in healthcare for racial and ethnic groups in the United States. Data gathered in school health offices could help meet the challenges of these problems and shape new national outcomes for children.

It is becoming apparent that the collection of health data is crucial to reach the full potential of the world's healthcare systems—the more health providers who support this goal, the greater the impact on clinical decision-making. If school nurses, in force, collect health data similarly across the nation, it will be possible to compare, for example, what happens in Ohio with what happens in Nebraska, making it easier to understand how differences in care affect health outcomes for children.

In 2018, the NASN put forth a data collection initiative that encourages school nurses to collect student health data that, they believe, "will connect school nursing with the greater healthcare system" (NASN, 2018). Data collection has the potential to identify relationships such as between student health office visits and test scores, office visits, and attendance; between inhaler use and school performance; or obesity and social-emotional development. School nurses also collect data from medical devices used by children in their care and have information about medication, including narcotics and opiates that are administered in school. The number of children who are absent from or late to school and the children who qualify for free lunch or medical insurance assistance are all valuable data points. School nurses keep vision, hearing, height, weight, blood pressure, and scoliosis records on well children. They have information on students with chronic conditions, and response data for students with asthma, allergies, seizure disorders, and diabetes. All these data, entered into a web-based interoperable information system, could be analyzed to see and understand the connections that exist between nurse intervention and student health outcomes and identify opportunities for improvement at all levels of care.

When one considers the combined data that can be collected by school nurses across the country, the far-reaching benefits for children are astounding. The widespread use of interoperable EHRs would realize those benefits.

Even on a smaller scale, school district-, county-, or state-level data collection can identify many school needs. Collected data can identify needs for teacher education, supplies, or extra staffing in the school health office. And they can point to the necessity for more significant mental health support, how chronic health conditions are affecting social-emotional wellness, whether health insurance is lacking, and how often children are seeing a primary care provider or dentist.

It is important to note that data are not only analyzed for statistics, although that information is always enlightening. Perhaps more important is that data can also be predictive by using past trends to predict future events. With predictive analytics, schools, or communities can calculate a potential risk posed and develop management plans to mitigate the risk. For example, the measles outbreak that began in 2018, in Rockland County, New York (New York State Department of Health, 2019), may have been avoided if data showing high rates of religious exemptions to vaccines for students in that county had been used as a predictor of the outbreak. Laws limiting medical and religious exemptions to immunizations that were enacted after the measles outbreak was full-blown could have been put in place ahead of the disaster and entirely averted the outbreak.

Privacy and Electronic Security

The highest standards of protection apply to information stored on computers in the health office. To ensure patient privacy, health records in the United States must comply with HIPAA, and FERPA. A database is an electronic system used by an organization as a method of storing, managing, and retrieving information. Since computerized health records require the storage of vast amounts of confidential patient data, the data must be stored in secure databases. In efforts to keep data secure, some healthcare settings have introduced security measures such as eye scans, bar codes, and wristbands to keep information safe.

Nurses working in schools have an equal responsibility to safeguard the privacy of student medical information. Laws are in place, with penalties, for those, including school nurses, who knowingly obtain or disclose individually identifiable health information. Information security is critical and should be addressed before any system is developed or installed in the school health office. The school nurse is possibly the only employee in the building or district with the education and understanding of the legal and ethical complexities of protecting health information, and the responsibility for security cannot be taken lightly. Employees should be trained and given copies of district security policies which they should be required to sign. Computers in the health office must be protected by a strong password, not easily guessed, and should be changed frequently. Substitute school nurses employed by the district should have their own password and should never sign in or chart using another nurse's password. Systems should offer overwrite protection, which ensures the creation of a legal record of charting. Student information on the screen must be shielded from view; a busy health office fills with students, teachers, staff, and parents, and it is easy to forget to shield or minimize the screen when a student comes in bleeding or gasping. Good, private computer positioning is essential.

Wearable Technology and Telemedicine

Wearable Technology

Since computers and the Internet have become so embedded in our lives, information is being fed by vast numbers of people and a huge system of interrelated computing devices. Common examples include home thermostats, security systems, smartphones, GPS devices, and hands-free voice controlled devices. These devices extend Internet connectivity beyond traditional devices like desktop or laptop computers to a diverse range of devices that use embedded technology to interact with the environment through the Internet. Wearable medical devices can monitor health by tracking daily steps, exercise levels, measuring heart rate and rhythm, and assessing sleep schedules. Some that are less common are body patches for EKG recording and cardiac monitoring, and skin sensors that monitor UV exposure. In 2017 the U.S. Food and Drug Administration approved a drug with a digital ingestion tracking system. The ingestible sensor embedded in the pill sends a message to verify that the medicine was actually taken. Information is transmitted to a mobile app so patients or caregivers can be sure the medication has been taken. Continuous glucose monitors and glucose sensors send blood glucose data to a computer or smartphone and update glucose data every 5 minutes, allowing students, parents, student aides, or school nurses to know a current glucose level. The monitor also displays up or down glucose trend arrows alerting users to rising or falling levels. There are wearable devices to detect seizures that include metal or silicone bracelets, wrist or ankle watches, body stickers, and necklaces. There are seizure sensitive mattresses, and seizure detecting cameras connected to computers. A single EKG lead attached to a smartphone has been developed to monitor episodic cardiac events in children. A smartphone app uses GPS and Wifi to remind a severely allergic person to bring their epinephrine when they leave home. There is now a bracelet to detect allergic reactions in children; the device uses light sensitive photodiodes to measure histamine levels so adult caregivers can treat a child's reaction before severe symptoms appear. Brain computer interface (BCI) systems are a technology that uses brain activity picked up by electrodes from a person's brain to control an external computer-driven device, for example, a prosthesis, to provide movement for a paralytic patient. All these devices are increasing the quality of patient care and bringing promise to people with health challenges. And, because school nurses are on the frontier of healthcare and often the first to see and use new devices or technologies, health offices must be supported with adequate technology and capable Wi-Fi access.

Telemedicine and Telehealth

Telemedicine and telehealth allow for medical advice, information, and some routine care remotely via smartphone messaging, online chat, or video conferencing. Telemedicine has evolved from chiefly being a way to bring medical care to rural areas to now becoming a way to offer care in urban and suburban areas as well. The goal of school-based telehealth, like all school health technology, is improved care and improved outcomes for children. Telemedicine brings a virtual doctor to the school, and in areas of South Carolina has shown decreases in students treated in the emergency department for asthma-related issues.

School nurses use a rolling cart with a high definition screen for videoconferencing and an array of digitally connected medical scopes that transmit sounds and pictures to the doctor via video. Telehealth extends the reach of healthcare and has the potential to keep more children in school and reduce time-consuming and expensive visits to the emergency department. The program requires a school nurse to be with the child at school, which increases nurse workflow. For this reason, already very busy school nurses sometimes resist the implementation of telemedicine into their schools.

Conclusion

The united power of school nurses across the nation, collecting and sharing data, would be unsurpassed in driving better health outcomes for children.

There is an enormous opportunity for school nurses to reshape school health practice and improve the delivery of care through technology. Academic success is unquestionably interwoven with the health and well-being of children, and with available technology, the school nurse can better impact both health and academic success. Evidence has shown that technology-driven data collection has the potential to transform the future of healthcare. The value and power of school nurses are enhanced when nurses recognize and acknowledge their unique contribution to childcare, and their role as an agent for change. The united power of school nurses across the nation, collecting and sharing data, would be unsurpassed in driving better health outcomes for children.

School nurses, invested in children's well-being, commit to continuous learning, skill development, and evidence-based practice; they are well-positioned to influence decisions and resource allocation for the health of children. The value of school nurses is closely related to their knowledge and confidence, which can give voice to necessary improvements in school healthcare. Decisions regarding technology to support school healthcare should be led by school nursing professionals committed to advancing the care of children into the future.

School districts that are budget constrained and often more focused on administrative and student technology than on health office technology may be swayed by professional school nurses when presented with well-researched information on the impact health office technology and related data collection could ultimately have on our nation's students' success.

References

Battelle for Kids. (n.d.). *Partnership for 21st century learning*. Retrieved from https://www.battelleforkids.org/networks/p21

Department of Health and Human Services, Office of the National Coordinator of Health Information Technology. (2018). *Justification of estimates for appropriations committee*. Retrieved from https://www.hhs.gov/sites/default/files/combined-onc.pdf

National Association of School Nurses. (2018). *National school health data set: Every student counts!* Retrieved from https://www.nasn.org/research/everystudentcounts

National Association of School Nurses. (2019). *Electronic health records: An essential tool for school nurses to keep students healthy* (Position Statement). Silver Spring, MD: Author. Retrieved from https://www.nasn.org/advocacy/professional-practice-documents/position-statements/ps-electronic-health-records

National Center for Education Statistics. (2019, August 13). *Back to school by the numbers: 2019–20 school year.* Retrieved from https://nces.ed.gov/blogs/nces/post/back-to-school-by-the-numbers-2019-20-school-year

New York State Department of Health. (2019, September). *Measles fact sheet.* Retrieved from https://www.health.ny.gov/publications/2170/

U.S. Census Bureau. (2013, September). *School enrollment in the United States:2011* (Report No. P20-571). Retrieved from https://www.census.gov/prod/2013pubs/p20-571.pdf

THE SHIFTING PARADIGM FOR SCHOOL HEALTH

LUCILLE A. JOEL

LEARNING OBJECTIVES

- Describe the meaning of population health to our practice.
- Appreciate the national and international impact of the Sustainable Development Goals (SDGs) and *Healthy People.*
- Identify approaches to instituting this new paradigm in professional education and school nursing practice.
- Anticipate the outcomes of a successful paradigm shift in school practice.

▊ Introduction

School nursing came into existence in 1902, at the encouragement of Lillian Wald, director of the Henry Street Settlement in New York City, later under her leadership to become the Visiting Nurse Service of New York. Early school nurses wore the medicalized uniforms associated with community nursing, but their concerns addressed a far broader agenda. Nursing currently finds itself in the midst of a paradigm shift for which those early days of school nursing may provide direction. Nursing curricula are deliberately moving toward the U.S. Department of Health, Education and Welfare's (DHEW) *Healthy People* initiative and the Sustainable Development Goals (SDGs) adopted by the United Nations as their focus since the year 2000 (UN, n.d.). These initiatives as well as population health are becoming the cornerstone for the study of nursing. The 17 goals (Box 25.1) of the SDGs and the Leading Health Indicators (LHIs; Box 25.2) of *Healthy People* set a broad multidimensional agenda that promises to impact social, economic, and political decision-making. Nurses are uniquely prepared to lead this work, bringing humanism to the clinical situation, as well as decision-making based on science and evidence. The need is to move past the linear assumptions and reductionist philosophy of our past to a new paradigm where clients are autonomous and empowered to participate on their own behalf with the support of family

BOX 25.1

2030 SUSTAINABLE DEVELOPMENT GOALS (SDGs), WORLD HEALTH ORGANIZATION
Goal 1: No poverty
Goal 2: Zero hunger
Goal 3: Good health and well-being
Goal 4: Quality education
Goal 5: Gender equality
Goal 6: Clean water and sanitation
Goal 7: Affordable and clean energy
Goal 8: Decent work and economic growth
Goal 9: Industry, innovation and infrastructure
Goal 10: Reduced inequalities
Goal 11: Sustainable cities and communities
Goal 12: Responsible consumption and production
Goal 13: Climate action
Goal 14: Life below water
Goal 15: Life on land
Goal 16: Peace, justice, and strong institutions
Goal 17: Partnerships for the goals

SOURCE: Reproduced with permission from the United Nations. *Sustainable development goals.* Retrieved from https://www.un.org/sustainabledevelopment/biodiversity/

and/or community and information technology. And the client may just as likely be a population as opposed to a single individual. Rising to this occasion requires new behaviors on the part of the caregiver, and introduction of this philosophy in the school, with parents, administration, and faculty socialized into this thinking.

Back to the Future

The early days of professional nursing practice were cast in the orientation of the public health, and there was a much more holistic understanding of community. This holistic view of community/population health grew out of the necessity to expand limited resources. Nurses were in the vanguard; they were relentless in their search for answers and willing to be creative in their inquisitiveness and risk-taking.

The first challenge is to define community/population. Populations may be geographically defined, defined by some common characteristic (membership in a health plan, employees of a specific corporation, congregants of a given church, or families in a specific school district), or by a common risk factor (smoker, low socioeconomic level,

BOX 25.2

LEADING HEALTH INDICATORS, *HEALTHY PEOPLE 2020*
- Access to health services
- Clinical preventive services
- Environmental quality
- Injury and violence
- Maternal, infant, and child health
- Mental health
- Nutrition, physical activity, and obesity
- Oral health
- Reproductive health
- Social determinants
- Substance abuse
- Tobacco

SOURCE: Office of Disease Prevention and Health Promotion. (n.d.). Leading health indicators development and framework. Retrieved from https://www.healthypeople.gov/2020/leading-health -indicators/Leading-Health-Indicators-Development-and-Framework

substance abuse, obesity). Population health is the distribution of health outcomes within a population, the determinants that influence distribution, and the policies and interventions that impact the determinants. The early nursing leaders in community and public health were also pioneers in population health. Margaret Sanger championed women's health among the immigrant population on New York's Lower East Side; Florence Wald focused her attention on the hospice population and the dying; Florence Nightingale dramatically reduced the mortality from battlefield wounds in the Crimea by introducing cleanliness and nutrition; Clara Maas made the yellow fever population the target of her practice and martyrdom; Dorothea Dix was the advocate for the mentally ill and established specialized hospitals for their care.

After two centuries of the progress of medical science, the dominant cultural bias of medicalization stresses a one-on-one priority in diagnosis and treatment driven by individual access not populations, and rendered by professionals trained for the job. The ensuing actions which have grown out of medicalization are rationing of health care resources (maybe not literally, but figuratively), the message to providers to "do what you are told," disruption of privileged relationships with caregivers, liability and distrust, and a crushing financial burden (both to government and individuals).

The Introduction of Systems Thinking

Today's practice environment is characterized as chaotic in its complexity and nurses claim to be overburdened by the myriad of factors which they must incorporate in their assessments, planning, interventions, and evaluation. But this need not be so, by breaking down the system into its parts, and viewing it as an open system as opposed to the mechanistic, linear paradigm of classical science, we can solve problems by looking at the relationships between those parts. All systems involved in a situation must be considered together, they are interdependent and interconnected, and what happens to one system has a ripple effect on all of the others. For example, intervening with a child's disruptive in-class behavior has implications for the child's school work and attendance, connectedness with peers, family relationships, perhaps mental/physical health, and other school-based and out-of-school activities. The child did not create this problem alone. Many people and factors were involved. All of the relevant parts must be identified, and their ownership or participation in the problem identified. They must own the problem, and adapt to change in order to find solutions. There is much you have to know about a child before you intervene. Nurses are comfortable with this style of thinking; it is no different than our understanding of the human body. Diabetes mellitus can forecast problems with vision, the heart, the liver, and the biliary system, and so on. The body is a fine-tuned system and problems with one system are often the precursor of multiple other problems which either preceded the primary problem or will surface over time. Leaning on one problem or the other can restore function, or realigning several may make the difference. The learning to take with you is that you can never look at one part of the puzzle in isolation. Is this too much to expect? No, this is nursing at its most holistic and comprehensive best.

History of Planning for Sustainability

Comprehensive planning for sustainable quality life experiences began in the environmental sector with the U.S. government's National Environmental Policy Act (NEPA) of 1969. This Act came largely in response to the 1969 Santa Barbara oil spill, which had a devastating impact on wildlife and the natural environment in the area. But NEPA was also the result of greater societal attention to the consequences of industrial pollution. Around the same time, and as a result of the push toward great concern for the environment, the Clean Water Act, the Water Quality Act, the push to ban DDT, and the institution of the National Wilderness Preservation System were all put into motion in the United States (University of Washington, 2015).

The last 50 years has witnessed a flurry of activity around the determinants/indicators of health and wellness. In the United States, there has been the *Healthy People* initiative, started in 1979 and currently in its fifth edition with *Health People 2030* (Centers for Disease Control and Prevention [CDC], 2019). The SDGs are the United Nation's blueprint for achieving a sustainable future. Consulting either of these documents will provide a comprehensive listing of determinants, and the challenges we face. The World Health Organization [WHO] offers an even simpler statement, "This unequal distribution of health-damaging experiences is not in any sense a 'natural' phenomenon but is the result of a toxic combination of poor social policies, unfair economic arrangements [where the already well-off and healthy become even richer and the poor who are already more likely to be ill become even poorer and sicker], and bad politics" (WHO, 2013).

Healthy People is a program for nationwide health-promotion and disease-prevention in response to an emerging consensus among scientists and health authorities that national health priorities should emphasize wellness (Healthy People 2020, n.d.). The *Healthy People* program was originally instituted by the DHEW, and later fell under the auspices of the CDC (2019). The first iteration contained goals for a 10-year period to reduce controllable health risks. The goals were subsequently updated every 10 years in *Healthy People 2000, Healthy People 2010, Healthy People 2020,* and *Healthy People 2030* (in process) each of which contained leading health indicators (LHIs) on which to focus.

As a natural companion to *Healthy People*, the government introduced the Healthy Communities program (HCP) in the last decades of the 20th century. Healthy Communities was designed to help with the work of *Healthy People* in state/regional/local communities, and to do this through coalitions of private and public sector entities and heavily promote volunteerism. By 2018, the CDC had funded 331 communities and 52 state and territorial health departments through the HCP with the intent of passing the "baton" to these local communities. As an outgrowth of Healthy Communities, a joint effort was established in 2018 between the regional Federal Reserve Banks and the Robert Wood Johnson Foundation to deepen collaboration across the sectors of community development, finance, population health, and public health (Build Healthy Places Network, n.d.). This is an excellent demonstration of the "American" way of partnering private and public sector resources to accomplish work which would otherwise remain dormant. The establishment of this country as a republic with deep commitment to states' rights and private investment for the public good suits this approach admirably.

All 50 states and the District of Columbia have been active participants in *Healthy People*. Many states have instituted their own reforms to eliminate self-identified health care disparities, and improve quality and value while managing cost. This is a direct result of prompting by the HCP initiative. A state-by-state summary of local initiatives can be found at: www.healthypeople.gov/2020/healthy-people-in-action/ State-and-Territorial-Healthy-People-Plans. Each State and Territory has a Healthy People Coordinator who serves as a liaison with the federal government. The Coordinator's job is to ensure their State or Territory's plan is in line with *Healthy People* goals and objectives. Most states have created data banks for surveillance of their own *Healthy People* profile, and have begun the work toward addressing inequities with an emphasis on primary care for needy populations, healthy living, and chronic disease management. In the State of Illinois, a network of 30 community-based health centers and free clinics deliver primary care to underserved populations. Other projects address dental health among HIV patients, the need for nutritious and affordable food, and rural and mobile primary care. Special projects in Maryland and Wisconsin direct their primary care efforts to the Latino and Hmong populations, respectively. New York State has dedicated a large part of its *Healthy People* resources to in-school education, making health literacy a priority, and accessing youth to information on HIV,

STD, and pregnancy. Hep Free Hawaii (HFH) is a collaborative effort of caregivers, community activists, and nonprofit organizations to increase awareness of, testing, and treatment for hepatitis and other liver diseases in Hawaii. Hawaii has the highest rate of liver cancer in the United States, a direct result of the disproportionately high rate of hepatitis infection in the Asian American, Native Hawaiian, and Pacific Islander populations in the state. By targeting this high risk population, HFH hopes to decrease liver cancer rates through prevention, early detection, and treatment of hepatitis.

In comparable fashion, the UN moved forward, beginning with the 1972 Stockholm Conference on Human Environment, to build an agenda on the rights of people to adequate food, sound housing, safe water, access to means of family planning, and much more. The term "sustainable development" was first coined by Gro Harlem Brundtland, who was to become Director-General of the World Health Organization (WHO) in 1998, and had long championed health as a human right. She put sustainable development on the international agenda (Norway in the UN, 2017).

The initial recognition to revitalize humanity's connection with nature ended in the ratification of the UN Millennium Development Goals and a target date for significant accomplishment by 2015. Realizing the enormity of this challenge, the action plan for the Millennium Goals was quickly vested in the 2030 Agenda for Sustainable Development and accepted by the General Assembly in September of 2015, signifying transition from a national to an international orientation. Earlier UN work in this area focused on undeveloped and developing countries. Now this latest initiative targeted all 191 geopolitical constituents of the UN. The 2030 Agenda consists of 17 SDGs with 169 associated targets which are integrated and indivisible, and will serve to evaluate progress (UN, n.d.).

Determinants of Health

And it is the distribution of determinants within populations that dictates health and equity. The determinants of health are simple, yet profound. They are a range of situations into which people are born, grow, live, work, worship, and age; and these circumstances are shaped by the distribution of money, power, and resources. Determinants fall into several broad categories: Policy-making, social factors, health services, individual behavior, biology, and genetics (CDC, 2019). In the United States they are first presented in the *Healthy People 2020* agenda. The *Healthy People* initiative provides 10 evidence-based national objectives per year for improving the health of all Americans. In December 2010, DHEW announced *Healthy People 2020*'s health promotion and disease prevention agenda. This adds to three previous *Healthy People* generations of work. For three decades, the *Healthy People* initiative has established benchmarks and monitored progress over time to encourage collaboration across communities and sectors, empower people to make informed health decisions, and measure the impact of prevention activities. The latest outcomes for the LHI in *Healthy People* can be found at: www.healthypeople.gov/2020/leading-health-in-dicators/LHI-Infographic-Gallery#Nov-2019. A comparability between the LHI of *Healthy People* and the SDGs is readily apparent. They should not operate at cross purposes, but be conceptualized as logical partners in population health.

Policies at the local, state, and federal levels affect individual and population health. Increasing taxes on tobacco sales, for example, can improve population health by reducing the number of people and the amount of tobacco products used. The same analogy applies to the Highway Safety Act and the National Traffic and Motor Vehicle Safety Acts, which authorized the federal government to set and regulate standards for motor vehicles and highways. This led to an increase in safety standards for cars, including seat belts, which in turn reduced rates of injuries and deaths from motor vehicle accidents. Similar statutes/rules and regulations are in place for food handling, protective gear to be used in children's sports and bike riding, and more. Those policies geared to environmental protection have already been mentioned.

Social determinants of health are conditions in the environments that affect a wide range of health, functioning, and quality-of-life outcomes and risks. Conditions (e.g., social, economic, and physical) in various environments and settings (e.g., school, church, workplace, and neighborhood) affect patterns of social engagement, one's sense of security, general well-being of people, and quality of life. In turn, these factors can have a significant influence on population health outcomes. Examples of these elements include safe and affordable housing, access to education, public safety, availability of healthy foods, local emergency/health services, and environments free of life-threatening toxins and pollutants. By working to establish policies that positively influence social, economic, and physical conditions and those that support changes in individual behavior, we can improve health for large numbers of people in ways that can be sustained over time. Improving the conditions in which we live, learn, work, and play and the quality of our relationships will create a healthier population, society, and workforce. These determinants are broken down much more finitely in www.healthypeople.gov/2020.

Both access to health services and the quality of health services can impact health. *Healthy People 2020* directly addressed access to health services as a topic area and incorporated quality of health services throughout a number of related topics. Lack of access, or limited access, to health services greatly impacts an individual's health status. When individuals do not have health insurance, they are less likely to participate in preventive care and are more likely to delay medical attention for problems. Much emphasis in this area is linked to the presence of a usual primary care provider (PCP) or "medical home" where health and wellness are monitored, collaborative relationships are facilitated, and a trusting relationship exists for the client. It is here that the client will find caregivers who will honor their role as an advocate. In 2019 data, there was a strong relationship between level of education and insurance status and the presence of a PCP or "medical home" (Arenson, Hudson, NaeHyung, & Lai, 2019).

Many public health and health care interventions focus on changing individual behaviors such as substance abuse, diet, and physical activity. Positive changes in individual behavior can reduce the rates of chronic disease in the population. The latest *Healthy People* indicator information shows gain or data exceeding the targets for environmental air quality, infant mortality, immunizations, graduation rates from high school, substance abuse among adolescents, screening for colorectal cancer, blood pressure control, physical activity among adults, injury and violence prevention, amphetamine/cocaine and alcohol use among 11th and 12th graders, and adolescent and adult tobacco use. On the negative side, mental health problems are growing in frequency and severity among youth. Latest available data show the percentage of adolescents aged 12 to 17 reporting having had a major depressive episode in the past 12 months increased about 10%, from 8.3% to 9.1%, moving away from the *Healthy People 2020* target of 7.5% (*Healthy People 2020*, 2014).

Some biological and genetic factors affect specific populations more than others. For example, older adults are biologically prone to being in poorer health than adolescents due to the physical and cognitive effects of aging. Sickle cell disease is a common example of a genetic determinant of health, and is inherited when both parents carry the gene for sickle cell. Similar patterns exist for hemophilia and vision/hearing and communication deficits. The importance of genetic history should not be overlooked. The establishment of a trusting relationship goes a long way in obtaining a complete and honest history.

There is emergent international and national consensus around what has to be accomplished to achieve equality in healthy living. The expansion of knowledge of these social determinants, including among healthcare workers, can by itself improve the quality and standard of life for people who are marginalized. This is the challenge for nursing today as it seeks to bring holistic care to populations. These are the times of a search for sanity and safety in the spirit of community. A cultural reform characterized by demands for personal responsibility and satisfaction and accomplished within a climate of autonomy, advocacy, and self-care is timely. Many of these indicators/determinants/goals are legislatively guaranteed, and should be reinforced in every school setting and to every citizen, regardless of affluence or seeming privilege.

And neither is *Healthy People* compartmentalized at the national level, or is the product of a static process. Each iteration of *Healthy People* (2000, 2010, 2020, 2030) has been reviewed by the Secretary's Advisory Committee on National Health Promotion and Disease Prevention for the coming decade. This Committee consists of subject matter experts and is a nonfederal advisory committee to the Secretary of the U.S. Department of Health and Human Service (DHHS). Focus is placed on the deficits of the last report, retaining what worked and editing where more precision in words or metrics is needed. A very visible factor in the process is the reliance on measurability and the use of scientific evidence. There is a noted focus on population health, elimination of disparities and promotion of health equity, and health literacy (Kearney-Nunnery, 2020).

Nontraditional Situations Which Challenge Role Execution

It is obvious that the health determinants overlap and interact in a complex manner, and that there is no one clear solution to many problems. School nurses are confronted with some very difficult situations that create the need for intervention of the law and challenge our personal values. You may be confronted by students exposed to violence and abuse, or other very difficult family situations. School victimization is also frequently common. The best advice is to know what is reportable and to whom, and follow the lines of authority, unless your intuition or experience tells you otherwise.

Nearly half of 5- to 17-year-olds have experienced trauma in the form of at-school victimization. Exposure to trauma increases students' risk for mental health disorders and school failure. Analyzing the California Healthy Kids Survey of 2010, we observe victimization on school grounds, substance use, and symptoms of depression and eating disorders among a sample of sixth to 12th graders ($N = 639,925$). Between 20% and 50% of students had experienced at least one type of victimizing event on school grounds, with the highest incidence in middle schools. A significantly higher share of victimized students reported using substances, having symptoms of depression, and having eating disorders when compared to nonvictimized students (Nash, 2019). School district investment in school nurses, social workers, and school-based health centers could increase preventive interventions to improve school climate, student well-being, and academic success. It is important that school nurses reach out to experts to verify their observations, seeking consultation when necessary. Access should exist to school psychologists, learning specialists, social workers, and physicians, at the very least.

At NASN 2019, the 51st NASN Annual Conference, Kim Nash, a forensic nursing specialist with the International Association of Forensic Nurses, shared her expertise on child trafficking (Nash, 2019). The brochure, *Look Beneath the Surface* (DHHS: Administration for Children & Families, 2018), provides crucial information school nurses need to support child victims of human trafficking. It addresses the exploitation of someone for the purpose of compelled labor or a commercial sex act through the use of force, fraud, or coercion. If a person younger than 18 is induced to engage in a sexual act for money or something else of value, it is a crime regardless of whether there is any force, fraud, or coercion. Victims can be anyone from around the world or right next door: women and men, adults and children, U.S. citizens and noncitizens. Some populations are at higher risk for human trafficking, including victims of other forms of violence, disconnected youth, and racial and ethnic minorities. Child victims of trafficking are often exploited for sexual purposes, including prostitution, pornography, and sex tourism. They are also exploited for forced labor, including domestic servitude, factory work, and farming.

Suicide is death caused by injuring oneself with the intent to die. A suicide attempt is when someone harms themselves with the intent to end their life, but they do not die as a result of their actions. School nurses will all too frequently find themselves confronted with such situations. Several factors can increase the risk for suicide and protect against it. Suicide is connected to other forms of injury and violence, and causes serious health and economic consequences. For example, suicide risk is higher among people who have experienced violence, including child abuse, bullying, or sexual violence. Protective factors like family and community support, and easy access to health care can help decrease the risk for suicidal thoughts and behavior. It is the second leading cause of death for people 10 to 34 years of age. Preventive strategies include creating "safe spaces(s)"; promoting connectedness with peers, supportive adults, and within communities; teaching coping and problem-solving skills; and identifying and supporting those at risk (National Center for Injury Prevention & Control, 2019). Perfecting these skills takes time, aptitude, and confronting your own feelings about such situations, but mostly it takes the motivation to make a difference.

When communicating with children who have experienced severe emotional trauma, it is important to remember that these children may have experienced other forms of trauma and abuse prior to or during this situation. Children may have normalized violence, often assume what has happened is their fault, react with hostility, and may not establish trust easily. They also may have been coached to answer your questions in a certain way. The first step when encountering these situations is to work to have the student develop acceptance and comfort in your presence.

Healthy People 2030 has an even more ambitious agenda than *Healthy People 2020* for school nurses and the school-aged child. It includes 63 pages of objectives; however, absent from those pages are goals related to addressing Adverse Childhood Experiences (ACEs), toxic stress, developmental trauma, and trauma-responsive practices (Merck, 2018). This is not only curious but also flies in the face of current science, which documents how the impact of exposure to adversity in childhood affects short- and long-term health outcomes, including school attendance and performance.

These situations together with emotionally charged areas such as sexual exploitation, transgender issues, and violence for the sake of violence, make other aspects of health and well-being seem mundane, but they are not. The fact exists that certain cultural patterns make obesity, inactivity, and poor diet acceptable. During the past 20 years, there has been a dramatic increase in obesity in the United States and, although there has been some leveling off in recent years, rates remain at historically high levels. How does this affect our children? Is the role modeling to their advantage? And the fact that certain children are genetically at high risk for disease only complicates the equation. This is where the school nurse assumes the role of teacher, and advocate for the child, and ideally for the family. This is when education for self-care becomes the priority, as your lifetime gift to a child.

Credentials for the Role of School Nurse

For school nurses, the challenge is not to reject individual students' needs, but to move forward with equal vigor to adopt populations as client, and to focus on the *Healthy People* Initiative and the United Nation's Sustainable Development Agenda. School Nurses require more sophistication and specialization than found in entry-level education for the registered nurse. There is clear need for national Certification as a School Nurse (NCSN) and ideally preparation as a School Nurse Practitioner, which is a hybrid of primary care of school-aged children, practice within the school system as a liaison to education, and community/public health nursing. School nursing is firmly grounded in community/public health. The goal of community/public health moves beyond the individual to focus on community health promotion and disease prevention and is one of the primary roles of the school nurse. School nurses must also feel competent to deliver culturally competent care in our culturally diverse communities.

Though national certification may be merited and desirable, under the Constitution and states' rights the requirements for school practice are deferred to each state. In exceptional situations, states' rights have been preempted by federal mandates. One example of this is the multi-state compact for state licensure of nurses. Such has not been the case for school nursing. Though school nurses have been proven leaders in improving the general well-being of school children, their credentialing and mandatory presence in schools varies according to state law. A few examples of school nurse pre-service requirements include:

■ Arizona: School nurses must obtain a school nurse certificate issued by the Department of Education, which requires a current RN license in Arizona and a bachelor's degree.

■ California: School nurses must be currently registered as an RN, possess a bachelor's degree, and must have a current credential in school nursing, which requires 26 units beyond the bachelor's degree.

■ Maine: School nurses in Maine must possess a current RN license in Maine and a bachelor's degree. Candidates for school nurse jobs must also have at least 3 years of experience as a nurse, with at least one of those years being within the 5 years immediately prior to their initial application.

■ New Mexico: School nurse professionals must possess an RN license and a bachelor's degree, while school nurse supervisors must possess an RN license and a master's degree. (National Association of State Boards of Education [NASBE], n.d.)

Most states require that a school nurse acquire and maintain certification through the state's Department of Health or the Department of Education. School nurses throughout the United States often pursue the National Certified School Nurse (NCSN) credential through the National Board for Certification of School Nurses (NBCSN). To earn the NCSN credential, applicants must take and pass an examination, offered as a computer examination that can be taken at testing centers located throughout the United States. To qualify to sit for the NCSN examination, candidates must possess the following:

■ At least 1,000 clinical hours within the past 3 years;

■ A current RN license; *and*

■ A bachelor's degree or higher in nursing; *or*

■ A bachelor's degree in a health-related field relevant to school nursing, which must include at least 6 credits in the following subjects (in any combination):

● Management of primary healthcare problems among children and/or adolescents;

● Health assessment of children and/or adolescents; and

● Public health/community health/epidemiology.

The NCSN certification is valid for a period of 5 years. To qualify for recertification, candidates must possess a current RN license and at least 2,000 hours of clinical practice in school nursing in the past 5 years, of which at least 750 hours must be in the past 3 years.

The purpose of the test is to measure a nurse's understanding of the type of health concerns typically encountered in a school setting and the interventions that help keep student populations healthy. Nurses are also tested on their understanding of the types of ethical issues unique to the school environment. Additionally, school nurses are required to complete a set number of hours of continuing education periodically, the number of which varies by state (RN to MSN, n.d.).

As with all legislation/regulation, the devil is in the detail. In the case of absenteeism, is the school administration allowed to hire noncredentialed RNs to substitute for RNs credentialed in school practice? Does the law allow for one certified school nurse per district, which may include many school locations, or is the requirement per school? In a district with many locations, is the school nurse expected to supervise health aides placed in some schools as an alternative to a fully qualified school nurse?

▒ Conclusion

The role of nursing in general, and school nursing in particular is moving toward the goal of servicing populations. This new frame of reference will demand system's thinking, and a much broader frame of reference than has been traditional in nursing practice. *Healthy People 2030*, and the 2030 Sustainable Development Goals of the United Nations provide a good starting point for our knowledge on determinants of health, but only manipulation of these determinants in our work will perfect our facility to direct our practice toward them.

▒ References

Arenson, M. A., Hudson, P. J., NaeHyung, L., & Lai, B. (2019). The evidence on school-based health centers: A review. *Global Pediatric Health*, *2019*, 6. doi: 10.1177/2333794X19828745

Build Healthy Places Network. (n.d.). *About us*. Retrieved from https://buildhealthyplaces .org/about-us/#NAC

Centers for Disease Control and Prevention. (2019). *Social determinants of health*. Retrieved from https://www.cdc.gov/socialdeterminants/index.htm

Healthy People 2020. (2014). *Healthy People 2020 leading health indicators: Progress update*. Retrieved from https://www.healthypeople.gov/2020/leading-health-indicators/ Healthy-People-2020-Leading-Health-Indicators%3A-Progress-Update

Healthy People 2020. (n.d.). *About Healthy People*. Retrieved from www.healthypeople .gov/2020/About-Healthy-People/

Kearney-Nunnery, R. (2020). *Advancing your career* (7th ed.). Philadelphia, PA: F.A. Davis.

Merck, A. (2018). Tell gov't: Address childhood trauma in Healthy People 2030! *Salud America*. Retrieved from https://salud-america.org/tell-govt-address-childhood-trauma -in-healthy-people-2030/

Nash, K. (2019). *Recognize child victims of human trafficking*. NASN Annual Conference, Denver, CO.

National Association of State Boards of Education. (n.d.). *School nurse qualifications*. Retrieved from https://statepolicies.nasbe.org/health/categories/health-services/school -nurse-qualifications

National Center for Injury Prevention and Control, Division of Violence Prevention. (2019). *Suicide: Prevention strategies*. Retrieved from https://www.cdc.gov/violenceprevention/suicide/prevention.html

Norway in the UN. (2017). *Mother of sustainable development*. Retrieved from https://www.norway.no/en/missions/un/norway-and-the-un/norways-rich-history-at-the-un/important-norwegians-in-un-history/gro/

Office of Disease Prevention and Health Promotion. (n.d.). *Leading health indicators development and framework*. Retrieved from https://www.healthypeople.gov/2020/leading-health-indicators/Leading-Health-Indicators-Development-and-Framework

RN to MSN. (n.d.). *How to become a school nurse*. Retrieved from https://www.rntomsnedu.org/school-nurse/

United Nations. (n.d.). *Sustainable development goals*. Retrieved from https://www.un.org/sustainabledevelopment/sustainable-development-goals/

University of Washington. (2015). *Center for Communication and Civic Engagement. Rethinking Prosperity*. Retrieved from http://rethinkingprosperity.org/a-shift-in-health-consciousness-leads-to-closure-of-many-mcdonalds-locations/

U.S. Department of Health and Human Services: Administration for Children & Families. (2018a). *Look beneath the surface*. Retrieved from https://www.acf.hhs.gov/otip/partnerships/look-beneath-the-surface

U.S. Department of Health and Human Services: Administration for Children & Families. (2018b). *Human trafficking: Look beneath the surface*. Retrieved from acf.hhs.gov/resource/look-beneath-the-surface.

U.S. Department of Health and Human Services: Administration for Children & Families. (n.d.). *What we do*. Retrieved from https://www.acf.hhs.gov/about/what-we-do

World Health Organization. (2013). *The economics of social determinants of health and health inequalities: A resource book (PDF)*. Retrieved from www.who.int/gho/publications/world_health/

PANDEMICS AND PLAGUES

JANICE LOSCHIAVO

LEARNING OBJECTIVES

- Distinguish between infection and infectious disease.
- Describe the function of the immune system.
- State three ways disease can be transmitted.
- Evaluate the effectiveness of Primary, Secondary and Tertiary Prevention.
- Define and contrast epidemic, pandemic, outbreak, plague, and novel diseases
- Distinguish among isolation, quarantine, and social distancing.
- Compare Coronavirus with other pandemics.
- Plan the safest strategies for the new school environment.

Introduction

In early May of 2020, when this chapter was written, the United States was still experiencing the primary wave of the Coronavirus Pandemic. We know that, eventually, it will pass and what we have experienced will forever influence our personal and professional lives. Issues that were once viewed significant are now seen as trivial. As a hypothetical fear became a reality, Americans began to understand that less is needed to be happy. We learned much in a very short period.

As we enter the next phase of this nightmare, people demand and deserve factual information. The difficult part is that along with other health professionals we are dealing with a unique crisis in *real-time*. News changes daily, sometimes hourly. There are conflicts among health specialists and those who make decisions based on economy. While most people passionately adhere to recommended restrictions, others minimize the problem and feel the health threat is exaggerated. Whether we choose to ignore or abide by recommendations, clearly one's actions impact those around us. As we prepare for the eventual reopening of our schools, there can be *no* arguments or compromises where the well-being of children is at stake.

Likewise, no one would dare to disagree with the essential role the nurse has played on the *front lines* throughout this catastrophe. As school nurses, our *front line* is the school and those who stand within. We face unprecedented challenges. Our contribution as nurses and health educators has never been more crucial. The school nurse is, and always will be, the heart of the school.

We must now join together in hopes that we can help restore our schools to the level of academic excellence we previously enjoyed and continue to provide education in the safe, happy refuge our students so desperately need.

History demands that we understand the past before planning the future. In this chapter, we look back at the history of other pandemics, evaluate the Coronavirus impact and strategize what we must do in the future. It is time to step into the trenches and do our jobs on the *front line*.

Infection Versus Infectious Diseases

If one takes an historical look back at plagues and pandemics it is clear that infectious diseases have wreaked havoc on people for centuries. Once a new infectious agent becomes established in a host it can easily spread from animal to person or person to person, and sustain itself in the new population that has no immunity to this unknown agent. This is what has occurred with the Coronavirus.

Infectious or communicable diseases are caused by pathogenic microorganisms such as bacteria, viruses, parasites, or fungi (World Health Organization [WHO], n.d.). An infectious disease differs from an infection in that with an infection, the organism invades the body, the tissues react but the infection does not alter the host's health. This is a subclinical infection. The host does not have an infectious disease unless symptoms present themselves. Most infections initiate in the mucous membranes of our body and the host manifests fever, diarrhea, fatigue, aches, and cough. Other, more specific signs and symptoms may present for a particular disease.

Immune Response

The immune system is our body's complex defense network comprised of trillions of immune cells. These cells protect us against substances that do not belong in our bodies and can cause infection and disease (Immune Response, n.d.).

When the person is initially exposed to an antigen or infectious agent, a primary response occurs. Immune cells are activated, and antibody levels rise then slowly decrease once the antigen has been eliminated from the host. After a latent period of several days, antibodies begin to appear in the blood. The dose or antigen correlates with the severity of the illness. A higher/longer exposure increases the risk of the immune response and death rates are naturally higher in densely populated areas.

The next and subsequent times the person encounters this same antigen, the immune response is much quicker, and response is even more powerful (New Health Advisor, n.d.).

Herd Immunity

Herd Immunity, or community Immunity, happens when so many people in a community become immune to an infectious disease either from vaccination or previous infections, that it stops the disease from spreading. In most cases 80% to 95% of the population must be immune to the disease to stop its spread (Healthline, 2020).

Modes of Disease Transmission

There are several ways in which disease is transmitted: airborne, contact (direct and indirect), vehicle (e.g., water, milk, food), vector, and transplacental.

- Airborne transmission: When a person breathes, sneezes, or coughs, particles/droplets are carried by the air to other people. Examples of airborne diseases are cold, influenza, and Coronavirus.
- Contact transmission: When a diseased person comes into close contact with another person. Smallpox and impetigo are spread by contact transmission.
- Vehicle transmission: Disease carried through water, milk, food, or blood. Cholera and typhoid fever are examples of diseases caused by vehicle transmission.
- Vector transmission: Caused by arthropods transmitting infection by inoculation into the skin or mucosa by biting or depositing of infectious material on the skin or food. This is how malaria and plagues are spread.
- Transplacental transmission: Disease is passed from mother to fetus in utero or during delivery. Examples of diseases spread in utero are measles and syphilis (Preserve Articles, n.d.).

Barriers to Infection

The two primary barriers to infection are the skin and mucous membranes. Skin coverage keeps out infections and protects our inner organs. It is the first defense mechanism in our immune system. Skin contains Langerhans cells. If these cells sense that a harmful bacterium has invaded the skin, they release a chemical signal that initiates a response from the white blood cells to that area to fight the infection (Johnson, 2018).

Mucous membranes protect the inside parts of the body that are exposed to air. Nasal membranes, for example, are lined with small blood vessels that warm and humidify air and cilia. They keep germs out of the body by trapping debris that you breath in. If the skin and mucous membranes are unable to ward-off the offending pathogen, then an infectious disease can invade the body and cause illness or death.

▨ Epidemic Versus Pandemic Versus Plagues

An epidemic is best described as increase in the number of cases of a disease which affects people that reside in a community or certain region. The incidence is more than what is typically anticipated for the population in that area and spreads rapidly. The onset of the epidemic is sudden and unexpected.

A pandemic is the worldwide spread of a new disease that involves many people. It is considered the highest possible level of disease. As noted by the Centers for Disease Control and Prevention (CDC), a pandemic is an epidemic that has spread over several countries or continents, usually affecting many people in an efficient and sustained manner causing many deaths. Both words have been used in reference to the Coronavirus outbreak but how they are used appears to be subjective (MPH Online, n.d.).

When an epidemic crosses over into pandemic, a major difference is that more governments are involved in attempting to treat the people who have it and to prevent the progression of the disease According to the CDC, once a pandemic is declared the Federal Drug Administration may begin issuing "emergency use authorizations" (EUAs) which allow doctors to prescribe medications outside of the FDA-approved use (Food and Drug Administration, n.d.).

In contrast, plagues are contagious bacterial diseases. For example, the Black Plague was transmitted by fleas once they had bitten an infected rodent. It is characterized by fever and buboes. Today, bacterial infections are successfully treated with antibiotics and do not represent the same health threat previously known to man.

Areas of the world have endemic diseases which are constantly present. It is a usual prevalence of a disease or infection within a geographic area. A novel disease is a virus not seen before. It is isolated from the primary host and spreads to an animal or human where it has not been previously identified.

See Table 26.1 for a timeline of plagues and pandemics experienced as far back as records can be deciphered. Data are approximate since much information varies according to source.

▨ The Coronavirus

On March 11, 2019, the WHO declared the Coronavirus a global pandemic and gave us the acronym COVID-19. The acronym was formed as follows: The pointed structures of the virus under a microscope resemble a crown: CO (corona in Spanish), V indicates virus, D indicates disease, and 2019 is the year it was first detected.

▨ Origin

There are several theories on where and how the pandemic actually started. The Coronavirus is believed to have originated in Wuhan, China, where people frequent what is known as Wet Markets. These are places where animals are slaughtered and sold with other food items. Sanitation measures are questionable. The culprit appears

TABLE 26.1 TIMELINE OF PLAGUES AND PANDEMICS

YEAR	PLAGUE/PANDEMIC	INFECTIOUS DISEASE	DEATH TOLL
165–180	Antonine Plague: Roman soldiers returned from war ill. It is believed to be cause by measles or smallpox and to have contributed to the fall of Rome.	Unknown	5 million
541–750	Plague of Justinian: This was the first plague outbreak that would be later become known as the Black Death, causing 10,000 deaths a day.	Bubonic Plague	30–50 million
1346–1351	Black Death: The deadliest pandemic of all time spread from Asia through trade ships by fleas feeding on infected rats. When rats died, the fleas switched to feeding on humans.	Bubonic Plague	200 million
1530–1600	New World Smallpox: Exploration of the new world led to trade of animals and plants. Native populations of South America had no immunities to Eurasian diseases. It contributed to the collapse of Aztec and Inca civilizations.	Smallpox	56 million
1629–1631	Great Plague of Milan: Ferrara in northern Italy was the only city that did not experience any deaths. The city immediately implemented border controls and sanitation laws.	Bubonic Plague	1 million
1817–present	Third Cholera Pandemic: Caused by contaminated water; it resurfaces in areas of India and Indonesia where water is contaminated and the sanitation system is poor.	Cholera	1 million
1885–1950	Third Plague of China: This plague prompted scientific research into the cause and led to the discovery of bacteria.	Bubonic Plague	12 million
1918–1920	Spanish Flu: One third of the global population was infected, 500,000 million. Had high mortality for all age groups.	Influenza	40–50 million
1968–1970	Hong Kong Flu: Our seasonal flu is one strain of the Hong Kong Flu.	Influenza	1–4 million
1981–present	HIV/AIDS Pandemic: Hypothesis is that the virus jumped from chimps to humans through bush hunting in central Africa.	HIV	36 million
2019–present	COVID-19: Spread by small droplets while coughing, sneezing, or talking. The droplets fall and do not travel through the air. Statistics are as of 5/28/20.	Coronavirus	356,000

COVID-19, Coronavirus 2019.

to be a bat coronavirus, altered through genetic sequencing. Bats are not sold but may have had contact with animals that had contact with people.

There is also a possibility that the disease spread was a result of a Chinese laboratory accident. The Chinese equivalent of our CDC is near the Wet Market. A worker may have accidentally become infected or some toxic waste may have not been disposed of properly. The lab was known to be involved in research on deadly bat virus illnesses (Ignatius, 2020).

Another theory is that the disease was spread from the bats to poultry and then to the pangolin (Sandoiu, 2020). The pangolin may have been the intermediate animal. It is similar to an anteater and the meat is considered a delicacy in China (Sandoiu, 2020).

Regardless of the origin, the deadly virus was passed into the new, human host who had no previous immunity. It is clearly impossible to predict what will be the ultimate outcome of the Coronavirus. What we can do is learn from the history of pandemics and hopefully determine the best course of action for today.

▨ Scope of the Coronavirus Pandemic

The impact of the Coronavirus has been wide spread and frightening. The toll it has taken on people will not be evaluated for many years to come but at the time of this writing (Andrew, 2020):

- Cases have been reported on every continent except Antarctica.
- The United States has had over 100,000 deaths (as of 5/28/20).
- Many hospitals reported severe shortages of ventilators, masks, gowns, and other personal protective equipment.
- 2.7 billion people have been placed on lock downs, curfews, or other restrictions.
- $2.3 trillion have been lost in the global economy.
- Most state and local governments closed schools from March until the end of June; no plans have been made for reopening.
- Bars, nightclubs, parks, and playgrounds were closed, and restaurants opened only for takeout food.
- People shopped for food and medicine practicing social distancing wearing gloves and masks.
- The summer Olympics in Tokyo was postponed until 2021.
- 22 million Americans applied for unemployment.
- Morgues were filled to capacity, so bodies were stored in refrigerated trucks.
- Funeral services were limited or postponed indefinitely.
- Sporting events, religious gatherings, political and cultural events were cancelled or postponed.

- Widespread shortages of food and household cleaning products were experienced.

- Hospitals were closed to all but the patient. Families were not permitted to be with loved ones.

- Hospitals converted dining areas and total floors just to accommodate COVID-19 patients.

Incubation Period

The incubation period is the time from when a person is exposed to a pathogen to when they develop symptoms. This can vary according to the wellness of the host and the virulence of the offending organism.

Typically, Coronvirus pathogens incubate from 2 to 14 days with an average of 5 days between exposure to symptoms appearing. Many individuals are infected but do not exhibit symptoms.

Researchers estimate that people who get infected can spread it to others 2 to 3 days before symptoms start and are most contagious 1 to 2 days before they feel sick. People remain infectious from 2 days prior to symptoms to 2 weeks (Hersh, 2020).

The Coronavirus enters the human host through the mouth, eyes, or nose and can go directly to the lungs once inhaled. After entering the body, the virus spreads to the back of the nasal passage and to the mucous membranes in the throat, attaching to the body's cell receptors. From there it enters the outer walls of the host's cells as it breaches the cell membrane making it possible for the virus to proliferate and infect other cells in the body. One cell can be replicated millions of times before it dies. From the back of the nasal passage, the infection can reach into the lungs, causing inflammation in the mucous membranes that line the passages and damaging the air sacs. This inhibits the lungs' ability to oxygenate the blood and remove carbon dioxide from the bloodstream. This can cause fluid retention, pus, and dead cells leading to pneumonia. Many patients require ventilators and some, even with intervention, will die of respiratory failure (Times of Israel, 2020). Those individuals with a history of lung disease are more vulnerable to the respiratory complications.

Specific, common symptoms include, dry cough, fatigue, increased sputum production, shortness of breath, and loss of sense of smell and taste (Smith, 2020). Of those infected with Coronavirus, one in five progress to shortness of breath and respiratory distress. These patients will need intervention through high levels of oxygen or be placed on a ventilator for many weeks.

Mutation

All viruses mutate or undergo small changes in their DNA composition. Mutations can make the virus more or less virulent. It is suspected that the Coronavirus has picked up several mutations since it first started infecting humans in late 2019.

The Coronavirus is believed to mutate at a slower rate than the flu virus which is why each year a different vaccine is needed. It is suggested that the vaccine, whenever it is developed, would be a single dose and not have to be repeated yearly (Beeman, 2020).

▓ Transmission

Scientists are still investigating specifically how COVID-19 is transmitted. It appears to occur when people are in close contact, less than 6 feet apart, and share small droplets while talking, coughing, or sneezing. The infected droplets can be inhaled by a healthy host, entering the lungs through the nose or mouth or landing on the other person's face. Hands easily spread the droplets to the mucous membranes of the eyes or nose.

If the droplet falls on a surface it can live up to 3 days, depending on the type of surface (Healthline, n.d.). A healthy person can easily touch a contaminated surface and transmit the virus to their eyes, nose, or mouth. Therefore, handwashing and masks are so important.

▓ Quarantine Versus Isolation Versus Social Distancing

Whether you are quarantined, isolated, or social distancing, you are attempting to stop the spread of a contagious disease. Each one of these techniques carries a different level of protective behavior.

Quarantines are for the well person or group that do not exhibit any symptoms but were exposed to the disease. It is useful during outbreaks, epidemics, or pandemics. *Isolation* is reserved for those who are already sick. The goal is to keep the infectious person away from healthy people to prevent disease from spreading (CDC, 2020). *Social distancing* involves avoiding large gatherings and close contact with others. It is suggested that you keep a minimum of 6 feet (2 meters) apart and avoid large gatherings of more than 10 people. When congregating is unavoidable, it is essential to wear a mask and gloves to protect yourself and others (Cleveland Clinic, Health Essentials, 2020).

▓ School Perspectives for Coronavirus

At this writing it is uncertain when schools will reopen. When they do open, the atmosphere will not be risk-free. Therefore, it is essential that we carefully plan the safest, most effective strategies to protect our children and staff plus give parents the reassurance they so need. All must appreciate that we are knowledgeable and in control of these most difficult times.

This section begins with information that is currently known and concludes with suggestions on how we can prepare for a future which, right now, is completely unknown.

▨ What School Nurses Should Expect

One is naïve if it is expected that we will return to the same school atmosphere we left in March. Know that we will be facing a new normal and the challenges will be many. Keep in mind the following strong possibilities:

- ▪ You will have added work, completing what you left in March and starting an unprecedented school year.
- ▪ Returning to school does not mean that the pandemic worries are behind us.
- ▪ Teachers and staff will be more vulnerable to the Coronavirus than students and will be frightened.
- ▪ Major issues such as the opioid crisis, violence, child abuse, and bullying will continue to cause concern and possibly exacerbate.
- ▪ Academic delays are inevitable. Most children lag after a summer recess. Special needs children suffer most since they require an environment tailored to educational and emotional needs and have missed related therapy sessions.
- ▪ Coronavirus may have an acute phase resurgence. We are only months into this pandemic. Other pandemics have lasted years or decades.
- ▪ Schools may have to offer interim closing and/or modified schedules.
- ▪ After prolonged social isolation, mental health must be a consideration. Children may manifest behavioral problems especially if their family has struggled with the loss of a loved one or decrease of income.
- ▪ Re-entry requirements and exclusions will be time-consuming and perhaps difficult to enforce.
- ▪ If virtual learning is to continue in some manner, lower income districts/ families may not have the means to purchase even one computer, much less two or more for larger families. Lack of parental technical skills will further contribute to inequity.
- ▪ Students have missed social milestones such as sporting events, field trips, proms, college orientations, so forth. Lack of these joyous events can have social implications for years to come.

▨ Prevention Concepts for Students, Staff, and the School Plant

If we look back at our public health roots, we are reminded that nurses entered schools in 1902 to help control the spread of disease. Even without COVID-19, this responsibility is an overwhelming task.

School nurses focus on prevention as opposed to intervention. The nurse in the hospital must intervene once the health problem has surfaced. The school nurse works to prevent it from occurring. To accomplish this, we address prevention at three levels: Primary, Secondary, and Tertiary. The following are mere suggestions for the school nurse to consider employing with the consent of public health officials and administration.

Primary Prevention

Primary prevention is accomplished during the period before a person is diseased by providing strategies designed to promote optimum health, and specific protection measures against the disease agent. Examples include health education, handwashing, and immunizations. This is the most efficient and cost-effective. Students must be taught and *retaught*, at least annually, the importance of handwashing, covering coughs and sneezes, and staying home when ill. Avoidance and education are essential. The following are appropriate suggestions.

Teachers and all staff, bus drivers, lunch personnel, custodians, aides, and so forth should be provided with educational opportunities on the nature and necessary actions needed to prevent disease spread. Teachers and staff must be reminded to self-isolate when ill and encouraged to refer children exhibiting symptoms immediately to the school nurse.

The school plant and grounds are to be cleaned and well ventilated prior to students and staff entering, throughout the day as needed and comprehensively at the end of the school day. Disinfecting procedures should include desk surfaces, doorknobs, phones commonly used, and classroom equipment.

Consideration should be given for schools to open with split shifts, so rooms, corridors and stairwells are not as congested. It would be helpful if, when moving through halls, social distancing is adhered to. Marking stairs and hallways in one direction would move the students efficiently. Another possibility is for teachers to change classes and allow students to remain in the classrooms with chairs arranged 6 feet apart.

Lunchroom gatherings and assemblies should be staggered and offered as necessary. Student activities that involve gatherings after school should be slowly introduced according to guidelines. Weather permitting, have students spend as much time outdoors as possible.

Reminders to cover coughs/sneezes and wash hands should be posted about the school.

Secondary Prevention

Once the disease process is established, either clinically or subclinically, secondary prevention is accomplished through early diagnosis and prompt treatment. The goal is to halt the process or lessen negative consequences of the disease. This is where screening is important. The following are appropriate suggestions.

Students and staff should be screened before entering the school bus or building. Staff, students, or parents should attest that they or their child have not been or are not currently ill, have not recently traveled or have any one in their home or close contacts exhibiting illness.

The person should be assessed for any apparent physical symptoms such as cough or anxiety and a temperature should be taken. This physical assessment can also include an oxygen level check. If there are any concerns about the individual's wellness, the individual should be excluded. Anyone complaining of a constitutional symptom during the school day should be excluded. Return policy should be determined by school health officials in compliance with the American Academy of Pediatrics and CDC Guidelines.

Tertiary Prevention

Tertiary prevention deals with disease outcomes. More than just stopping the progress is needed. The goal is to return the person to a useful place in society with maximum use of remaining capabilities. If a student has been excluded, virtual instruction should be provided by the teacher. Any teacher with a diagnosis of COVID-19 should be permitted sick time as needed.

Keep detailed records of number of health office visits, absentees, exclusions, and confirmed cases. If there is a significant rise in the number of confirmed COVID-19 illnesses, or a sudden rise in cases, school closure should be considered by school officials.

Resources

In most school settings, the school nurse functions independently. However, when a problem is larger than we can handle within the resources of our school, we must work as a team with other health professionals. The goal is to protect the students and staff, adequately prepare the school plant, and enforce sanitation measures in concert with local and state officials.

It took a global pandemic to highlight the importance of coordination of resources in our healthcare delivery system. The stronger the system the better the overall outcome will be. Table 26.2 lists public health officials and agencies that are working to control and ultimately eliminate COVID-19.

Testing Procedures

Currently there are two forms of testing for COVID-19: viral tests and antibody tests.

The viral test determines if you have an infection. This is a diagnostic test done by looking for the virus's genetic material which would be found during an active infection (CDC, n.d.). If you are ill with symptoms identified with COVID-19, then you should have a viral test. It is performed by placing a swab in the nose and taking a specimen from the back of the throat.

The antibody test tells you if you had a previous infection or exposure and if you have responded to the infection by building antibodies. It does not determine immunity though some might be comforted in feeling they have some protection. It is *not* a test for the virus itself. The antibodies can take up to 3 weeks after exposure to show up in the blood. No one knows yet if the presence of antibodies to the virus protects one from getting infected again or how long the protection might last.

TABLE 26.2 COVID-19 RESOURCES: AGENCIES, ASSOCIATIONS, AND ORGANIZATIONS

AGENCIES, ASSOCIATIONS, AND ORGANIZATIONS	ROLE/RESOURCES
American Academy of Pediatrics (AAP)	The professional association of pediatricians. The Academy offers continuing medical education programs and publishes position statements on major issues affecting children.
Centers for Disease Control and Prevention (CDC)	The CDC is the leading national public health institute of the United States. The CDC is a U.S. federal agency under the Department of Health and Human Services. Its main goal is to protect public health and safety through the control and prevention of disease, injury, and disability in the United States and internationally.
Center for Infectious Disease Research and Policy (CIDRAP)	CIDRAP is a center within the University of Minnesota that focuses on addressing public health preparedness and emerging infectious disease response. CIDRAP works to prevent illness and death from targeted infectious disease threats.
Federal Emergency Management Agency (FEMA)	FEMA is an agency of the U.S. Department of Homeland Security created in 1979. It created the system in place today by which a presidential disaster declaration of an emergency triggers financial and physical assistance and has the responsibility for coordinating government-wide relief efforts.
Food and Drug Administration (FDA)	The FDA is responsible for protecting the public health by ensuring the safety, efficacy, and security of human and veterinary drugs, biological products, and medical devices. This is the agency that approves the different types of COVID-19 tests.
Health Insurance Portability and Accountability Act (HIPAA)	This federal law restricts access to individuals' private medical information. HIPAA required the creation of national standards to protect sensitive patient health information from being disclosed without the patient's consent or knowledge. On March 18, 2020, HIPAA announced disclosure of information concerning COVID-19 victims for treatment purposes to family and friends involved in the infected person's care in circumstances suggesting imminent danger (Hagen, 2020).
Local Departments of Health	Play a central role in providing essential public health services in communities by monitoring for outbreaks of infectious diseases, health promotion, nutrition programs, home visits, personal health services, immunizations, sexually transmitted infections, testing, counseling, and well-baby services.

(continued)

TABLE 26.2 COVID-19 RESOURCES: AGENCIES, ASSOCIATIONS,
AND ORGANIZATIONS (*CONTINUED*)

AGENCIES, ASSOCIATIONS, AND ORGANIZATIONS	ROLE/RESOURCES
National Association of School Nurses (NASN)	Provides school nurses with the Framework for 21st Century School Nursing Practice. Through position statements, NASN gives us structure and focus for the key principles and components of current day, evidence-based school nursing practice. It is aligned with the Whole School, Whole Community, Whole Child model that calls for a collaborative approach to learning and health. The key principle of community/public health includes population-based care.
National Institutes of Health (NIH)	The NIH is the primary agency of the United States government responsible for biomedical and public health research. It was founded in the 1870s and is part of the U.S. Department of Health and Human Services.
School Medical Advisor	Most schools employ a chief medical inspector or school physician. Together, the school nurse and physician develop standards of care for the students in concert with recommendations from credited resources.
State Departments of Health	Regulate a wide range of healthcare settings for quality of care such as hospitals, nursing homes, assistive living, and medical day care facilities.
Department of Health and Human Services (DHHS)	The DHHS is also referred to as the Health Department. It is a cabinet-level executive branch department of the U.S. federal government. Its goal is to protect the health of all Americans and provide essential human services.
Worls Health Organization (WHO)	Established on April 7, 1948, WHO is a specialized agency of the United Nations that is concerned with international public health and is headquartered in Geneva, Switzerland. WHO describes its job as the global guardian of health.

According to a May 20, 2020 report from a University of Minnesota policy center, unless there is a local COVID-19 outbreak, workforces and hospitals should *not* be doing universal testing of asymptomatic patients. No one should use antibody testing to issue *immunity passports* because the tests can deliver inaccurate results, and no one yet knows how protective the antibodies are. According to Michael Osterholm, director of the University of Minnesota Center for Infectious Disease Research and Policy:

> Biomedical researchers are focused now on the need for a test to detect not just antibodies but "neutralizing antibodies" which are tiny proteins that block the virus from penetrating into the host cell. These neutralizing antibodies could confer at least some level of protection, but it does not appear to be conclusive at this time. (Carlson, n.d.)

▧ Contact Tracing

Contact tracing tracks down the individual who might have been infected by a person who had been positively diagnosed. The recent contacts of that person should quarantine themselves and prevent further spread. The trained interviewer speaks with the recently diagnosed to help them recall everyone with whom they have had close contact during the time frame they may have been infectious. Those people are then closely monitored (Fink, 2020).

▧ Vaccine Hopes

A vaccine to prevent Coronavirus disease is our best hope for controlling and eventually ending this pandemic. Currently, we have no vaccine available and we have conflicting reports on when one will be developed. Clearly, there are several steps that must be enacted. Researchers are working hard to create a vaccine for what has now been termed SARS-CoV-2 because of its similarity to the virus that causes SARS.

Vaccines are given as a live or weakened form of the organism causing the disease. This prompts the immune system to respond without causing the disease. It is referenced as attenuated because the ability to cause disease has been reduced. Inactivated vaccines use a killed or inactive, version of the germ that causes disease. This causes just the immune response but no actual disease or infection. This does not provide the same level of protection as the live vaccine.

Once a vaccine has been developed, there is a timeline before it is available for use. This usually takes years. Animal testing is conducted which usually takes 3 to 6 months. This is followed by clinical trials: phase 1 includes testing the vaccine in humans; phase 2 deals with formulation and doses to prove effectiveness; and phase 3 includes a larger sample of people. In all probability it will take 12 to 18 months or longer to test in human clinical trials and we still cannot be certain an effective vaccine is possible for this virus.

The final steps involve production, distribution, and administration to the global population. Since we do not have any immunity to COVID-19 we do not know if one or two doses are needed, or if the vaccine will be live or inactive. Lastly, immunity must be confirmed with follow-up testing. Yes, much work needs to be done, yet the many pharmaceutical companies, governments, and private agencies working on this gives us hope (Mayo Clinic, 2020).

▧ Notable Concerns Related to COVID-19

Pediatric Multi-Symptom Inflammatory Syndrome

Experts believe that the Coronavirus primarily affects adults yet a rare, serious complication of COVID-19 has been identified in children in at least 19 states—pediatric multisymptom inflammatory syndrome (PMIS). Many children with this syndrome had the same virus that causes COVID-19 or have been in contact with someone who has (PMIS).

PMIS resembles Kawasaki disease and can affect the heart but lacks the typical COVID-19 symptoms of cough and shortness of breath. PMIS has appeared in approximately 100 children under 15 years of age (Breen, 2020).

Children have a developing immune system which quickly responds to fight off infection. Of importance is the duration and severity of common symptoms such as high temperature, red tongue, cracked lips, abdominal pain, systemic rash. *This is a very serious illness. Refer immediately if a child presents with symptoms or if a parent shares concerns with you.*

Academic Lag

Most would agree that our teachers have done a wonderful job in implementing virtual learning experiences for children. Keep in mind, school closed abruptly, and teachers were left to deal with technology issues for which they may not have been prepared. In most cases this has proven even more challenging and time-consuming than a routine classroom experience. Despite the gallant efforts, all would agree that children have lost academic progress.

Suggestion: Students could begin the new year in their previous classrooms, with the teacher they left in March. Students would have an opportunity to review work with the teacher that knows them. Last year's teacher would be able to assess needs. Given several weeks of academic and social support, students would move into the next grade with greater confidence. Students would also have an opportunity to emotionally reconnect with the teacher, classmates, and complete the grade-closing activities.

Mental Health Issues

Everyone reacts differently when placed in a stressful situation. How one responds will depend on background, the things that make you different, and the community. Older people and those chronically ill are at higher risk for severe illness, as are children, teens, substance abusers, and those with mental health conditions. There are families that struggle with the normal hours of togetherness. Add the increase in time and financial issues, many will suffer even more.

Suggestion: Note if the individual seems excessively worried or sad. If the person has increased the use of alcohol or drugs, experienced unexplained headaches, began unhealthy eating or sleeping habits and now has difficulty completing tasks, the person needs counseling. Listen carefully, ask questions, and immediately refer. Do not try to counsel (CDC, n.d.).

Routine Healthcare

Since well visits and elective care was suspended, children may be deficient in immunizations and have health issues that were not previously addressed.

Suggestion: Assist as needed in updating children's health requirements. With administrative support, be lenient when feasible and exclude when the situation warrants caution.

Evolving and Inconsistent Information

We have already witnessed the many different and changing recommendations from the credited sources included in this chapter. It is understandable since so much is still unknown. In most cases information is given based on the facts known at the time. As these facts are updated, recommendations will be altered. School nurses should continue to follow scientific data and respect that it will not give us one simple answer. Using current, available information, experts will refine, change, and ask us to adapt as we move forward.

Suggestion: As we strive to resume our daily routines, it is far too easy to blame and politicize. It is much harder to confront the problem and help find solutions. As nurses, this is what we do.

◼ The Expanded Role of the School Nurse

Nurses are prepared to deal with emergency situations. However, as emergency department or intensive care workers we respond to the acute care atmosphere, work alongside the physician and our nursing colleagues to intervene and stop the progression of the illness.

School nurses work in an educational setting, as opposed to a crisis-driven, intervention atmosphere. Primary prevention, through education, is how we differ from the hospital nurse. Under the care of the school nurse, children who have chronic conditions are well-managed and seldom need intervention. Our job is to keep people out of the hospital through education. Acutely ill people are not brought to school in an ambulance. On the rare occasion that someone reports to school very ill or becomes acutely sick during the school day, we are responsible to recognize and respond appropriately. Fortunately, these occasions are rare.

Now the school atmosphere has changed. Our role will be expanded to detect and isolate the infectious child or adult. This will mean evaluating every person as a potential victim of COVID-19. We must triage as is done in the emergency department.

Following the Nursing Process, each person complaining of constitutional symptoms should have a careful history as previously recommended before they enter the building. Their vital signs, blood pressure, temperature, pulse, lung assessment, and oxygen saturation level (pulse oxygen) should also be taken.

In addition to the normal supplies of bandages, ice packs, splints, and screening equipment, every nursing office should now include adequate supplies of protective equipment such as face masks, face shields, gowns, gloves, and bonnets. A good source of light is essential so keep adequate pen lights or a goose-neck light for checking throats.

There should be several thermometers available along with sphygmomanometer with pediatric and adult blood pressure cuffs. A dual-head stethoscope is essential to listen to cardiac as well as lung sounds. Important now is that we also stock a pulse oximeter. Some schools may choose to stock oxygen; however, caution is urged since oxygen is highly combustible. Before purchasing, check if the local police carry oxygen and what their response time typically is.

The school health office must continue to be a safe refuge for all. There should be a procedure for separating the child who comes to you with contagious disease symptoms and those who need an ice pack or emotional support. If the office is too small to accommodate separation of students, consider setting up an area in the hall for quick visits. There must be an adequate ventilation system or accessible window. A clean sink with antibacterial soap must be available for you and anyone who enters and leaves your office. Eye-wash stations should probably not be used unless the container and cups can be properly sanitized. Alert administration if what you are working in is not adequate.

Suggestions

- *Be an active participant in formulating plans to reopen the schools.* With a background in public health, the school nurse is an essential member of the team in preparing for crises and must be included in the team planning for reopening of schools. Partner with colleagues and appropriate agencies while practicing within the Framework for the 21st Century School Nursing Practice.

- *Consider offering a virtual health office.* Open your *office* an hour before and/or after school to speak with parents and teachers on non-urgent questions and advise when the individual should stay home. You could also use this time to alert parents of immune-compromised children when the absentee rate is high. This should cut down on health office traffic, texting, and phone calls during the school day.

- *Clarify, in advance, whom you are to take directions from.* Most schools have layers of administrators and you cannot spend your day worrying about who you told what and conflicting directions. You are to take care of the ill person and let those in authority take care of each other.

- *Continue to keep abreast of updated information including new restrictions, state and local guidelines, and the prevalence of COVID-19 cases in the community.* Access the CDC and AAP recommendations for school re-entry.

- *Suggest that only authorized people enter the school.* Visitors who have a legitimate need to enter the building should be screened as others are.

- *Confirm the accessibility of emergency respondents.* If you need to summon help, will police arrive first? Will they be carrying oxygen? Will the paramedics come? How long is the response time?

- *Follow recommendations for those who are to be immunized for COVID-19.* When the vaccine is made available, revisit those who have been granted religious, medical, or provisional exclusions and see if they are also to be an exclusion for COVID-19.

- *Employ the Nursing Process to evaluate each person who complains of constitutional symptoms.* Remember, you are working in a different mode now. Consider each person as possibly infected.

New Rules

At the time of this writing, all are looking for a collaborative decision on when schools will reopen from reliable national, local, administrative sources. This decision no doubt will be based on data. The data presented will determine the date. Please consider following these few new rules.

Rule 1: Put Your Own Oxygen Mask on First

You have heard this before. Today we say, put your own N95 mask on first but the symbolism is the same. You must take care of yourself before you will be capable of caring for others. Wear protective equipment and insist that others do as well. Purchase for yourself or ask your district to provide scrubs for you to wear only at schools. Leave your office for lunch. Take a coffee break. Walk outside for fresh air every day. Remember to prioritize tasks as you see appropriate. Consider student staff needs first. Paperwork can wait.

Rule 2: Work Collaboratively With Administration, National/State/Local Officials, and Colleagues

Do not forget the chain of command. Inform administration if you feel it necessary to make a call to an agency or outside source. Now, more than ever, do not get involved with non-nursing tasks. You should be expected to do the jobs that only a nurse *can* do, not what no one else *wants* to do.

Rule 3: Be Discreet

Do not speak to anyone outside of school without seeking permission first from administration. People still have the right to privacy.

■ Conclusion

As we move forward in this frightening, uncharted territory remember that people have suffered from deadly plagues and pandemics for centuries. Some pandemics have lasted many years and still have not been eradicated. We do not know what the future impact will be, but history has taught us that it will pass, and other, novel diseases will continue to emerge.

By the end of May 2020, we started becoming more comfortable with the Coronavirus threat. Cities started reopening. Beach goers were at least permitted to sunbathe. Many fear that by gathering again we will have an increase in cases and deaths. We must recognize that when there is a dramatic threat such as we have experienced, it does not suddenly disappear. The risk might have lessened, but there is still a lot of infection throughout the country. Testing has not been done on every person so many have not been diagnosed. If schools do open in September, we must also be prepared for the flu season to strike. Do not minimize the impact seasonal flu has on our health status.

In December of 2019, well before the first case of Coronavirus was diagnosed, the Gallop Poll, for the 18th consecutive year, designated nurses as the most trusted professionals; 2020 has been declared "The Year of the Nurse." It is safe to anticipate that the current level of trust and respect will undoubtedly exist for many years to come.

No one will dispute the fact that nurses have played an essential role on the *front lines* of care dealing with the Coronavirus. Once schools reopen, the *front line* will move into schools and this deadly virus will threaten to harm our students and staff. As a most trusted professional, with courage, confidence, and compassion, school nurses will take their place on this new *front line*.

▨ References

Andrew, S. (2020, April). *Here's the devastating impact of the coronavirus pandemic.* Retrieved from www.cnn.com/2020/04/20/health/coronavirus-impact

Beeman, A. (2020). *Coronavirus mutations suspected, but that's not necessarily a bad thing.* Retrieved from https://heavy.com/news/2020/05/coronavirus-mutations-suspected -not-necessarily-bad/

Breen, K. (2020, May). *Pediatric multi-symptom inflammatory syndrome: What are the symptoms?* Retrieved from www.today.com/health/pediatric-multi-symptom

Carlson, J. (n.d.). *U's infectious disease center urges better use of virus testing.* Retrieved from www.msn.com/en-us/health/medical/us-infectious

Centers for Disease Control and Prevention. (2020, April). *How coronavirus spreads.* Retrieved from www.kron4.com/health/coronavirus/cdc-covid-19

Centers for Disease Control and Prevention. (n.d.). *Testing for COVID-19.* Retrieved from www.cdc.gov/coronavirus/2019-ncov/symptoms

Centers for Disease Control and Prevention. (n.d.). *Mental health and coping during COVID-19.* Retrieved from www.cdc.gov/coronavirus/2019-ncov/daily-life

Cleveland Clinic, Health essentials. (2020, April). *COVID-19: Understanding quarantine, isolation and social distancing.* Retrieved from health.clevelandclinic.org/covid-19

Fink, J. (2020, May). *Newsweek. What is Contact tracing?* Retrieved from www.newsweek .com/robert-redfield-cdc-contact

Food and Drug Administration. (n.d.). *Emergency use authorization.* Retrieved from www .fda.gov/.../emergency-use-authorization

Hagen, K. (2020, March). *COVID-19 and patient disclosure and reporting. HIPAA.* Retrieved from www.schwabe.com/newsroom-publications-covid-19

Healthline. (2020). *Herd immunity: What it means for COVID-19.* Retrieved from www .healthline.com/health/herd-immunity

Hersh, E. (2020, March). *Coronavirus Incubation Period: How long before symptoms appear?* Retrieved from www.healthline.com/.../coronavirus-incubation-period

Ignatius, D. (2020). How did covid-19 begin? *Washington Post.* Retrieved from www.washingtonpost.com/opinions/global-opinions/

Immune Response. (n.d.). *Your bodies first line of defense.* Retrieved from www.immuneresponse.org

Johnson, J. (2018, December). *How does skin prevent disease?* Retrieved from healthfully.com/how-does-skin-prevent-disease

Mayo Clinic. (2020, May). *COVID-19 vaccine: Get the facts.* Retrieved from www.mayoclinic.org/diseases-conditions/corona

MPH Online. (n.d.). *Outbread: 10 of the worst pandemics in history.* Retrieved from www.mphonline.org/worst-pandemics-in-history

New Health Advisor. (n.d.). *Primary immune response and secondary immune response.* Retrieved from www.newhealthadvisor.org/Primary-Immune-Response

Preserve Articles. (n.d.). *What are the different modes of disease transmission.* Retrieved from www.preservearticles.com/health/what-are-the

Sandoiu, A. (2020, February). *Coronavirus: Pangolins may have spread the disease to humans.* Retrieved from www.medicalnewstoday.com/articles/coronavirus

Smith, C. (2020, May). *The most bizarre coronavirus symptom may be the key to early diagnosis.* Retrieved from https://bgr.com/2020/05/13/coronavirus-symptoms-loss-of-smell-may-be-a-key-covid-19-sign/

Times of Israel. (2020, March). *How does the coronavirus enter the body.* Retrieved from www.timesofisrael.com/how-does-the-coronavirus

World Health Organization. (n.d.). *Infectious diseases.* Retrieved from www.who.int/topics/infectious_diseases

Further Readings

Dailymail. (2020, May). *Huge NYC morgue opens in Brooklyn with bodies stored.* Retrieved from www.dailymail.co.uk/news/article-8300519/Huge

Fairbank, R. (n.d.). *The different COVID-19 test explained.*

Health. (2020, March). *Epidemic vs. Pandemic.* Retrieved from www.health.com/.../epidemic-vs-pandemic

Live Science. (2020, May). *20 Of the worst epidemics and pandemics in history.* Retrieved from www.health.com/.../epidemic-vs-pandemic

McNeill William, H. (1976). *Plagues and peoples.* New York, NY: Random House.

Outbreak: 10 of the Worst Pandemics in history (n.d.). Retrieved from www.mphonline.org/worst-pandemics-in-histo

Prevention. (n.d.). *Pediatric multi-symptom inflammatory syndrome in children.* Retrieved from www.prevention.com/health/a32446882/pediatric

WebMD. (2020, January). *Coronavirus incubation period: How long and when most contagious.* Retrieved from www.webmd.com/lung/coronavirus-incubation-period

INDEX